# METHODS IN MOLECULAR BIOLOGY

*Series Editor*
John M. Walker
School of Life and Medical Sciences
University of Hertfordshire
Hatfield, Hertfordshire, UK

For further volumes:
http://www.springer.com/series/7651

For over 35 years, biological scientists have come to rely on the research protocols and methodologies in the critically acclaimed *Methods in Molecular Biology* series. The series was the first to introduce the step-by-step protocols approach that has become the standard in all biomedical protocol publishing. Each protocol is provided in readily-reproducible step-by-step fashion, opening with an introductory overview, a list of the materials and reagents needed to complete the experiment, and followed by a detailed procedure that is supported with a helpful notes section offering tips and tricks of the trade as well as troubleshooting advice. These hallmark features were introduced by series editor Dr. John Walker and constitute the key ingredient in each and every volume of the *Methods in Molecular Biology* series. Tested and trusted, comprehensive and reliable, all protocols from the series are indexed in PubMed.

# Ribosome Biogenesis

## Methods and Protocols

Edited by

## Karl-Dieter Entian

*Institute for Molecular Biosciences, Goethe University Frankfurt, Frankfurt am Main, Hessen, Germany*

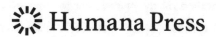 Humana Press

*Editor*
Karl-Dieter Entian
Institute for Molecular Biosciences
Goethe University Frankfurt
Frankfurt am Main, Hessen, Germany

ISSN 1064-3745          ISSN 1940-6029   (electronic)
Methods in Molecular Biology
ISBN 978-1-0716-2503-3          ISBN 978-1-0716-2501-9   (eBook)
https://doi.org/10.1007/978-1-0716-2501-9

This Humana imprint is published by the registered company Springer Science+Business Media, LLC, part of Springer Nature.
The registered company address is: 1 New York Plaza, New York, NY 10004, U.S.A.

# Dedication

This book is dedicated to my wife Heike Grüter and my son Christoph Grüter for all their great support and understanding.

# Preface

Ribosomes are the organelles that synthesize proteins according to the genetically encoded information. Whereas prokaryotic ribosomes were even reconstituted in vitro, eukaryotic ribosomes are more complex. In yeast—as a eukaryotic model organism—about 5–10% of the genomic capacity is needed for the biogenesis of a ribosome. Worldwide a remarkable number of laboratories is investigating all aspects of ribosome biogenesis. As shown by the increasing number of participants in the respective meetings, approximately 3,000 scientists are working on structural, functional, and biomedical aspects of ribosome biogenesis. This book covers most of the significant steps during eukaryotic ribosome biogenesis. The research areas are introduced by reviews followed by chapters covering the respective methods of investigation.

A comparative survey about the unity and diversity of ribosome biogenesis in pro- and eukaryotic cells is provided in Part I (Chapter 1). The genomic organization of eukaryotic rDNA and the role of RNA polymerase I in ribosome biogenesis are summarized in Part II (Chapters 2 and 3). *In vitro* methods to study RNA polymerase I structure and its function are outlined in Part III (Chapters 4–6). Ribosome assembly in the nucleolus and a method to analyze the nucleo-cytoplasmic transport of assembled ribosomes and RNP complexes are dealt with in Part IV (Chapters 7 and 8). Various modifications increasing the complexity of rRNAs and the methods to analyze these modifications are given in Part V (Chapters 9–12). Finally, Part VI provides a review of eukaryotic translation and several methods to analyze translation *in vivo* (Chapters 13–16). Remarkably, for the first time a fully reconstituted eukaryotic yeast translation system is described together with the methods to purify the respective proteins.

This book is a valuable resource for scientists and all those interested in key questions in ribosome biogenesis. It provides an overview of the abundant literature and is supposed to stimulate collaborations.

*Frankfurt am Main, Hessen, Germany*                              *Karl-Dieter Entian*

# Acknowledgments

The majority of articles was supported by Deutsche Forschungsgemeinschaft SFB 960 (RNP Biogenesis: Assembly of *Ribosomes* and Non-*ribosomal* RNPs and Control of their Function) and SPP 1784 (Chemical Biology of Natural Nucleic Acid Modifications). The editor is extremely grateful to his scientific teachers and friends Friedrich K. Zimmermann, Darmstadt, Dieter Mecke, Tübingen, Michael Ciriacy, Düsseldorf, James A. Barnett, Norwich, Piotr Slonimski, Gif-sur-Yvette, Jim Matoon, Colorado Springs, and Bernhard Prior, Stellenbosch for all their support and stimulating scientific discussions. I also thank John Walker, Anna Rakowski, Patrick Marton and Tessy Pria for their excellent support during editing this book.

The majority of articles in this book were supported by Deutsche Forschungsgemeinschaft. Collaborative network SFB 960 "Biogenesis of Ribosomes" and priority programme SPP1784 "Chemical Biology of Native Nucleic Acid Modifications". I also acknowledge the great computing support of Christoph Grüter.

# Contents

PART I   RIBOSOME BIOGENESIS

PART II   GENOMIC ORGANIZATION

PART III   RNA POLYMERASES

# Contributors

MARTIN ALTVATER • *Institute of Biochemistry, ETH Zurich, Zurich, Switzerland*

SANDRA BLANCHET • *Department of Physical Biochemistry, Max Planck Institute for Biophysical Chemistry, Goettingen, Germany*

CHRISTINA BRAUN • *Biochemistry III—Institute for Biochemistry, Genetics and Microbiology, University of Regensburg, Regensburg, Germany*

EVA DOSKOCIL • *Institute for Biochemistry, Genetics and Microbiology, University of Regensburg, Regensburg, Germany*

CHRISTOPH ENGEL • *Regensburg Center for Biochemistry (RCB), University of Regensburg, Regensburg, Germany*

KARL-DIETER ENTIAN • *Institute of Molecular Biosciences, J.W. Goethe University, Frankfurt/M., Germany*

SÉBASTIEN FERREIRA-CERCA • *Biochemistry III–Regensburg Center for Biochemistry–Institute for Biochemistry, Genetics and Microbiology, University of Regensburg, Regensburg, Germany*

UTE FISCHER • *Institute of Biochemistry, ETH Zurich, Zurich, Switzerland*

JOACHIM GRIESENBECK • *Universität Regensburg, Regensburg Center for Biochemistry (RCB), Lehrstuhl Biochemie III, Regensburg, Germany*

FLORIAN B. HEISS • *Regensburg Center for Biochemistry (RCB), University of Regensburg, Regensburg, Germany*

KRISTIN HERGERT • *Universität Regensburg, Regensburg Center for Biochemistry (RCB), Lehrstuhl Biochemie III, Regensburg, Germany*

CLAUDIA HÖBARTNER • *Institute of Organic Chemistry, Julius-Maximilians-University Würzburg, Würzburg, Germany*

MONA HÖCHERL • *Regensburg Center for Biochemistry (RCB), University of Regensburg, Regensburg, Germany*

MICHAEL JÜTTNER • *Biochemistry III–Regensburg Center for Biochemistry–Institute for Biochemistry, Genetics and Microbiology, University of Regensburg, Regensburg, Germany*

MICHAEL KERN • *Biochemistry III—Regensburg Center for Biochemistry—Institute for Biochemistry, Genetics and Microbiology, University of Regensburg, Regensburg, Germany*

ROBERT KNÜPPEL • *Biochemistry III—Institute for Biochemistry, Genetics and Microbiology, University of Regensburg, Regensburg, Germany*

SEBASTIAN KRUSE • *Universität Regensburg, Regensburg Center for Biochemistry (RCB), Lehrstuhl Biochemie III, Regensburg, Germany*

GERNOT LÄNGST • *Universität Regensburg, Regensburg Center for Biochemistry (RCB), Lehrstuhl Biochemie III, Regensburg, Germany*

ANAM LIAQAT • *Institute of Organic Chemistry, Julius-Maximilians-University Würzburg, Würzburg, Germany*

PHILIPP E. MERKL • *Universität Regensburg, Regensburg Center for Biochemistry (RCB), Lehrstuhl Biochemie III, Regensburg, Germany; TUM ForTe, Technische Universität München, Munich, Germany*

PHILIPP MILKEREIT • *Universität Regensburg, Regensburg Center for Biochemistry (RCB), Lehrstuhl Biochemie III, Regensburg, Germany*

MICHAELA OBORSKÁ-OPLOVÁ • *Institute of Biochemistry, ETH Zurich, Zurich, Switzerland; Institute of Medical Microbiology, University of Zurich, Zurich, Switzerland*

ULI OHMAYER • *Regensburg Center for Biochemistry (RCB), Institut für Biochemie, Genetik und Mikrobiologie, Universität Regensburg, Regensburg, Germany; Evotec München GmbH, Martinsried, Germany*

VIKRAM GOVIND PANSE • *Institute of Medical Microbiology, University of Zurich, Zurich, Switzerland; Faculty of Science, University of Zurich, Zurich, Switzerland*

JORGE PEREZ-FERNANDEZ • *Biochemistry III—Institute for Biochemistry, Genetics and Microbiology, University of Regensburg, Regensburg, Germany; Department of Experimental Biology, University of Jaen, Jaén, Spain*

MICHAEL PILSL • *Universität Regensburg, Regensburg Center for Biochemistry (RCB), Lehrstuhl Biochemie III, Regensburg, Germany*

SOPHIA PINZ • *Institute for Biochemistry, Genetics and Microbiology, University of Regensburg, Regensburg, Germany*

GISELA PÖLL • *Regensburg Center for Biochemistry (RCB), University of Regensburg, Regensburg, Germany*

NAMIT RANJAN • *Department of Physical Biochemistry, Max Planck Institute for Biophysical Chemistry, Goettingen, Germany*

CHRISTOPHER SCHÄCHNER • *Universität Regensburg, Regensburg Center for Biochemistry (RCB), Lehrstuhl Biochemie III, Regensburg, Germany*

CATHARINA SCHMID • *Universität Regensburg, Regensburg Center for Biochemistry (RCB), Lehrstuhl Biochemie III, Regensburg, Germany*

KATRIN SCHWANK • *Universität Regensburg, Regensburg Center for Biochemistry (RCB), Lehrstuhl Biochemie III, Regensburg, Germany*

MAKSIM V. SEDNEV • *Institute of Organic Chemistry, Julius-Maximilians-University Würzburg, Würzburg, Germany*

WOLFGANG SEUFERT • *Institute for Biochemistry, Genetics and Microbiology, University of Regensburg, Regensburg, Germany*

SUNNY SHARMA • *Department of Cell Biology and Neurosciences, Rutgers University, Piscataway, NJ, USA*

FABIAN TEUBL • *Regensburg Center for Biochemistry (RCB), Institut für Biochemie, Genetik und Mikrobiologie, Universität Regensburg, Regensburg, Germany*

HERBERT TSCHOCHNER • *Universität Regensburg, Regensburg Center for Biochemistry (RCB), Lehrstuhl Biochemie III, Regensburg, Germany*

PETER WATZINGER • *Institute of Molecular and Cellular Biology, Goethe University, Frankfurt am Main, Germany*

JUN YANG • *Department of Cell Biology and Neurosciences, Rutgers University, Piscataway, NJ, USA*

# Part I

**Ribosome Biogenesis**

# Chapter 1

# A Comparative Perspective on Ribosome Biogenesis: Unity and Diversity Across the Tree of Life

Michael Jüttner and Sébastien Ferreira-Cerca ⓘⒹ

## Abstract

Ribosomes are universally conserved ribonucleoprotein complexes involved in the decoding of the genetic information contained in messenger RNAs into proteins. Accordingly, ribosome biogenesis is a fundamental cellular process required for functional ribosome homeostasis and to preserve satisfactory gene expression capability.

Although the ribosome is universally conserved, its biogenesis shows an intriguing degree of variability across the tree of life. These differences also raise yet unresolved questions. Among them are (a) what are, if existing, the remaining ancestral common principles of ribosome biogenesis; (b) what are the molecular impacts of the evolution history and how did they contribute to (re)shape the ribosome biogenesis pathway across the tree of life; (c) what is the extent of functional divergence and/or convergence (functional mimicry), and in the latter case (if existing) what is the molecular basis; (d) considering the universal ribosome conservation, what is the capability of functional plasticity and cellular adaptation of the ribosome biogenesis pathway?

In this review, we provide a brief overview of ribosome biogenesis across the tree of life and try to illustrate some potential and/or emerging answers to these unresolved questions.

**Key words** Ribosome biogenesis, Ribosome assembly, rRNA, Maturation, RNA modifications, Eukaryotes, Archaea, Bacteria, Tree of life, Comparative biology, Evolution, Adaptation

## 1 In Search of Unity?

From an historical perspective, the search for unifying concepts in Science in general and in Biology in particular has been a key step to our fundamental and general understanding of molecular processes across the tree of life [1–7]. This idea can be easily grasped by famous aphorism variations around this theme: "From the elephant to butyric acid bacterium—it is all the same!" ([8], cited in [2]) or "Anything found to be true of *E. coli* must also be true of elephants" (attributed to Jacques Monod, 1954 [2]). However, there are also valid arguments to think that elephants and bacteria are characterized, to some extent, by distinguishable biological properties. Accordingly, molecular processes, including ribosome

Karl-Dieter Entian (ed.), *Ribosome Biogenesis: Methods and Protocols*, Methods in Molecular Biology, vol. 2533, https://doi.org/10.1007/978-1-0716-2501-9_1, © The Author(s) 2022

biogenesis, have been dissected from two albeit different and in part contra intuitively but cross-fertilizing viewpoints: a unifying and a dividing functional perspective [9–11]. As such comparative—ribosome biogenesis—biology may be torn apart between defining the real weight of functional similarities and differences which biological systems may adopt. In any case, these similarities and differences can only be appreciated in the light of detailed knowledge about the scrutinized biological system across a larger number of entities.

In this chapter, we attempt to provide a short comparative overview on the molecular principles required for ribosome biogenesis. In addition, we like to highlight few challenges and surprises that may alter our unifying/differential view on ribosome biogenesis across the tree of life.

## 2 Ribosome Biogenesis

### 2.1 Once Upon a Time … Ribosome Basic Facts

Ribosomes are universally conserved ribonucleoprotein particles allowing the decoding of the genetic information carried within messenger RNAs into amino-acid chains, the proteins [12]. Cytosolic ribosomes are composed of two ribosomal subunits, the small and the large ribosomal subunit (SSU and LSU, respectively) [12]. Strikingly, ribosomes are formed around a universally conserved structural core composed of three ribosomal RNA (rRNAs) molecules and 33 universally conserved ribosomal proteins (r-proteins) [13, 14]. Cytosolic ribosomes isolated from prokaryotic and eukaryotic organisms differ by the numbers and composition of their structural components, the r-proteins and rRNAs. Typically, cytosolic bacterial and archaeal 70S ribosomes are formed by the 30S (SSU) and 50S (LSU) ribosomal subunits [15–17]. Those are themselves composed of varying amounts of r-proteins (Figs. 1 and 2) which interact with the SSU 16S rRNA and LSU 23S and 5S rRNAs. These rRNAs also present various degree of organism's specific sequence size variations [54–56].

In eukaryotic cells, cytosolic 80S ribosomes are formed by the 40S (SSU) and 60S (LSU) ribosomal subunits [57, 58]. Concerning the amounts of ribosomal proteins, eukaryotic ribosomal subunits show also some, however less pronounced intra domain variations, compared to those observed across the bacterial and archaeal kingdoms (Figs. 1 and 2) [13, 14]. A striking feature of eukaryotic ribosomes is the presence of longer and additional rRNAs, the SSU 18S rRNA and the LSU 25/28S, 5.8S and 5S rRNAs [44, 59, 60].

In eukaryotes, rRNAs size expansion occurs by virtue of incorporation of additional rRNA sequences, the expansion segments, within the universally conserved prokaryotic-like rRNA core [23, 24, 61]. These expansion segments are varying in size and composition across eukaryotes [23, 24, 61, 62] and may have

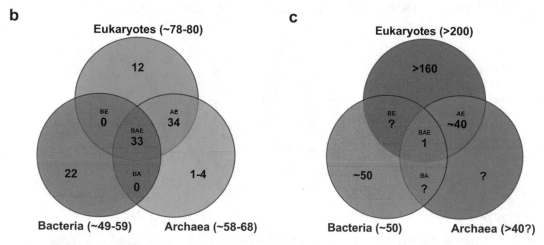

**a**

| | Bacteria | Archaea | Eukarya |
|---|---|---|---|
| rDNA repeats numbers [1] | 1-16 | 1-4 | 150-200 (> 1,000 in plants) |
| rRNAs | 16S, 23S and 5S | 16S, 23S and 5S | 18S, 25/28S, 5.8S and 5S |
| rRNA expansion segments [2] | yes (uncommon) | yes (variable - only few) | yes (variable amounts and length) |
| ribosomal proteins [3] | | 33 universal r-proteins | |
| | ≈49-59 44 ubiquitous | ≈58-68 54 ubiquitous / 71 described | ≈78-80 78 ubiquitous |
| in vitro reconstitution [4] | yes | yes | no* |
| rRNA modifications [5] | protein-based ( ≈36 modif) | protein- and sRNP-based | protein- and sRNP-based |
| 2´O-Methylation / Pseudourydilation | 4/11 | Sso (67/9); Hv (4/2) 7-127 C/D box sRNA | Sc (55/49); Hs (94/95) |
| additional "stand-alone" base modifications | ≈ 20 | Hv (7)/Tko (>100) | 12 |
| Ribosome biogenesis factors [6] | ≈ 50 | >40? | >200 |

**b**

Eukaryotes (~78-80)

12

BE 0    AE 34

BAE 33

22    BA 0    1-4

Bacteria (~49-59)    Archaea (~58-68)

**c**

Eukaryotes (>200)

>160

BE ?    AE ~40

BAE 1

~50    BA ?    ?

Bacteria (~50)    Archaea (>40?)

**Fig. 1** | Ribosome and ribosome biogenesis key features overview across the tree of life. (**a**) Summary of ribosome and ribosome biogenesis key features. Modified from [18] according to [1] [19–22]; [2] [23–27]; [3] [13, 14, 28]; [4] [29–35]; [5] [36–43]; [6] [10, 44–48]. Sso—*Saccharolobus solfataricus*; Hv—*Haloferax volcanii*; Tko—*Thermococcus kodakarensis*; Hs—*Homo sapiens*; Sc—*Saccharomyces cerevisiae*. (**b, c**) Summary of shared ribosomal proteins (**b**) and ribosome biogenesis factors (**c**) across the three domains of life. Numbers of r-proteins and putative ribosome biogenesis factors sequence homologues shared between bacteria, archaea, and eukarya (BAE); bacteria, archaea (BA), archaea and eukarya (AE), bacteria and eukarya (BE), or unique to bacteria (B), or archaea (A), or eukarya (E), are indicated [based on [10, 13, 14, 28, 41, 44–51] and our unpublished results]. (Modified from Londei and Ferreira-Cerca [52])

originated early on during rRNA evolution, since some progenitors of these expansion segments have been traced within modern archaeal but also in some case in bacterial rRNAs [23–25, 63–66].

The diverse composition of r-proteins which is, up to now, apparently more predominant in bacteria and archaea [13, 14, 55], could indicate that in these cellular contexts, ribosome assembly, that is, the assembly of r-proteins with the rRNAs, and ribosome function may tolerate a higher degree of flexibility than in most eukaryotes. It is also interesting that reductive evolution (loss) of r-proteins seems to prevail in archaea [13, 14, 25].

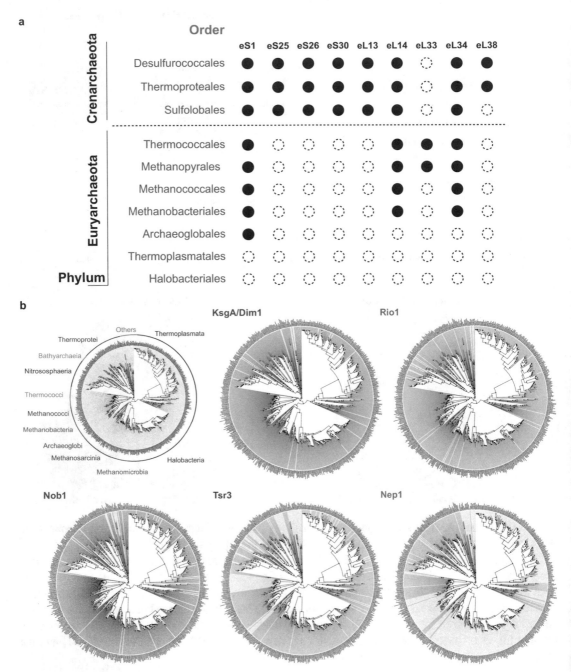

**Fig. 2** | Exemplary conservation of selected ribosomal proteins and putative ribosome biogenesis factors involved in small ribosomal subunit biogenesis in archaea. (**a**) Exemplary repartition of selected archaeal ribosomal proteins shared between archaea and eukaryotes across two major archaeal Phyla. Black circle denotes the presence, and open circle denotes the absence of sequence homologue for the indicated ribosomal protein of the small (S) or large (L) ribosomal subunits, respectively (adapted from [13, 14] using the nomenclature proposed in [49]). (**b**) Phylogenetic conservation profile of the indicated known or putative small ribosomal subunit ribosome biogenesis factors across 1500 archaeal genomes were generated using AnnoTree (http:/annotree.uwaterloo.ca) [53]. Archaeal classes are annotated in a phylogenetic tree (upper left) as provided by AnnoTree. Note the absence of significant homology for Nep1 (e.g., Thermoplasmata, Halobacteria and more) or Tsr3 (e.g., Thermococcales) in a large group of organisms, in contrast to the more widespread distribution of KsgA/Dim1, Rio1, and Nob1 archaeal homologs. Modified from Londei and Ferreira-Cerca [52]

From a compositional point of view archaea and eukaryotes do share common r-proteins which are absent in bacteria, whereas bacteria do possess domain specific r-proteins [49, 61]. This correlates with the increased structural similarities between archaeal and eukaryotic ribosomal subunits in comparison to their bacterial counterparts [25, 61, 67].

This structural similarity has been observed early on by the group of James Lake, using electron microscopy, thereby, suggesting a closer evolutionary relationship of archaea and eukaryotes [15, 67, 68]. Recent phylogenetic analysis [69–71] and higher resolution structure analysis of ribosomal subunits [25, 61, 67] essentially confirm this idea but also provide additional insights into structural differences between the different domains of life, like for example differences in the peptide exit tunnel geometry [72], or species-specific structural alteration which may be related to organism-specific environmental adaptations [62, 73].

# 3 The Ribosome Assembly Process

The ribosome assembly process, that is, the assembly of r-proteins with rRNAs, has been analyzed very early in the history of ribosome research. Early work from the Nomura laboratory in the 1960–1970s aiming to understand the individual contribution of the r-proteins/rRNA to the protein synthesis process, has led to the first in vitro reconstitution of bacterial ribosomal subunits from its isolated structural components [29, 30, 74–77]. These studies were then followed by r-proteins omission experiments which culminated in the establishment of the first ribosomal proteins assembly maps describing r-proteins assembly dependencies [29–31]. Beyond being biochemical masterpieces, these studies have revealed key features of the ribosomal assembly process in bacteria. Notably, the self-assembling nature of ribosomal subunit formation, and the fact that ribosome assembly proceeds via a combination of cooperative and hierarchical mechanisms [29–31, 78, 79]. However, these in vitro assembly experiments have been mitigated by the fact that they occur under nonphysiological conditions, thereby suggesting the existence of in vivo facilitating mechanisms which were discovered later [29–31, 78, 79]. Remarkably, in vitro reconstitution of ribosomal subunits has not only been achieved using structural components isolated from different bacterial sources, but also from two evolutionary divergent representative archaea [32–34]. In contrast, similar in vitro reconstitution of eukaryotic ribosomal subunits solely using purified structural components has not been accomplished to date.

Despite this fundamental biochemical difference, some aspects of ribosome assembly in bacteria and eukaryotes follow rather similar molecular principles, for example the hierarchical and cooperative assembly, or stepwise stabilization of r-proteins [18, 78–87]. Together these similarities suggest that ribosome assembly has likely evolved around a self-assembling (presumably self-replicating) ancestor ribosome [26, 88], which has retained some of its original assembly properties and constraints. Not surprisingly, some of these ancestral properties/constraints are most probably universally shared. In addition, existing molecular mechanisms have been modified (adapted or optimized), new ones implemented, or some maybe lost, due to organisms or common ancestor specific requirements. All these evolutionary contributions are not trivial to disentangle, but functional and structural analysis of the ribosome assembly pathway, in model and probably most importantly in nonmodel organisms, will help us to further clarify the inherited molecular constraints and properties underlying the assembly of ribosomal subunits.

## 4   Facilitating Ribosome Assembly

As mentioned above, efficient ribosome assembly in vivo depends on ribosome biogenesis factors which are collectively believed to facilitate various aspects of the ribosome biogenesis process [44, 59, 60, 78, 79]. These ribosome biogenesis factors can be subdivided into different protein classes according to their respective structural organization and/or enzymatic activity. For example, ribosome biogenesis progression depends on the presence of energy consuming enzymes, like GTPases, ATPases (AAA ATPase, RNA helicase, etc.). However, it is important to note that the ensemble of ribosome biogenesis factors differs in numbers and nature from bacteria to eukaryotes [10, 18, 44, 59, 60, 78, 79] (Fig. 1). Accordingly, the relative domain-specific repartition of structural features and/or enzyme activities implicated in ribosome biogenesis progression may vary considerably between different groups and may reflect functional adaptations within the different domains of life. For example, GTPases seem to be enriched in the bacterial ribosome biogenesis pathway, whereas ATP-dependent processes, or β-propeller containing proteins are enriched in the eukaryotic ribosome biogenesis context [10, 18, 44, 59, 60, 78, 79].

In fact, and with the exception of the (almost) universally conserved dimethyl-transferase KsgA/Dim1 [89, 90], ribosome biogenesis factors are not well conserved between bacteria and archaea or between bacteria and eukaryotes [18, 45]. In contrast, a substantial portion of eukaryotic ribosome biogenesis factors are found in archaeal genomes even though our understanding of their respective functions in archaea remains still limited [45]. Nevertheless, we and others could demonstrate some functional analogy with their eukaryotic counterparts in vivo and/or in vitro [18, 91–93]. These observations suggest that probably more (if not most) of these eukaryotic-like ribosome biogenesis sequence signatures present in archaea might be authentic ribosome biogenesis factors shared between archaea and eukaryotes. In comparison, eukaryotic ribosome biogenesis is characterized by a large increase of eukaryotes-specific ribosome biogenesis factors (>200) [46, 59, 60]. The functional requirements for this "sudden" increased complexity of eukaryotic ribosome biogenesis remains to be fully understood (Fig. 1).

In addition, to composition and number variations observed in bacteria, archaea, and eukaryotes, organisms specific variations can be observed [18, 36, 45, 90, 94, 95]. For example, the set of ribosome biogenesis factors vary across the archaeal phylum and seems to follow the general trend of reductive evolution previously observed for archaeal r-proteins (Fig. 2) [13, 14, 52]. In eukaryotes, ribosome biogenesis factors diversity further increases from unicellular to multicellular eukaryotes with the addition of factors implicated in ribosome biogenesis [46, 59, 60]. Moreover, recent studies have provided new insights into ribosome biogenesis plasticity thereby suggesting that the order of functional requirement of some assembly factors/r-proteins can vary or be functionally bypassed in some conditions [90, 96–100].

These observations have various implications for our understanding of ribosome biogenesis evolution and plasticity. For one, the presence/absence of certain molecular components can be tolerated owing that the proper rescue mechanisms are implemented (coevolving). Furthermore, these imply a higher functional plasticity of the order of events within the ribosome biogenesis pathway, whereby an alternative assembly landscape might be used or kinetically favored depending on the cellular context [81, 87, 98, 101]. However, it should be noted that this apparent diversity/plasticity may still converge to the formation of essential assembly intermediates that are functionally and/or structurally equivalent, thereby fulfilling critical inherited molecular events required for ribosome biogenesis.

Accordingly, and despite differences in the nature and amounts of the ribosome biogenesis factor ensemble, it is conceivable that the core function supported by some or all ribosome biogenesis factors are functionally equivalent across the tree of life, thereby suggesting evolutionary constraints which would have favored the establishment of dedicated functional mimicry rather than functional divergence around the universal ribosome core [18]. It is for example striking, that some divergent ribosome biogenesis factors implicated in the formation of the SSU in model bacteria, archaea and eukaryotes, are binding at very similar locations within the nascent pre-ribosomal subunits and may fulfill similar molecular tasks (see further discussion in [18]). For instance, the SSU rRNA 3' end processing follows a very similar pattern which involves a KH-domain containing ribosome biogenesis factor which interact and presumably stabilized the 3′ end of the 16S/18S rRNA, thereby enabling efficient and presumably controlled endonucleolytic cleavage. In *E. coli*, the Era GTPase, which contains a KH-domain [102–104] interact with the endonuclease YbeY and the r-protein uS11 [105], thereby facilitating 3′ end maturation. In eukaryotes, Pno1/Dim2, a KH-domain containing protein, interacts with the endonuclease Nob1 and both are located in proximity of uS11. Moreover, mutational analysis revealed functional implication of uS11, Pno1/Dim2 and Nob1 for 18S rRNA maturation [106–110]. Furthermore, archaeal homologues for Pno1/Dim2, Nob1 and uS11 are present in most archaeal genomes [111]. Considering that both the endonucleases and KH-domains (type I vs. type II) are evolutionary distinct and presumably unrelated, these observations suggest a functional convergence/mimicry at the basis of the maturation of the 16S/18S rRNA 3′ end. Whereas, the origin of this divergence at the molecular level is poorly understood, evolutionary constraints have remarkably selected a very similar mode of action in its principle (see further discussion in [18]).

Further supporting the existence of functional convergence enabling ribosomal subunit synthesis, we and others have proposed that pseudocircularization events might represent an early common feature of ribosomal subunits biogenesis [82, 112, 113]. However, the implicated molecular machineries are to some extent very different.

In prokaryotic organisms, stabilization of the 5′-3′ mature ends of the nascent rRNA precursors in a topologically limited environment is enabled by the formation of double-stranded RNA structures, the processing stems [114–121]. In all archaeal organisms analyzed so far, this environment is further stabilized by the formation of a true covalent circularization of the pre-rRNA, in form of precircular rRNA intermediates [112, 122, 123]. Finally, in eukaryotes, recent cryo-EM studies have revealed stabilization of a pseudocircular intermediate of the pre-LSU [124]. The formation of this intermediate requires the participation of a distinct eukaryotes-specific ribosome biogenesis subcomplex which may stabilize the LSU root helix bundle prior to the assembly of the universally conserved r-protein uL3 [124, 125]. Noteworthy, early maturation of the pre-23S rRNA by mini-RNase III, which liberates the nascent 23S rRNA from its processing stem in *B. subtilis*, is stimulated by the presence of uL3 [126]. In addition, uL3 is critical to initiate in vitro assembly of bacterial 50S [127, 128].

In the case of the SSU, the snoRNA U3 and its associated proteins provide a scaffold that brings distant rRNA elements in close proximity within an encapsulated environment described as for the 90S/SSU Processome [129–131]. However, the relative orientation of the future mature 5′-3′ ends in these structures is not resolved.

Finally, the formation of the SSU central pseudoknot is a universal feature required for SSU biogenesis and function [132, 133]. In eukaryotes, its formation is facilitated by the snoRNA U3, which is not present in bacteria and archaea [44, 59, 60, 134, 135]. However alternative (U3-independent) mechanisms, enabling the formation of the SSU central pseudoknot in these cellular contexts have been proposed [135–138]. For example, sequences present in the 5' end of the pre-16S rRNA show potential complementarity, similar to U3, which could hybridize with the region required for central pseudoknot formation [136, 139–141].

## 5  Processing and Modifications of Ribosomal RNA

Concomitantly to the assembly process, rRNAs are matured by ribonuclease activities and modified at various positions [18, 37, 44, 59, 60, 78, 79, 114, 142].

Despite billion years of independent evolution most rRNAs are predominantly transcribed as a polycistronic operon [19]. It is believed that this organization is required for the efficient coordinated assembly of ribosomal subunits. However, this idea has been challenged on the one hand by the presence of naturally occurring independent rDNA production units, and on the other hand, by early genetic engineering experiments which have successfully separated the polycistronic eukaryotic SSU and LSU rRNAs [143, 144]. The immature precursor-rRNA contains flanking regions that need to be matured by the action of various ribonucleases. These maturations events are timely ordered during the ribosomal subunit biogenesis process. This relative ordering presumably depends on specific ribosomal subunit assembly statuses which in turn control substrate accessibility or its relative positioning [18, 37, 44, 59, 60, 78, 79, 114, 143, 145]. The inherent irreversible property of these processing steps may also impose various degrees of "quality control" constraints to the ribosome biogenesis process in order to avoid the irreparable formation of improperly assembled pre-ribosomal subunits.

Similar to the ribosome biogenesis factors, the set of ribonucleases used in bacteria, eukaryotes and presumably in archaea are not well conserved between these domains [18, 37, 44, 59, 60, 78, 79, 94, 114, 142]. In bacteria, whereas promiscuous ribonucleases are used, eukaryotic cells have developed a set of specific enzymes to mature their rRNAs, some of which are also present in archaea [18, 37, 44, 52, 59, 60, 78, 79, 94, 114, 142]. Based on our current knowledge, it is difficult to properly extract functional similarities between the different biological systems. However, we have previously noticed some peculiar common molecular principles required for the maturation of the SSU rRNA 3′-end (see above and [18]). However, additional structural and functional information capturing these events "in action" will be necessary to provide invaluable insights into the structural properties of their respective substrates [145].

Since the 1950s, ribosomal RNA modifications, which are mostly concentrated within or closed to the ribosomal subunit functional centers, have been known [37, 146, 147]. These modified rRNAs residues are found, to various extents, in all domains of life [37–40]. However, the mechanisms by which these modifications are added diverge across the tree of life. On the one hand, bacterial rRNAs are modified by stand-alone enzymes that are dependent on a specific assembly status to recognize and modify their respective substrates. On the other hand, and in addition to stand-alone enzymes, archaea and eukaryotic organisms utilize an RNA-guided modification machinery, whereby RNA-protein complexes carrying methyltransferase or pseudouridylation activity are formed (C/D and H/ACA snoRNPs, respectively). In this context, the RNA part, which contains a sequence complementary to the targeted rRNA region, guides the enzymatic activity to its substrate [37, 39, 40, 148–150] (Fig. 1).

These different modes of action have important consequences regarding substrate recognition, timing of modifications and structural constraints that may be imposed by the formation of snoRNA::rRNA duplexes during ribosome assembly, and have thereby probably (re)shaped several aspects of the ribosome biogenesis pathway [18, 37]. Whereas the relative positions of the conserved modified residues are usually similar, the nature of the modification itself may vary across the tree of life [18, 151]. Finally, rRNA modifications appear to be dynamic across the tree of life, whereby significant variation in nature and number of modifications is observed, and may also vary during the organisms life time [36, 38, 39, 41, 90, 152, 153]. These variations may not only influence ribosome function but also the ribosome biogenesis pathway itself [18, 38, 39, 90, 154].

## 6    Learning from Organelle Ribosome Biogenesis?

Eukaryotic organelles also contain ribosomes, which are very distinct from cytoplasmic ribosomes. Organelle's ribosomes and their ribosome biogenesis pathways, which have not been discussed so far, may represent important resources to better extricate key ribosomal subunits biogenesis features. Organelle ribosomal subunits are interesting from several perspectives. First, the ribosomal subunits composition is rather diverse across different organisms. Second and in contrast to cytosolic ribosomal subunits, organelle ribosomal subunits contain a reduced amount of rRNA over r-proteins. Third, organelle ribosomal subunits contain organelle-specific ribosomal proteins, expending the possible diversity of the ribosome assembly landscape. These r-proteins may replace lost rRNA elements or stabilize the reduced rRNA core. Fourth, organelle ribosomal subunits have followed complicated independent evolutionary trajectories enabling the formation of ribosomal subunits optimized for the translation of a limited set of mRNAs [49, 155–157]. In addition to ribosome biogenesis factors shared between bacteria and organelles, recent studies have revealed the existence of specific dedicated multiprotein machineries required for the progression of organelle ribosome biogenesis [155, 158–166]. Despite this apparent sequence/structural specificity, intriguing functional similarity between cytosolic and organelle ribosome biogenesis pathway has been proposed. Altogether, these results suggest that despite very different evolutionary path ribosomal subunits biogenesis may proceed via functionally equivalent assembly intermediates and requires similar but diverse functional innovations facilitating ribosomal subunits assembly [155, 158–166]. Lessons from these and future studies will certainly reveal new insights on the evolution and adaptation of ribosomal subunit biogenesis.

# 7  Concluding Remarks

Despite undeniable differences between the ribosome biogenesis pathways as known from various model organisms, it is striking that some (key) ribosome biogenesis features have been maintained across billions of years of evolution. However, the evolutionary events which have led to components diversification while conserving functional similarities instead of consolidating a core of conserved ribosome biogenesis components remain rather enigmatic. Moreover, the extent of true functional divergence or functional convergence, along the ribosome biogenesis pathway, needs to be properly identified, promising exciting perspectives and challenges for comparative ribosome biology analysis in the future. Correspondingly, in the recent years metagenomics have revealed an unexpected microbial biodiversity [167], which awaits its biochemical and functional examination, and will certainly provide new insights into conserved principles of ribosome biogenesis.

In addition, our increased understanding of supposedly simplified ribosome biogenesis pathway present in symbionts, organelles, and organisms harboring reduced genomes, which for simplicity is not discussed in depth, will provide supplementary functional insights into common and specific principles of ribosome biogenesis [47, 55, 62, 160–162, 168].

Finally, thanks to the massive development in the field of genetic engineering we are probably at the very beginning of a massive biological revolution, which will ease the characterization of nonmodel organisms, to develop synthetic biology approaches, and to uncover some of the most fundamental secrets of life. How we will deal with this information will however be crucial to leverage the significance of these discoveries for our understanding of ribosome biogenesis. When reaching this point, emphasis toward functional similarity and diversity of the ribosome biogenesis process, or its plasticity, will have to be carefully appreciated and will require to understand the genuine functional implication of these molecular features across different organisms' lifestyle and organisms' specific evolutionary history [169].

## Acknowledgments

We are indebted to our many colleagues for their writing and/or invaluable discussions without which this essay would not have been possible. We also sincerely apologize to our colleagues, whose work we failed to discuss or highlight. We are grateful to Prof. Dr. Karl-Dieter Entian (University of Frankfurt, Germany), Dr. Brigitte Pertschy (University of Graz, Austria) and Dr. Robert Knüppel (University of Regensburg, Germany) for comments and suggestions.

Work in the Ferreira-Cerca laboratory is supported by the Chair of Biochemistry III "House of the Ribosome"—University of Regensburg, by the DFG-funded collaborative research center CRC/SFB960 "RNP biogenesis: assembly of ribosomes and non-ribosomal RNPs and control of their function" (SFB960-B13) and by an individual DFG grant to S.F.-C. (FE1622/2-1; Project Nr. 409198929).

## References

1. Einstein A (1916) Die Grundlage der allgemeinen Relativitätstheorie. Ann Phys 354: 769–822. https://doi.org/10.1002/andp.19163540702

2. Friedmann H (2004) From butyribacterium to E. coli: an essay on unity in biochemistry. Perspect Biol Med 47:47–66. https://doi.org/10.1353/pbm.2004.0007

3. Huxley J (1942) Evolution, the modern synthesis. G. Allen & Unwin Limited, Crows Nest

4. Laland KN, Uller T, Feldman MW et al (2015) The extended evolutionary synthesis: its structure, assumptions and predictions. Proc R Soc B Biol Sci 282:20151019. https://doi.org/10.1098/rspb.2015.1019

5. McElroy WD (1976) The unity in biochemistry. Trends Biochem Sci 1:93. https://doi.org/10.1016/0968-0004(76)90009-8

6. Pace NR, Sapp J, Goldenfeld N (2012) Phylogeny and beyond: scientific, historical, and conceptual significance of the first tree of life. Proc Natl Acad Sci 109:1011–1018. https://doi.org/10.1073/pnas.1109716109

7. Thauer R (1997) Biodiversity and unity in biochemistry. Antonie Van Leeuwenhoek 71: 21–32. https://doi.org/10.1023/A:1000149705588

8. Kluyver HJ, Donker HJL (1926) Die Einheit der Biochemie. Chem Zelle Gewebe 13:134–190

9. Crother B, Parenti L (2017) Assumptions inhibiting progress in comparative biology. CRC Press, Boca Raton

10. Hage AE, Tollervey D (2004) A surfeit of factors: why is ribosome assembly so much more complicated in eukaryotes than bacteria? RNA Biol 1:9–14. https://doi.org/10.4161/rna.1.1.932

11. Martinez P (2018) The comparative method in biology and the essentialist trap. Front Ecol Evol 6:130. https://doi.org/10.3389/fevo.2018.00130

12. Ramakrishnan V (2009) The ribosome: some hard facts about its structure and hot air about its evolution. Cold Spring Harb Symp Quant Biol 74:25–33. https://doi.org/10.1101/sqb.2009.74.032

13. Lecompte O, Ripp R, Thierry J et al (2002) Comparative analysis of ribosomal proteins in complete genomes: an example of reductive evolution at the domain scale. Nucleic Acids Res 30:5382–5390. https://doi.org/10.1093/nar/gkf693

14. Yutin N, Puigbò P, Koonin EV, Wolf YI (2012) Phylogenomics of prokaryotic ribosomal proteins. PLoS One 7:e36972. https://doi.org/10.1371/journal.pone.0036972

15. Lake JA, Henderson E, Oakes M, Clark MW (1984) Eocytes: a new ribosome structure indicates a kingdom with a close relationship to eukaryotes. Proc Natl Acad Sci 81:3786–3790

16. Tissières A, Watson JD (1958) Ribonucleoprotein particles from Escherichia coli. Nature 182:778–780. https://doi.org/10.1038/182778b0

17. Tissières A, Watson JD, Schlessinger D, Hollingworth BR (1959) Ribonucleoprotein particles from Escherichia coli. J Mol Biol 1:221–233. https://doi.org/10.1016/S0022-2836(59)80029-2

18. Ferreira-Cerca S (2017) Life and death of ribosomes in archaea. In: Clouet-d'Orval B (ed) RNA metabolism and gene expression in Archaea. Springer International Publishing, Cham, pp 129–158

19. Klappenbach JA, Saxman PR, Cole JR, Schmidt TM (2001) Rrndb: the ribosomal RNA operon copy number database. Nucleic Acids Res 29:181–184

20. Hadjiolov AA (1985) The nucleolus and ribosome biogenesis. Springer-Verlag, Wien

21. Stoddard SF, Smith BJ, Hein R et al (2015) rrnDB: improved tools for interpreting rRNA gene abundance in bacteria and archaea and a new foundation for future development. Nucleic Acids Res 43:D593–D598. https://doi.org/10.1093/nar/gku1201

22. Warner JR (1999) The economics of ribosome biosynthesis in yeast. Trends Biochem Sci 24:437–440. https://doi.org/10.1016/S0968-0004(99)01460-7

23. Gerbi S (1996) Expansion segments: regions of variable size that interrupt the universal core secondary structure of ribosomal RNA. In: Ribosomal RNA structure, evolution, processing, and function in protein biosynthesis, vol 71. CRC Press, Boca Raton, p 87

24. Gerbi SA (1986) The evolution of eukaryotic ribosomal DNA. Biosystems 19:247–258. https://doi.org/10.1016/0303-2647(86)90001-8

25. Armache J-P, Anger AM, Márquez V et al (2013) Promiscuous behaviour of archaeal ribosomal proteins: implications for eukaryotic ribosome evolution. Nucleic Acids Res 41:1284–1293. https://doi.org/10.1093/nar/gks1259

26. Petrov AS, Gulen B, Norris AM et al (2015) History of the ribosome and the origin of translation. Proc Natl Acad Sci 112:15396–15401. https://doi.org/10.1073/pnas.1509761112

27. Parker MS, Sallee FR, Park EA, Parker SL (2015) Homoiterons and expansion in ribosomal RNAs. FEBS Open Bio 5:864–876. https://doi.org/10.1016/j.fob.2015.10.005

28. Nakao A, Yoshihama M, Kenmochi N (2004) RPG: the ribosomal protein gene database. Nucleic Acids Res 32:D168–D170. https://doi.org/10.1093/nar/gkh004

29. Culver GM (2003) Assembly of the 30S ribosomal subunit. Biopolymers 68:234–249. https://doi.org/10.1002/bip.10221

30. Nierhaus KH, Lafontaine DL (2004) Ribosome assembly. In: Protein synthesis and ribosome structure. Wiley-VCH Verlag GmbH & Co. KGaA, Weinheim, pp 85–143

31. Nierhaus KH (1991) The assembly of prokaryotic ribosomes. Biochimie 73:739–755. https://doi.org/10.1016/0300-9084(91)90054-5

32. Londei P, Teixidò J, Acca M et al (1986) Total reconstitution of active large ribosomal subunits of the thermoacidophilic archaebacterium Sulfolobus solfataricus. Nucleic Acids Res 14:2269–2285

33. Sanchez EM, Londei P, Amils R (1996) Total reconstitution of active small ribosomal subunits of the extreme halophilic archaeon

Haloferax mediterranei. Biochim Biophys Acta Protein Struct Mol Enzymol 1292: 140–144. https://doi.org/10.1016/0167-4838(95)00179-4

34. Sanchez ME, Urena D, Amils R, Londei P (1990) In vitro reassembly of active large ribosomal subunits of the halophilic archaebacterium *Haloferax mediterranei*. Biochemistry 29:9256–9261. https://doi.org/10.1021/bi00491a021

35. Mangiarotti G, Chiaberge S (1997) Reconstitution of functional eukaryotic ribosomes from Dictyostelium discoideum ribosomal proteins and RNA. J Biol Chem 272:19682–19687. https://doi.org/10.1074/jbc.272.32.19682

36. Sas-Chen A, Thomas JM, Matzov D et al (2020) Dynamic RNA acetylation revealed by quantitative cross-evolutionary mapping. Nature 583:638–643. https://doi.org/10.1038/s41586-020-2418-2

37. Sloan KE, Warda AS, Sharma S et al (2016) Tuning the ribosome: the influence of rRNA modification on eukaryotic ribosome biogenesis and function. RNA Biol 14(9):1138–1116. https://doi.org/10.1080/15476286.2016.1259781

38. Dennis PP, Tripp V, Lui L et al (2015) C/D box sRNA-guided 2′-O-methylation patterns of archaeal rRNA molecules. BMC Genomics 16:632. https://doi.org/10.1186/s12864-015-1839-z

39. Grosjean H, Gaspin C, Marck C et al (2008) RNomics and modomics in the halophilic archaea Haloferax volcanii: identification of RNA modification genes. BMC Genomics 9:470. https://doi.org/10.1186/1471-2164-9-470

40. Lafontaine DLJ, Tollervey D (1998) Birth of the snoRNPs: the evolution of the modification-guide snoRNAs. Trends Biochem Sci 23:383–388. https://doi.org/10.1016/S0968-0004(98)01260-2

41. Coureux P-D, Lazennec-Schurdevin C, Bourcier S et al (2020) Cryo-EM study of an archaeal 30S initiation complex gives insights into evolution of translation initiation. Commun Biol 3:58. https://doi.org/10.1038/s42003-020-0780-0

42. Grünberger F, Knüppel R, Jüttner M, et al (2020) Exploring prokaryotic transcription, operon structures, rRNA maturation and modifications using nanopore-based native RNA sequencing. bioRxiv 2019.12.18.880849. https://doi.org/10.1101/2019.12.18.880849

43. Sharma S, Lafontaine DLJ (2015) 'View from a bridge': a new perspective on eukaryotic rRNA base modification. Trends Biochem Sci 40:560–575. https://doi.org/10.1016/j.tibs.2015.07.008

44. Thomson E, Ferreira-Cerca S, Hurt E (2013) Eukaryotic ribosome biogenesis at a glance. J Cell Sci 126:4815. https://doi.org/10.1242/jcs.111948

45. Ebersberger I, Simm S, Leisegang MS et al (2014) The evolution of the ribosome biogenesis pathway from a yeast perspective. Nucleic Acids Res 42:1509–1523. https://doi.org/10.1093/nar/gkt1137

46. Henras AK, Plisson-Chastang C, O'Donohue M-F et al (2015) An overview of pre-ribosomal RNA processing in eukaryotes. Wiley Interdiscip Rev RNA 6:225–242. https://doi.org/10.1002/wrna.1269

47. Grosjean H, Breton M, Sirand-Pugnet P et al (2014) Predicting the minimal translation apparatus: lessons from the reductive evolution of mollicutes. PLoS Genet 10:e1004363. https://doi.org/10.1371/journal.pgen.1004363

48. Woolford JL, Baserga SJ (2013) Ribosome biogenesis in the yeast Saccharomyces cerevisiae. Genetics 195:643–681. https://doi.org/10.1534/genetics.113.153197

49. Ban N, Beckmann R, Cate JHD et al (2014) A new system for naming ribosomal proteins. Curr Opin Struct Biol 24:165–169. https://doi.org/10.1016/j.sbi.2014.01.002

50. Nürenberg-Goloub E, Kratzat H, Heinemann H et al (2020) Molecular analysis of the ribosome recycling factor ABCE1 bound to the 30S post-splitting complex. EMBO J 39:e103788. https://doi.org/10.15252/embj.2019103788

51. Márquez V, Fröhlich T, Armache J-P et al (2011) Proteomic characterization of archaeal ribosomes reveals the presence of novel archaeal-specific ribosomal proteins. J Mol Biol 405:1215–1232. https://doi.org/10.1016/j.jmb.2010.11.055

52. Londei P, Ferreira-Cerca S (2021) Ribosome biogenesis in archaea. Front Microbiol 12:1476. https://doi.org/10.3389/fmicb.2021.686977

53. Mendler K, Chen H, Parks DH et al (2019) AnnoTree: visualization and exploration of a functionally annotated microbial tree of life. Nucleic Acids Res 47:4442–4448. https://doi.org/10.1093/nar/gkz246

54. Cannone JJ, Subramanian S, Schnare MN et al (2002) The comparative RNA web

(CRW) site: an online database of comparative sequence and structure information for ribosomal, intron, and other RNAs. BMC Bioinform 3:2–2. https://doi.org/10.1186/1471-2105-3-2

55. Nikolaeva DD, Gelfand MS, Garushyants SK (2020) Simplification of ribosomes in bacteria with tiny genomes. bioRxiv 755876. https://doi.org/10.1101/755876

56. Quast C, Pruesse E, Yilmaz P et al (2012) The SILVA ribosomal RNA gene database project: improved data processing and web-based tools. Nucleic Acids Res 41:D590–D596. https://doi.org/10.1093/nar/gks1219

57. Chao FC (1957) Dissociation of macromolecular ribonucleoprotein of yeast. Arch Biochem Biophys 70:426–431. https://doi.org/10.1016/0003-9861(57)90130-3

58. Chao F-C, Schachman HK (1956) The isolation and characterization of a macromolecular ribonucleoprotein from yeast. Arch Biochem Biophys 61:220–230. https://doi.org/10.1016/0003-9861(56)90334-4

59. Baßler J, Hurt E (2019) Eukaryotic ribosome assembly. Annu Rev Biochem 88:281–306. https://doi.org/10.1146/annurev-biochem-013118-110817

60. Klinge S, Woolford JL (2019) Ribosome assembly coming into focus. Nat Rev Mol Cell Biol 20:116–131. https://doi.org/10.1038/s41580-018-0078-y

61. Melnikov S, Ben-Shem A, Garreau de Loubresse N et al (2012) One core, two shells: bacterial and eukaryotic ribosomes. Nat Struct Mol Biol 19:560–567. https://doi.org/10.1038/nsmb.2313

62. Barandun J, Hunziker M, Vossbrinck CR, Klinge S (2019) Evolutionary compaction and adaptation visualized by the structure of the dormant microsporidian ribosome. Nat Microbiol 4:1798–1804. https://doi.org/10.1038/s41564-019-0514-6

63. Penev PI, Fakhretaha-Aval S, Patel VJ et al (2020) Supersized ribosomal RNA expansion segments in Asgard archaea. Genome Biol Evol 12:1694–1710. https://doi.org/10.1093/gbe/evaa170

64. Tirumalai MR, Kaelber JT, Park DR et al (2020) Cryo-electron microscopy visualization of a large insertion in the 5S ribosomal RNA of the extremely halophilic archaeon Halococcus morrhuae. FEBS Open Bio 10:1938–1946. https://doi.org/10.1002/2211-5463.12962

65. Stepanov VG, Fox GE (2021) Expansion segments in bacterial and archaeal 5S ribosomal

RNAs. RNA 27:133–150. https://doi.org/10.1261/rna.077123.120

66. Bowman JC, Petrov AS, Frenkel-Pinter M et al (2020) Root of the tree: the significance, evolution, and origins of the ribosome. Chem Rev 120:4848–4878. https://doi.org/10.1021/acs.chemrev.9b00742

67. Lake JA (1985) Evolving ribosome structure: domains in Archaebacteria, eubacteria, eocytes and eukaryotes. Annu Rev Biochem 54:507–530. https://doi.org/10.1146/annurev.bi.54.070185.002451

68. Lake JA (2015) Eukaryotic origins. Philos Trans R Soc Lond Ser B Biol Sci 370:20140329. https://doi.org/10.1098/rstb.2014.0321

69. Spang A, Saw JH, Jorgensen SL et al (2015) Complex archaea that bridge the gap between prokaryotes and eukaryotes. Nature 521:173–179

70. Williams TA, Foster PG, Nye TMW et al (2012) A congruent phylogenomic signal places eukaryotes within the archaea. Proc Biol Sci 279:4870. https://doi.org/10.1098/rspb.2012.1795

71. Zaremba-Niedzwiedzka K, Caceres EF, Saw JH et al (2017) Asgard archaea illuminate the origin of eukaryotic cellular complexity. Nature 541(7637):353–358

72. Dao Duc K, Batra SS, Bhattacharya N et al (2019) Differences in the path to exit the ribosome across the three domains of life. Nucleic Acids Res 47:4198–4210. https://doi.org/10.1093/nar/gkz106

73. Melnikov S, Manakongtreecheep K, Söll D (2018) Revising the structural diversity of ribosomal proteins across the three domains of life. Mol Biol Evol 35:1588–1598. https://doi.org/10.1093/molbev/msy021

74. Dohme F, Nierhaus KH (1976) Total reconstitution and assembly of 50S subunits from Escherichia coli ribosomes in vitro. J Mol Biol 107:585–599. https://doi.org/10.1016/S0022-2836(76)80085-X

75. Mizushima S, Nomura M (1970) Assembly mapping of 30S ribosomal proteins from E. coli. Nature 226:1214–1218. https://doi.org/10.1038/2261214a0

76. Nomura M, Erdmann VA (1970) Reconstitution of 50S ribosomal subunits from dissociated molecular components. Nature 228:744–748. https://doi.org/10.1038/228744a0

77. Traub P, Nomura M (1968) Structure and function of E. coli ribosomes. V. Reconstitution of functionally

active 30S ribosomal particles from RNA and proteins. Proc Natl Acad Sci U S A 59:777–784. https://doi.org/10.1073/pnas.59.3.777

78. Davis JH, Williamson JR (2017) Structure and dynamics of bacterial ribosome biogenesis. Philos Trans R Soc Lond Ser B Biol Sci 372(1716):20160181. https://doi.org/10.1098/rstb.2016.0181

79. Shajani Z, Sykes MT, Williamson JR (2011) Assembly of bacterial ribosomes. Annu Rev Biochem 80:501–526. https://doi.org/10.1146/annurev-biochem-062608-160432

80. de la Cruz J, Karbstein K, Woolford JL (2015) Functions of ribosomal proteins in assembly of eukaryotic ribosomes in vivo. Annu Rev Biochem 84:93–129. https://doi.org/10.1146/annurev-biochem-060614-033917

81. Duss O, Stepanyuk GA, Puglisi JD, Williamson JR (2019) Transient protein-RNA interactions guide nascent ribosomal RNA folding. Cell 179:1357–1369.e16. https://doi.org/10.1016/j.cell.2019.10.035

82. Ferreira-Cerca S, Pöll G, Kühn H et al (2007) Analysis of the in vivo assembly pathway of eukaryotic 40S ribosomal proteins. Mol Cell 28:446–457. https://doi.org/10.1016/j.molcel.2007.09.029

83. Gamalinda M, Ohmayer U, Jakovljevic J et al (2014) A hierarchical model for assembly of eukaryotic 60S ribosomal subunit domains. Genes Dev 28:198–210. https://doi.org/10.1101/gad.228825.113

84. Ohmayer U, Gamalinda M, Sauert M et al (2013) Studies on the assembly characteristics of large subunit ribosomal proteins in S. cerevisae. PLoS One 8:e68412. https://doi.org/10.1371/journal.pone.0068412

85. Ohmayer U, Gil-Hernández Á, Sauert M et al (2015) Studies on the coordination of ribosomal protein assembly events involved in processing and stabilization of yeast early large ribosomal subunit precursors. PLoS One 10:e0143768. https://doi.org/10.1371/journal.pone.0143768

86. Pöll G, Braun T, Jakovljevic J et al (2009) rRNA maturation in yeast cells depleted of large ribosomal subunit proteins. PLoS One 4:e8249. https://doi.org/10.1371/journal.pone.0008249

87. Rodgers ML, Woodson SA (2019) Transcription increases the cooperativity of ribonucleoprotein assembly. Cell 179:1370–1381.e12. https://doi.org/10.1016/j.cell.2019.11.007

88. Fox GE (2010) Origin and evolution of the ribosome. Cold Spring Harb Perspect Biol 2: a003483. https://doi.org/10.1101/cshperspect.a003483

89. Connolly K, Rife JP, Culver G (2008) Mechanistic insight into the ribosome biogenesis functions of the ancient protein KsgA. Mol Microbiol 70:1062–1075. https://doi.org/10.1111/j.1365-2958.2008.06485.x

90. Seistrup KH, Rose S, Birkedal U et al (2016) Bypassing rRNA methylation by RsmA/Dim1during ribosome maturation in the hyperthermophilic archaeon Nanoarchaeum equitans. Nucleic Acids Res 45(4):2007–2015. https://doi.org/10.1093/nar/gkw839

91. Hellmich UA, Weis BL, Lioutikov A et al (2013) Essential ribosome assembly factor Fap7 regulates a hierarchy of RNA–protein interactions during small ribosomal subunit biogenesis. Proc Natl Acad Sci U S A 110:15253–15258. https://doi.org/10.1073/pnas.1306389110

92. Knüppel R, Christensen RH, Gray FC et al (2018) Insights into the evolutionary conserved regulation of Rio ATPase activity. Nucleic Acids Res 46:1441–1456. https://doi.org/10.1093/nar/gkx1236

93. Veith T, Martin R, Wurm JP et al (2012) Structural and functional analysis of the archaeal endonuclease Nob1. Nucleic Acids Res 40:3259–3274. https://doi.org/10.1093/nar/gkr1186

94. Clouet-d'Orval B, Batista M, Bouvier M et al (2018) Insights into RNA-processing pathways and associated RNA-degrading enzymes in Archaea. FEMS Microbiol Rev 42:579–613. https://doi.org/10.1093/femsre/fuy016

95. Knüppel R, Trahan C, Kern M et al (2021) Insights into synthesis and function of KsgA/Dim1-dependent rRNA modifications in archaea. Nucleic Acids Res 49(3):1662–1687. https://doi.org/10.1093/nar/gkaa1268

96. Ameismeier M, Cheng J, Berninghausen O, Beckmann R (2018) Visualizing late states of human 40S ribosomal subunit maturation. Nature 558:249–253. https://doi.org/10.1038/s41586-018-0193-0

97. Bubunenko M, Korepanov A, Court DL et al (2006) 30S ribosomal subunits can be assembled in vivo without primary binding ribosomal protein S15. RNA 12:1229–1239. https://doi.org/10.1261/rna.2262106

98. Mulder AM, Yoshioka C, Beck AH et al (2010) Visualizing ribosome biogenesis: parallel assembly pathways for the 30S subunit.

Science 330:673. https://doi.org/10.1126/science.1193220

99. Pratte D, Singh U, Murat G, Kressler D (2013) Mak5 and Ebp2 act together on early pre-60S particles and their reduced functionality bypasses the requirement for the essential pre-60S factor Nsa1. PLoS One 8:-e82741. https://doi.org/10.1371/journal.pone.0082741

100. Zorbas C, Nicolas E, Wacheul L et al (2015) The human 18S rRNA base methyltransferases DIMT1L and WBSCR22-TRMT112 but not rRNA modification are required for ribosome biogenesis. Mol Biol Cell 26:2080–2095. https://doi.org/10.1091/mbc.E15-02-0073

101. Talkington MWT, Siuzdak G, Williamson JR (2005) An assembly landscape for the 30S ribosomal subunit. Nature 438:628–632. https://doi.org/10.1038/nature04261

102. Sharma MR, Barat C, Wilson DN et al (2005) Interaction of era with the 30S ribosomal subunit: implications for 30S subunit assembly. Mol Cell 18:319–329. https://doi.org/10.1016/j.molcel.2005.03.028

103. Tu C, Zhou X, Tropea JE et al (2009) Structure of ERA in complex with the 3' end of 16S rRNA: implications for ribosome biogenesis. Proc Natl Acad Sci U S A 106:14843–14848. https://doi.org/10.1073/pnas.0904032106

104. Tu C, Zhou X, Tarasov SG et al (2011) The era GTPase recognizes the GAUCACCUCC sequence and binds helix 45 near the 3' end of 16S rRNA. Proc Natl Acad Sci U S A 108:10156–10161. https://doi.org/10.1073/pnas.1017679108

105. Vercruysse M, Köhrer C, Shen Y et al (2016) Identification of YbeY-protein interactions involved in 16S rRNA maturation and stress regulation in Escherichia coli. mBio 7:e01785-16. https://doi.org/10.1128/mBio.01785-16

106. Jakovljevic J, de Mayolo PA, Miles TD et al (2004) The carboxy-terminal extension of yeast ribosomal protein S14 is necessary for maturation of 43S preribosomes. Mol Cell 14:331–342. https://doi.org/10.1016/S1097-2765(04)00215-1

107. Lamanna AC, Karbstein K (2009) Nob1 binds the single-stranded cleavage site D at the 3'-end of 18S rRNA with its PIN domain. Proc Natl Acad Sci U S A 106:14259–14264. https://doi.org/10.1073/pnas.0905403106

108. Lebaron S, Schneider C, van Nues RW et al (2012) Proof reading of pre-40S ribosome maturation by a translation initiation factor and 60S subunits. Nat Struct Mol Biol 19:744–753. https://doi.org/10.1038/nsmb.2308

109. Pertschy B, Schneider C, Gnädig M et al (2009) RNA helicase Prp43 and its co-factor Pfa1 promote 20 to 18S rRNA processing catalyzed by the endonuclease Nob1. J Biol Chem 284:35079–35091. https://doi.org/10.1074/jbc.M109.040774

110. Woolls HA, Lamanna AC, Karbstein K (2011) Roles of Dim2 in ribosome assembly. J Biol Chem 286:2578–2586. https://doi.org/10.1074/jbc.M110.191494

111. Jia MZ, Horita S, Nagata K, Tanokura M (2010) An archaeal Dim2-like protein, aDim2p, forms a ternary complex with a/eIF2α and the 3' end fragment of 16S rRNA. J Mol Biol 398:774–785. https://doi.org/10.1016/j.jmb.2010.03.055

112. Jüttner M, Weiß M, Ostheimer N et al (2019) A versatile cis-acting element reporter system to study the function, maturation and stability of ribosomal RNA mutants in archaea. Nucleic Acids Res 48(4):2073–2090. https://doi.org/10.1093/nar/gkz1156

113. Veldman GM, Klootwijk J, van Heerikhuizen H, Planta RJ (1981) The nucleotide sequence of the intergenic region between the 5.8S and 26S rRNA genes of the yeast ribosomal RNA operon. Possible implications for the interaction between 5.8S and 26S rRNA and the processing of the primary transcript. Nucleic Acids Res 9:4847–4862. https://doi.org/10.1093/nar/9.19.4847

114. Bechhofer DH, Deutscher MP (2019) Bacterial ribonucleases and their roles in RNA metabolism. Crit Rev Biochem Mol Biol 54:242–300. https://doi.org/10.1080/10409238.2019.1651816

115. Bubunenko M, Court DL, Refaii AA et al (2013) Nus transcription elongation factors and RNase III modulate small ribosome subunit biogenesis in E. coli. Mol Microbiol 87:382–393. https://doi.org/10.1111/mmi.12105

116. Condon C (2007) Maturation and degradation of RNA in bacteria. Curr Opin Microbiol 10:271–278. https://doi.org/10.1016/j.mib.2007.05.008

117. Deutscher MP (2009) Chapter 9: Maturation and degradation of ribosomal RNA in bacteria. In: Progress in molecular biology and translational science. Academic Press, Cambridge, pp 369–391

118. Gegenheimer P, Apirion D (1975) Escherichia coli ribosomal ribonucleic acids are not cut from an intact precursor molecule. J Biol Chem 250:2407–2409

119. Gegenheimer P, Watson N, Apirion D (1977) Multiple pathways for primary processing of ribosomal RNA in Escherichia coli. J Biol Chem 252:3064–3073

120. Srivastava AK, Schlessinger D (1990) Mechanism and regulation of bacterial ribosomal RNA processing. Annu Rev Microbiol 44:105–129. https://doi.org/10.1146/annurev.mi.44.100190.000541

121. Young RA, Steitz JA (1978) Complementary sequences 1700 nucleotides apart form a ribonuclease III cleavage site in *Escherichia coli* ribosomal precursor RNA. Proc Natl Acad Sci U S A 75:3593–3597

122. Danan M, Schwartz S, Edelheit S, Sorek R (2012) Transcriptome-wide discovery of circular RNAs in archaea. Nucleic Acids Res 40:3131–3142. https://doi.org/10.1093/nar/gkr1009

123. Tang TH, Rozhdestvensky TS, d'Orval BC et al (2002) RNomics in Archaea reveals a further link between splicing of archaeal introns and rRNA processing. Nucleic Acids Res 30:921–930

124. Kater L, Thoms M, Barrio-Garcia C et al (2017) Visualizing the assembly pathway of nucleolar pre-60S ribosomes. Cell 171:1599–1610.e14. https://doi.org/10.1016/j.cell.2017.11.039

125. Joret C, Capeyrou R, Belhabich-Baumas K et al (2018) The Npa1p complex chaperones the assembly of the earliest eukaryotic large ribosomal subunit precursor. PLoS Genet 14:e1007597. https://doi.org/10.1371/journal.pgen.1007597

126. Redko Y, Condon C (2009) Ribosomal protein L3 bound to 23S precursor rRNA stimulates its maturation by Mini-III ribonuclease. Mol Microbiol 71:1145–1154. https://doi.org/10.1111/j.1365-2958.2008.06591.x

127. Nowotny V, Nierhaus KH (1982) Initiator proteins for the assembly of the 50S subunit from Escherichia coli ribosomes. Proc Natl Acad Sci U S A 79:7238–7242. https://doi.org/10.1073/pnas.79.23.7238

128. Spillmann S, Dohme F, Nierhaus KH (1977) Assembly in vitro of the 50S subunit from Escherichia coli ribosomes: proteins essential for the first heat-dependent conformational change. J Mol Biol 115:513–523. https://doi.org/10.1016/0022-2836(77)90168-1

129. Chaker-Margot M, Barandun J, Hunziker M, Klinge S (2017) Architecture of the yeast small subunit processome. Science 355:eaal1880. https://doi.org/10.1126/science.aal1880

130. Kornprobst M, Turk M, Kellner N et al (2016) Architecture of the 90S pre-ribosome: a structural view on the birth of the eukaryotic ribosome. Cell 166:380–393. https://doi.org/10.1016/j.cell.2016.06.014

131. Sun Q, Zhu X, Qi J et al (2017) Molecular architecture of the 90S small subunit pre-ribosome. eLife 6:e22086. https://doi.org/10.7554/eLife.22086

132. Gutell RR, Larsen N, Woese CR (1994) Lessons from an evolving rRNA: 16S and 23S rRNA structures from a comparative perspective. Microbiol Rev 58:10–26

133. Powers T, Noller HF (1991) A functional pseudoknot in 16S ribosomal RNA. EMBO J 10:2203–2214

134. Hughes JM (1996) Functional base-pairing interaction between highly conserved elements of U3 small nucleolar RNA and the small ribosomal subunit RNA. J Mol Biol 259:645–654. https://doi.org/10.1006/jmbi.1996.0346

135. Lackmann F, Belikov S, Burlacu E et al (2018) Maturation of the 90S pre-ribosome requires Mrd1 dependent U3 snoRNA and 35S pre-rRNA structural rearrangements. Nucleic Acids Res 46:3692–3706. https://doi.org/10.1093/nar/gky036

136. Dennis PP, Russell AG, Moniz De Sá M (1997) Formation of the 5′ end pseudoknot in small subunit ribosomal RNA: involvement of U3-like sequences. RNA 3:337–343

137. Lundkvist P, Jupiter S, Segerstolpe A et al (2009) Mrd1p is required for release of base-paired U3 snoRNA within the preribosomal complex. Mol Cell Biol 29:5763–5774. https://doi.org/10.1128/MCB.00428-09

138. Sashital DG, Greeman CA, Lyumkis D et al (2014) A combined quantitative mass spectrometry and electron microscopy analysis of ribosomal 30S subunit assembly in E. coli. eLife 3:e04491. https://doi.org/10.7554/eLife.04491

139. Besançon W, Wagner R (1999) Characterization of transient RNA-RNA interactions important for the facilitated structure formation of bacterial ribosomal 16S RNA. Nucleic Acids Res 27:4353–4362. https://doi.org/10.1093/nar/27.22.4353

140. Pardon B, Wagner R (1995) The Escherichia coli ribosomal RNA leader nut region interacts specifically with mature 16S RNA.

Nucleic Acids Res 23:932–941. https://doi.org/10.1093/nar/23.6.932

141. Theissen G, Behrens SE, Wagner R (1990) Functional importance of the Escherichia coli ribosomal RNA leader box A sequence for post-transcriptional events. Mol Microbiol 4:1667–1678. https://doi.org/10.1111/j.1365-2958.1990.tb00544.x

142. Venema J, Tollervey D (1995) Processing of pre-ribosomal RNA in Saccharomyces cerevisiae. Yeast 11:1629–1650. https://doi.org/10.1002/yea.320111607

143. Brewer TE, Albertsen M, Edwards A et al (2020) Unlinked rRNA genes are widespread among bacteria and archaea. ISME J 14:597–608. https://doi.org/10.1038/s41396-019-0552-3

144. Liang W-Q, Fournier MJ (1997) Synthesis of functional eukaryotic ribosomal RNAs in trans: development of a novel in vivo rDNA system for dissecting ribosome biogenesis. Proc Natl Acad Sci U S A 94:2864–2868

145. Neueder A, Jakob S, Pöll G et al (2010) A local role for the small ribosomal subunit primary binder rpS5 in final 18S rRNA processing in yeast. PLoS One 5:e10194. https://doi.org/10.1371/journal.pone.0010194

146. Littlefield JW, Dunn DB (1958) Natural occurrence of thymine and three methylated adenine bases in several ribonucleic acids. Nature 181:254–255. https://doi.org/10.1038/181254a0

147. Littlefield JW, Dunn DB (1958) The occurrence and distribution of thymine and three methylated-adenine bases in ribonucleic acids from several sources. Biochem J 70:642–651

148. Omer AD, Ziesche S, Decatur WA et al (2003) RNA-modifying machines in archaea. Mol Microbiol 48:617–629. https://doi.org/10.1046/j.1365-2958.2003.03483.x

149. Breuer R, Gomes-Filho J-V, Randau L (2021) Conservation of archaeal C/D box sRNA-guided RNA modifications. Front Microbiol 12:496. https://doi.org/10.3389/fmicb.2021.654029

150. Czekay DP, Kothe U (2021) H/ACA small ribonucleoproteins: structural and functional comparison between archaea and eukaryotes. Front Microbiol 12:488. https://doi.org/10.3389/fmicb.2021.654370

151. Piekna-Przybylska D, Decatur WA, Fournier MJ (2008) The 3D rRNA modification maps database: with interactive tools for ribosome analysis. Nucleic Acids Res 36:D178–D183. https://doi.org/10.1093/nar/gkm855

152. Hebras J, Krogh N, Marty V et al (2019) Developmental changes of rRNA ribose methylations in the mouse. RNA Biol 17(1):150–164. https://doi.org/10.1080/15476286.2019.1670598

153. Krogh N, Jansson MD, Häfner SJ et al (2016) Profiling of 2'-O-Me in human rRNA reveals a subset of fractionally modified positions and provides evidence for ribosome heterogeneity. Nucleic Acids Res 44:7884–7895. https://doi.org/10.1093/nar/gkw482

154. Decatur WA, Fournier MJ (2002) rRNA modifications and ribosome function. Trends Biochem Sci 27:344–351. https://doi.org/10.1016/S0968-0004(02)02109-6

155. Greber BJ, Ban N (2016) Structure and function of the mitochondrial ribosome. Annu Rev Biochem 85:103–132. https://doi.org/10.1146/annurev-biochem-060815-014343

156. Sulima OS, Dinman DJ (2019) The expanding riboverse. Cell 8(10):1205. https://doi.org/10.3390/cells8101205

157. Tomal A, Kwasniak-Owczarek M, Janska H (2019) An update on mitochondrial ribosome biology: the plant mitoribosome in the spotlight. Cells 8(12):1562. https://doi.org/10.3390/cells8121562

158. Bogenhagen DF, Ostermeyer-Fay AG, Haley JD, Garcia-Diaz M (2018) Kinetics and mechanism of mammalian mitochondrial ribosome assembly. Cell Rep 22:1935–1944. https://doi.org/10.1016/j.celrep.2018.01.066

159. De Silva D, Tu Y-T, Amunts A et al (2015) Mitochondrial ribosome assembly in health and disease. Cell Cycle 14:2226–2250. https://doi.org/10.1080/15384101.2015.1053672

160. Karbstein K (2019) Mitochondria teach ribosome assembly. Science 365:1077–1078. https://doi.org/10.1126/science.aay7771

161. Saurer M, Ramrath DJF, Niemann M et al (2019) Mitoribosomal small subunit biogenesis in trypanosomes involves an extensive assembly machinery. Science 365:1144–1149. https://doi.org/10.1126/science.aaw5570

162. Zeng R, Smith E, Barrientos A (2018) Yeast mitoribosome large subunit assembly proceeds by hierarchical incorporation of protein clusters and modules on the inner membrane. Cell Metab 27:645–656.e7. https://doi.org/10.1016/j.cmet.2018.01.012

163. Ramrath DJF, Niemann M, Leibundgut M et al (2018) Evolutionary shift toward protein-based architecture in trypanosomal mitochondrial ribosomes. Science 362:eaau7735. https://doi.org/10.1126/science.aau7735

164. Jaskolowski M, Ramrath DJF, Bieri P et al (2020) Structural insights into the mechanism of mitoribosomal large subunit biogenesis. Mol Cell 79:629–644.e4. https://doi.org/10.1016/j.molcel.2020.06.030

165. Maiti P, Lavdovskaia E, Barrientos A, Richter-Dennerlein R (2021) Role of GTPases in driving mitoribosome assembly. Trends Cell Biol 31:284–297. https://doi.org/10.1016/j.tcb.2020.12.008

166. Soufari H, Waltz F, Parrot C et al (2020) Structure of the mature kinetoplastids mitoribosome and insights into its large subunit biogenesis. Proc Natl Acad Sci U S A 117:29851–29861. https://doi.org/10.1073/pnas.2011301117

167. Castelle CJ, Banfield JF (2018) Major new microbial groups expand diversity and alter our understanding of the tree of life. Cell 172:1181–1197. https://doi.org/10.1016/j.cell.2018.02.016

168. Liu Z, Gutierrez-Vargas C, Wei J et al (2016) Structure and assembly model for the Trypanosoma cruzi 60S ribosomal subunit. Proc Natl Acad Sci U S A 113:12174–12179. https://doi.org/10.1073/pnas.1614594113

169. Jüttner M, Ferreira-Cerca S (2022) Looking through the Lens of the Ribosome Biogenesis Evolutionary History: Possible Implications for Archaeal Phylogeny and Eukaryogenesis. Mol Biol Evol 39:msac054. https://doi.org/10.1093/molbev/msac054

# Part II

## Genomic Organization

# Chapter 2

## Establishment and Maintenance of Open Ribosomal RNA Gene Chromatin States in Eukaryotes

Christopher Schächner, Philipp E. Merkl, Michael Pilsl, Katrin Schwank, Kristin Hergert, Sebastian Kruse, Philipp Milkereit, Herbert Tschochner, and Joachim Griesenbeck

### Abstract

In growing eukaryotic cells, nuclear ribosomal (r)RNA synthesis by RNA polymerase (RNAP) I accounts for the vast majority of cellular transcription. This high output is achieved by the presence of multiple copies of rRNA genes in eukaryotic genomes transcribed at a high rate. In contrast to most of the other transcribed genomic loci, actively transcribed rRNA genes are largely devoid of nucleosomes adapting a characteristic "open" chromatin state, whereas a significant fraction of rRNA genes resides in a transcriptionally inactive nucleosomal "closed" chromatin state. Here, we review our current knowledge about the nature of open rRNA gene chromatin and discuss how this state may be established.

**Key words** Nucleolus, Nucleolar organizer region (NOR), Ribosomal DNA, Ribosomal RNA genes, RNA polymerase I, Transcription, Chromatin, Nucleosome, Preinitiation complex (PIC), High mobility group (HMG) box proteins, Upstream binding factor (UBF), Hmo1, Psoralen cross-linking, Chromatin immunoprecipitation (ChIP), Chromatin endogenous cleavage (ChEC), Electron microscopy (EM)

## 1 Introduction

This short review aims at summarizing research which has contributed to our current understanding of characteristic chromatin states at eukaryotic rRNA gene loci sharing many conserved features from yeast to human. This subject has also (partly) be covered by other reviews in the past, which are recommended for further reading [1–5]. The regulation of RNAP I transcription by epigenetic mechanisms (including posttranslational covalent modifications of histones and other components of the RNAP I transcription machinery, as well as DNA-methylation) has been reviewed in great detail in the past [6–9] and will not be subject of this article.

Karl-Dieter Entian (ed.), *Ribosome Biogenesis: Methods and Protocols*, Methods in Molecular Biology, vol. 2533, https://doi.org/10.1007/978-1-0716-2501-9_2, © The Author(s) 2022

In the nucleus of eukaryotic cells, the genetic information encoded in the DNA is assembled in the structure of chromatin. The basic unit of chromatin is called the nucleosome and consists of approximately 146 bp of DNA wrapped around a histone octamer (reviewed in [10–12]). The tight wrapping of the nucleic acid around the protein core renders the DNA in part inaccessible which plays an important role for the regulation of essential nuclear processes like replication, DNA-repair, and transcription. To deal with nucleosomal DNA, eukaryotic cells developed mechanisms altering chromatin structure at distinct loci in specific situations (reviewed in [13, 14]). Accordingly, characteristic changes in chromatin structure and posttranslational covalent modification state of chromatin components correlate with transitions in the transcriptional status of individual genes. Understanding the relationship between chromatin structure and transcription will be essential to fully comprehend the complex process of eukaryotic gene expression.

## 2    Visualization of rRNA Transcription

### 2.1 Actively Transcribed rRNA Genes Are Prominent Structures in Nuclear Chromatin Spreads

In eukaryotes, there are at least three different nuclear RNAPs, numbered I–III, each of which has a distinct set of target genes (reviewed in [15], see also short reviews by Merkl et al. and Pilsl et al., this issue). Whereas RNAP II transcribes all protein coding genes, RNAP III is dedicated to the synthesis of small noncoding RNAs including the 5S rRNA and tRNAs. In all organisms—with only one known exception [16]—RNAP I has only one acknowledged genomic target locus from which it synthesizes a large precursor transcript encompassing the sequences of three out of four rRNAs (hereafter called rRNA gene). Remarkably, rRNAs produced by RNAP I account for more than 60% of cellular RNA synthesis in exponentially growing *S. cerevisiae* cells (hereafter called yeast, reviewed in [17]). This is achieved by a strong promoter with a stably bound preinitiation complex (PIC) (reviewed in [18]), as well as the multimerization of the genomic templates (reviewed in [19]). Thus, rRNA genes exist as clusters of repeated transcription units, the so-called nucleolar organizer regions (NORs), at one or more genomic locations depending on the organism. Actively transcribed NORs are part of the nucleolus, the dominant nuclear substructure of early ribosome biogenesis, whereas inactive NORs do not associate with nucleoli (reviewed in [20]).

Even slightly before the different nuclear RNAPs were biochemically defined [21, 22], it was possible to visualize the enzymes transcribing their target loci in chromatin spreads by electron microscopy (EM) [23–25]. The first transcription units that were unambiguously identified by this method were the actively transcribed extrachromosomal ribosomal RNA genes isolated from amphibian oocytes [25]. These transcription units showed a characteristic "Christmas-tree" like appearance with tightly packed elongating RNAPs forming the stem, and protein-coated nascent rRNAs extending from the polymerases forming the branches of the trees. Depending on the preparation, Christmas trees can be decorated with "terminal balls" representing preribosomal assembly intermediates [26]. Ever since, rRNA gene Christmas-trees have been observed in chromatin spreads from different cell types of many organisms (reviewed in [27, 28]). These studies yielded important insights in aspects of RNAP I transcription at the single molecule level. More recently, the spreading technique combined with cryo-EM tomography allowed to obtain more detailed structural information about yeast RNAP I transcribing its native template [29]. In fact, shortly after the first Christmas trees had been described, the conserved repeated "beads-on-the-string" nature of nontranscribed eukaryotic chromatin came into the focus of the researchers [30, 31]. The beads-on-the-string seen in EM were biochemically defined as complexes of DNA and histone octamers, the fundamental units of chromatin named nucleosomes [32–34].

**2.2  rRNA Genes Transcribed by RNAP I Are Nucleosome Depleted**

The above analyses of chromatin spreads provided first insights into how different RNAPs deal with the chromatin template (reviewed in [27]). Thus, nonribosomal chromatin moderately transcribed by (presumably) RNAP II remained at least partially covered with nucleosomes [35–37]. This indicated that nucleosomes may either persist or are reestablished upon RNAP II transcription. In contrast, there was evidence that RNAP I and RNAP III transcription occurred exclusively on nucleosome depleted templates even in situations when transcription rate was reduced (reviewed in [27, 38–40]). Complementing EM analyses, endonucleases were used as molecular probes to investigate chromatin structure (reviewed in [41–43]). Endonucleases can only poorly access DNA assembled into a nucleosome. Therefore, endonuclease cleavage at a genomic region of interest can be used to deduce information about local nucleosome occupancy. In such assays, DNA in actively transcribed rRNA gene chromatin was more accessible than DNA in nontranscribed rRNA gene chromatin, supporting the view of nucleosome depletion at RNAP I transcribed regions [44, 45]. This notion was corroborated by in vivo and in vitro cross-linking of chromosomal DNA with psoralen (reviewed in [46] and references therein). Psoralen is a parent compound of naturally occurring substances which can intercalate in DNA (reviewed in [47] and references therein). Upon exposure to long-wave ultraviolet (UVA) radiation, psoralen incorporation leads to DNA-interstrand cross-links. As observed for nucleases, nucleosome formation prevents psoralen intercalation into nucleosomal DNA tightly interacting with the histone octamer

[48, 49]. Therefore, psoralen cross-links are restricted to accessible nucleosome-free DNA regions. After DNA isolation from psoralen cross-linked chromatin, nucleosomes leave a characteristic footprint of approximately 146 bp of non–cross-linked DNA surrounded by cross-linked linker DNA. This can be analyzed by EM of the cross-linked DNA under denaturing conditions, in which the non–cross-linked DNA regions are visualized as single stranded DNA bubbles. Consistent with nucleosome depletion, DNA isolated from psoralen treated actively transcribed rRNA gene chromatin was heavily cross-linked and largely devoid of single-stranded DNA bubbles [50].

### 2.3 rRNA Genes Coexist in At Least Two Different Chromatin States

Psoralen cross-linking alters the mobility of deproteinized DNA fragments in native agarose gel electrophoresis [50]. A high-degree of psoralen incorporation in nucleosome-depleted DNA leads to a strong retardation of the corresponding fragment, whereas lower psoralen incorporation in nucleosomal DNA yields faster migrating fragments. In combination with Southern blot analysis this technique can be used to monitor nucleosome occupancy at specific restriction fragments obtained from psoralen cross-linked chromosomal DNA [50–52]. DNA-fragments deriving from psoralen cross-linked transcribed regions of rRNA genes from a human cell line and yeast cells migrated as two major bands with low and high mobility in native agarose gel electrophoresis, indicating that these genes adapt at least two different chromatin states [51, 52]. Nascent RNA was exclusively cross-linked to the fragment of low mobility, suggesting that nucleosome occupancy at actively transcribed rRNA genes is strongly decreased [51, 52]. This led to the model that rRNA genes may coexist at least in a nucleosome depleted, "open" chromatin state and a transcriptionally inactive nucleosomal "closed" chromatin state. It should be noted, that psoralen cross-linking measures nucleosome occupancy at selected loci, but does not allow straightforward conclusions about the transcriptional state of a gene (reviewed in [2, 3] and references therein). Therefore, open rRNA genes are not necessarily actively transcribed, although actively transcribed rRNA genes appear to be always in an open chromatin state. To date, no other chromosomal locus with a psoralen accessibility similar to open rRNA genes has been identified. Strikingly, psoralen cross-linking of heavily transcribed RNAP II-dependent genes did not yield fragments with the low mobility expected for fully cross-linked DNA [53]. This may corroborate the observations in EM that RNAP II transcribed gene regions retain a significant number of nucleosomal particles [35, 37]. Thus, the open rRNA gene chromatin state is probably unique regarding the extent of nucleosome depletion and the size of the nucleosome depleted region.

With the advent of chromatin immunoprecipitation (ChIP) the nucleosome-depleted nature of actively transcribed rRNA genes was challenged (reviewed in [2, 3]). In ChIP experiments, histone molecules coprecipitated rRNA gene fragments from extracts obtained from yeast cells carrying a reduced number of rRNA gene copies [54]. Because under these conditions, the majority of rRNA genes were transcribed [55], it was concluded that RNAP I transcribes a dynamic, nucleosomal chromatin template. A subsequent study based on chromatin endogenous cleavage (ChEC) experiments in yeast supported rather the model of robust histone/nucleosome depletion at actively transcribed rRNA genes [56]. ChEC is performed in yeast strains in which a protein of interest is expressed in fusion with Micrococcal nuclease (MNase) from *Staphylococcus aureus* [57]. MNase is a secreted DNA and RNA endo- and exonuclease which has long been used to study chromatin structure (reviewed in [41, 43], see chapter of Teubl et al. in this issue). MNase activity strictly depends on calcium. Thus, due to the low intracellular calcium concentrations recombinantly expressed MNase fusion proteins are not active. After isolation of crude nuclei from cells expressing MNase-fusion proteins and addition of calcium, the tethered nuclease will cut neighboring DNA. Specific cleavage events in genomic DNA can be monitored by Southern blot analysis, primer extension or high-throughput sequencing to reveal which DNA regions were in the proximity of the MNase fusion proteins [58, 59]. ChEC experiments can also be performed in combination with psoralen cross-linking to determine if a factor of interest preferentially associates with the open or the closed rRNA gene chromatin state [56, 60]. Using this method, it could be shown that RNAP I subunits fused to MNase specifically degraded the highly psoralen cross-linked fragments derived from open rRNA gene chromatin in yeast. In contrast, histone-MNase fusion proteins preferentially degraded the poorly psoralen cross-linked fragments derived from closed rRNA gene chromatin. These results supported the hypothesis that RNAP I transcribes a histone/nucleosome depleted chromatin template [56]. The apparent contradiction of these results to the conclusions derived from ChIP experiments [54] may be explained by the notion that the term histone depletion does not exclude that a few histone molecules occasionally associate with open rRNA gene chromatin. Additionally, even in yeast cells with a lower rRNA gene copy number, a small subpopulation of rRNA genes resides in the closed nontranscribed nucleosomal chromatin state [55, 61]. This nucleosomal subpopulation might then be detected in ChIP analyses, which—unlike the combination of ChEC with psoralen cross-linking analyses—does not distinguish between DNA fragments derived from open or closed rRNA gene chromatin. In higher eukaryotes ChEC combined with psoralen cross-linking analyses have not been conducted so far. Nevertheless, endonuclease accessibility of human rRNA gene loci combined with high throughput sequencing (HTS) suggested that nucleosome occupancy is reduced at rRNA genes when compared to intergenic regions [62]. More recently, a deconvolution histone ChIP-HTS analysis combined with genetic manipulation of RNAP I transcription in mice strongly supported that histone depletion at active rRNA genes is conserved from yeast to mammals [63, 64].

**2.4 HMG-Box Proteins Are Architectural Components of Open rRNA Gene Chromatin States**

The high mobility group (HMG) box is a structural motif first described in eukaryotic proteins with a high electrophoretic mobility (reviewed in [65]). HMG box proteins are involved in the regulation of many important DNA-dependent processes in the nucleus presumably due to their acknowledged function as architectural chromatin components. Along these lines, HMG-box proteins are conserved constituents of open rRNA gene chromatin (reviewed in [2, 63, 66, 67]). In vertebrates, the upstream binding factor (UBF) was initially identified to be required for proper recruitment of the basal RNAP I PIC at the rRNA gene promoter [68–70]. UBF has a characteristic arrangement of up to six tandemly repeated HMG-boxes (reviewed in [71]). Upon dimerization UBF may wrap DNA in one single loop in a structure called the "enhancesome" in vitro [72]. It was suggested that this structure establishes a characteristic architecture at the rRNA gene promoter (reviewed in [71]). In vivo, UBF molecules spread along the entire rRNA gene region transcribed by RNAP I [62, 63, 66, 73, 74]. Additionally, UBF is preferentially recruited to repetitive enhancer DNA elements preceding the rRNA gene promoter in higher eukaryotes [62, 63, 69, 73, 74]. UBF was shown to localize to NORs harboring active rRNA genes [75]. During the cell division cycle, UBF stays associated with NORs which have been transcriptionally active even upon RNAP I transcription shutdown at mitosis [76–78]. In this condition, UBF likely maintains NORs bearing active rRNA gene clusters in a hypocondensed, open chromatin state leading to "secondary constrictions" visualized by light microscopy in plant mitotic chromosomes early in the twentieth century [79–81]. Yeast contains a bona fide UBF homologue Hmo1 [82, 83]. As UBF, Hmo1 is a chromatin component of actively transcribed rRNA gene regions but has only one HMG-box and—in contrast to UBF—no reported role in RNAP I PIC formation [56, 84–86]. Both murine UBF and yeast Hmo1 are required to maintain the nucleosome depleted open rRNA gene chromatin state in the absence of RNAP I transcription [61, 63]. In agreement, both UBF and Hmo1 can destabilize nucleosomal templates in vitro [87, 88]. Furthermore, Hmo1 mediated DNA compaction, bridging and looping observed in vitro was suggested to be implicated in the maintenance of the nucleosome depleted rRNA gene chromatin state in vivo [89]. UBF and Hmo1 bind to various DNA sequences in vitro [90–92] and genome wide ChIP analyses suggested that both proteins additionally associate with nucleosome depleted promoter regions of highly transcribed RNAP II dependent genes [84–86, 93]. This indicates that UBF and Hmo1 may generally recognize structures associated with highly transcribed DNA templates. This hypothesis was substantiated in in vitro studies in which Hmo1 bound preferentially to DNA templates thought to mimic transcription intermediates [91]. Along these lines it has also been suggested that Hmo1 protects negatively supercoiled DNA at gene boundaries in vivo [94], indicating that (r)DNA topology may be important for Hmo1 recruitment. Whereas there is evidence that recruitment of Hmo1 to rRNA gene sequences is dependent on prior RNAP I transcription [61, 86], RNAP I transcription may not be required to recruit UBF to the rRNA gene promoter or enhancer elements [95]. Thus, integration of rRNA gene enhancer repeats from *Xenopus laevis* at different loci in human chromosomes led to the formation of "pseudo-NORs" resulting in secondary constrictions in mitotic chromosomes (reviewed in [67, 96]). These structures were bound by human UBF, other components of the basal RNAP I transcription machinery and ribosome biogenesis factors [95, 97] but appear to be transcriptional inactive. Although, psoralen accessibility at pseudo-NOR sequences has not been tested to date, it is assumed that they reside in an open chromatin structure. Taken together, both Hmo1 and UBF are architectural proteins of open rRNA gene chromatin and involved in the maintenance of the nucleosome depleted state [56, 61, 63, 73]. Additionally, UBF binding at the rRNA gene promoter (and likely at enhancer regions) is likely related to its role in RNAP I PIC formation (reviewed in [18, 66]). As an essential PIC component, UBF—but not Hmo1—is required for the establishment of the open rRNA gene chromatin state in vivo [56, 63, 73].

**2.5 Molecular Requirements to Establish the Open rRNA Gene Chromatin State**

As indicated above, there is a tight correlation between RNAP I transcription and the establishment of the open chromatin state. In fact, studies in yeast indicated that the equilibrium of open and closed chromatin states observed in asynchronously dividing cells may be explained as the result of RNAP I transcription dependent opening and replication dependent closing of rRNA genes [61]. In each synthesis phase of the cell division cycle, replication leads to nucleosome deposition and chromatin closing at rRNA genes on both sister chromatids [98]. After rRNA genes have been replicated, opening of rRNA genes correlates with the onset of RNAP I transcription. In higher eukaryotes, cell division cycle dependent rRNA gene chromatin transitions were likely dismissed in early psoralen cross-linking studies in which interphase cells were compared with metaphase cells [51]. However at least in one study, time course experiments during the cell division cycle in a human cell line revealed very similar rRNA gene chromatin state transitions to those observed in yeast [99]. In agreement with a requirement for RNAP I transcription for establishment of the open rRNA gene chromatin state in replicating yeast cells, all rRNA genes adapt the closed chromatin state when RNAP I transcription is impaired [61]. In addition, there was good correlation between downregulation of RNAP I transcription and closing of rRNA gene chromatin in various physiological relevant situations. Thus, rRNA gene chromatin closing occurs when cells grow to stationary phase [51, 52, 100, 101], upon UV-damage [102, 103], or when cells differentiate [104]. On the other hand, upregulation of RNAP I transcription upon transfer of stationary yeast cells in fresh growth media correlates with rapid opening of rRNA genes [100, 101]. Furthermore, the observed opening of rRNA genes when replication-mediated chromatin closing was prevented strictly depends on ongoing RNAP I transcription [61].

It remains unclear if RNAP I transcription alone suffices to establish open, nucleosome-depleted rRNA gene chromatin. Thus, additional factors may assist RNAP I to convert genes from the closed to the open chromatin state. The "Facilitates Chromatin Transcription" (FACT) complex, known to support RNAP II transcription, was shown to associate with rRNA genes in yeast and human, copurified with human RNAP I and enhanced RNAP I nonspecific transcription from chromatin templates in vitro [39, 105]. In yeast, the chromatin remodeling factors Ino80, Isw1, and Isw2, as well as the Swi/Snf complex associate with rRNA genes in vivo and ex vivo and may modulate rRNA gene chromatin structure [106–108]. Furthermore, bona fide RNAP II transcription (elongation) factors TFIIH, Paf1, Spt4/5, Spt6, and THO were reported to support RNAP I transcription [109–114]. In addition, early ribosome biogenesis factors might be components of rRNA gene chromatin in yeast and higher eukaryotes perhaps supporting efficient RNAP I transcription [97, 115]. Finally, a constantly growing number of factors which are involved in (epigenetic) posttranslational covalent modifications of chromatin components (including proteins and nucleic acids), as well as noncoding RNAs may influence RNAP I transcription and the establishment of rRNA gene chromatin states (reviewed in [6–9]). Since most of the above factors have acknowledged roles in various nuclear processes, it is, however, often difficult to distinguish between direct and indirect effects on RNAP I transcription and rRNA gene chromatin structure.

## 3   Conclusions

Our current knowledge of molecular mechanisms required for establishment of the open rRNA gene chromatin state is mostly based on in vivo observations or ex vivo analyses of relatively crude cellular fractions. In the future, analyses with defined in vitro reconstituted chromatin will probably allow to stringently test current hypotheses and to describe molecular mechanisms which are responsible for chromatin opening (see [116] and chapter by Merkl et al., this issue). One promising approach may involve the investigation of isolated native rRNA gene chromatin templates. Chromosomal rRNA gene domains in their native chromatin context can be purified from yeast, and initial analyses indicate that important features of the in vivo chromatin structure are maintained upon isolation [107]. The purified chromatin can be subjected to functional biochemical assays, or single molecule structural analyses [107, 117]. The reconstitution of transcription using highly purified components of the RNAP I transcription machinery and the native chromatin template in vitro might closely reflect the in vivo situation. Together, these studies may help to derive a detailed understanding about the interplay between chromatin structure and transcription on a molecular level. Given the tight connection between RNAP I transcription and early steps in ribosome biogenesis [115], it should be attempted to include selected ribosome biogenesis factors in the purified system. Perhaps, this may lead us soon to the first Christmas trees "grown" in vitro.

# Acknowledgments

We are grateful to all scientists who contributed to this exciting field of research and apologize to those colleagues whose work has not been cited. We thank the members of the department of Biochemistry III for constant support and discussion. This work was funded by the Deutsche Forschungsgemeinschaft (DFG) in the context of the SFB960. P. E. M. was partly supported by a fellowship of the German National Academic Foundation.

# References

1. Birch JL, Zomerdijk JCBM (2008) Structure and function of ribosomal RNA gene chromatin. Biochem Soc Trans 36:619–624

2. Hamperl S, Wittner M, Babl V, Perez-Fernandez J, Tschochner H, Griesenbeck J (2013) Chromatin states at ribosomal DNA loci. Biochim Biophys Acta 1829:405–417

3. Moss T, Mars J-C, Tremblay MG, Sabourin-Felix M (2019) The chromatin landscape of the ribosomal RNA genes in mouse and human. Chromosome Res 27(1–2):31–40. https://doi.org/10.1007/s10577-018-09603-9

4. Németh A, Längst G (2008) Chromatin organization of active ribosomal RNA genes. Epigenetics 3:243–245

5. Schöfer C, Weipoltshammer K (2018) Nucleolus and chromatin. Histochem Cell Biol 150:209–225

6. Drygin D, Rice WG, Grummt I (2010) The RNA polymerase I transcription machinery: an emerging target for the treatment of cancer. Annu Rev Pharmacol Toxicol 50:131–156

7. Grummt I, Längst G (2013) Epigenetic control of RNA polymerase I transcription in mammalian cells. Biochim Biophys Acta 1829:393–404

8. Srivastava R, Srivastava R, Ahn SH (2016) The epigenetic pathways to ribosomal DNA silencing. Microbiol Mol Biol Rev 80:545–563

9. Sharifi S, Bierhoff H (2018) Regulation of RNA polymerase I transcription in development, disease, and aging. Annu Rev Biochem 87:51–73

10. Andrews AJ, Luger K (2011) Nucleosome structure(s) and stability: variations on a theme. Annu Rev Biophys 40:99–117

11. Kornberg RD, Lorch Y (1999) Twenty-five years of the nucleosome, fundamental particle of the eukaryote chromosome. Cell 98:285–294

12. Olins DE, Olins AL (2003) Chromatin history: our view from the bridge. Nat Rev Mol Cell Biol 4:809–814

13. Lai WKM, Pugh BF (2017) Understanding nucleosome dynamics and their links to gene expression and DNA replication. Nat Rev Mol Cell Biol 18:548–562

14. Rando OJ, Winston F (2012) Chromatin and transcription in yeast. Genetics 190:351–387

15. Vannini A, Cramer P (2012) Conservation between the RNA polymerase I, II, and III transcription initiation machineries. Mol Cell 45:439–446

16. Günzl A, Bruderer T, Laufer G, Schimanski B, Tu L-C, Chung H-M, Lee P-T, Lee MG-S (2003) RNA polymerase I transcribes procyclin genes and variant surface glycoprotein gene expression sites in Trypanosoma brucei. Eukaryot Cell 2:542–551

17. Warner JR (1999) The economics of ribosome biosynthesis in yeast. Trends Biochem Sci 24:437–440

18. Moss T, Langlois F, Gagnon-Kugler T, Stefanovsky V (2007) A housekeeper with power of attorney: the rRNA genes in ribosome biogenesis. Cell Mol Life Sci 64:29–49

19. Long EO, Dawid IB (1980) Repeated genes in eukaryotes. Annu Rev Biochem 49:727–764

20. McStay B (2016) Nucleolar organizer regions: genomic "dark matter" requiring illumination. Genes Dev 30:1598–1610

21. Kedinger C, Gniazdowski M, Mandel JL, Gissinger F, Chambon P (1970) Alpha-amanitin: a specific inhibitor of one of two DNA-pendent RNA polymerase activities from calf thymus. Biochem Biophys Res Commun 38:165–171

22. Roeder RG, Rutter WJ (1969) Multiple forms of DNA-dependent RNA polymerase in eukaryotic organisms. Nature 224:234–237

23. Miller OL, Beatty BR (1969) Extrachromosomal nucleolar genes in amphibian oocytes. Genetics 61(Suppl):133–143

24. Miller OL, Beatty BR (1969) Portrait of a gene. J Cell Physiol 74(Suppl 1):225+

25. Miller OL, Beatty BR (1969) Visualization of nucleolar genes. Science 164:955–957

26. Mougey EB, O'Reilly M, Osheim Y, Miller OL, Beyer A, Sollner-Webb B (1993) The terminal balls characteristic of eukaryotic rRNA transcription units in chromatin spreads are rRNA processing complexes. Genes Dev 7:1609–1619

27. Scheer U (1987) Contributions of electron microscopic spreading preparations ("Miller spreads") to the analysis of chromosome structure. Results Probl Cell Differ 14:147–171

28. Trendelenburg MF, Zatsepina OV, Waschek T, Schlegel W, Tröster H, Rudolph D, Schmahl G, Spring H (1996) Multiparameter microscopic analysis of nucleolar structure and ribosomal gene transcription. Histochem Cell Biol 106:167–192

29. Neyer S, Kunz M, Geiss C, Hantsche M, Hodirnau V-V, Seybert A, Engel C, Scheffer MP, Cramer P, Frangakis AS (2016) Structure of RNA polymerase I transcribing ribosomal DNA genes. Nature 540(7634):607–610. https://doi.org/10.1038/nature20561

30. Olins AL, Olins DE (1974) Spheroid chromatin units (v bodies). Science 183:330–332

31. Woodcock CL, Safer JP, Stanchfield JE (1976) Structural repeating units in chromatin. I. Evidence for their general occurrence. Exp Cell Res 97:101–110

32. Kornberg RD (1974) Chromatin structure: a repeating unit of histones and DNA. Science 184:868–871

33. Kornberg RD, Thomas JO (1974) Chromatin structure; oligomers of the histones. Science 184:865–868

34. Oudet P, Gross-Bellard M, Chambon P (1975) Electron microscopic and biochemical evidence that chromatin structure is a repeating unit. Cell 4:281–300

35. Foe VE, Wilkinson LE, Laird CD (1976) Comparative organization of active transcription units in Oncopeltus fasciatus. Cell 9:131–146

36. Laird CD, Chooi WY (1976) Morphology of transcription units in Drosophila melanogaster. Chromosoma 58:193–218

37. Laird CD, Wilkinson LE, Foe VE, Chooi WY (1976) Analysis of chromatin-associated fiber arrays. Chromosoma 58:169–190

38. French SL, Osheim YN, Schneider DA, Sikes ML, Fernandez CF, Copela LA, Misra VA, Nomura M, Wolin SL, Beyer AL (2008) Visual analysis of the yeast 5S rRNA gene transcriptome: regulation and role of La protein. Mol Cell Biol 28:4576–4587

39. Johnson JM, French SL, Osheim YN, Li M, Hall L, Beyer AL, Smith JS (2013) Rpd3- and spt16-mediated nucleosome assembly and transcriptional regulation on yeast ribosomal DNA genes. Mol Cell Biol 33:2748–2759

40. Scheer U (1978) Changes of nucleosome frequency in nucleolar and non-nucleolar chromatin as a function of transcription: an electron microscopic study. Cell 13:535–549

41. Reeves R (1984) Transcriptionally active chromatin. Biochim Biophys Acta 782: 343–393

42. Tsompana M, Buck MJ (2014) Chromatin accessibility: a window into the genome. Epigenetics Chromatin 7:33

43. Voong LN, Xi L, Wang J-P, Wang X (2017) genome-wide mapping of the nucleosome landscape by micrococcal nuclease and chemical mapping. Trends Genet 33:495–507

44. Reeves R (1978) Nucleosome structure of Xenopus oocyte amplified ribosomal genes. Biochemistry 17:4908–4916

45. Reeves R (1978) Structure of Xenopus ribosomal gene chromatin during changes in genomic transcription rates. Cold Spring Harb Symp Quant Biol 42(Pt 2):709–722

46. Toussaint M, Levasseur G, Tremblay M, Paquette M, Conconi A (2005) Psoralen photocrosslinking, a tool to study the chromatin structure of RNA polymerase I--transcribed ribosomal genes. Biochem Cell Biol Biochim Biol Cell 83:449–459

47. Hearst JE (1981) Psoralen photochemistry and nucleic acid structure. J Invest Dermatol 77:39–44

48. Hanson CV, Shen CK, Hearst JE (1976) Cross-linking of DNA in situ as a probe for chromatin structure. Science 193:62–64

49. Wieshahn GP, Hyde JE, Hearst JE (1977) The photoaddition of trimethylpsoralen to Drosophila melanogaster nuclei: a probe for chromatin substructure. Biochemistry 16: 925–932

50. Sogo JM, Ness PJ, Widmer RM, Parish RW, Koller T (1984) Psoralen-crosslinking of DNA as a probe for the structure of active nucleolar chromatin. J Mol Biol 178: 897–919

51. Conconi A, Widmer RM, Koller T, Sogo JM (1989) Two different chromatin structures coexist in ribosomal RNA genes throughout the cell cycle. Cell 57:753–761

52. Dammann R, Lucchini R, Koller T, Sogo JM (1993) Chromatin structures and transcription of rDNA in yeast Saccharomyces cerevisiae. Nucleic Acids Res 21:2331–2338

53. Cavalli G, Thoma F (1993) Chromatin transitions during activation and repression of galactose-regulated genes in yeast. EMBO J 12:4603–4613

54. Jones HS, Kawauchi J, Braglia P, Alen CM, Kent NA, Proudfoot NJ (2007) RNA polymerase I in yeast transcribes dynamic nucleosomal rDNA. Nat Struct Mol Biol 14: 123–130

55. French SL, Osheim YN, Cioci F, Nomura M, Beyer AL (2003) In exponentially growing Saccharomyces cerevisiae cells, rRNA synthesis is determined by the summed RNA polymerase I loading rate rather than by the number of active genes. Mol Cell Biol 23: 1558–1568

56. Merz K, Hondele M, Goetze H, Gmelch K, Stoeckl U, Griesenbeck J (2008) Actively transcribed rRNA genes in S. cerevisiae are organized in a specialized chromatin associated with the high-mobility group protein Hmo1 and are largely devoid of histone molecules. Genes Dev 22:1190–1204

57. Schmid M, Durussel T, Laemmli UK (2004) ChIC and ChEC; genomic mapping of chromatin proteins. Mol Cell 16:147–157

58. Schmid M, Arib G, Laemmli C, Nishikawa J, Durussel T, Laemmli UK (2006) Nup-PI: the nucleopore-promoter interaction of genes in yeast. Mol Cell 21:379–391

59. Zentner GE, Kasinathan S, Xin B, Rohs R, Henikoff S (2015) ChEC-seq kinetics discriminates transcription factor binding sites by DNA sequence and shape in vivo. Nat Commun 6:8733

60. Griesenbeck J, Wittner M, Charton R, Conconi A (2012) Chromatin endogenous cleavage and psoralen crosslinking assays to analyze rRNA gene chromatin in vivo. Methods Mol Biol Clifton NJ 809:291–301

61. Wittner M, Hamperl S, Stöckl U, Seufert W, Tschochner H, Milkereit P, Griesenbeck J (2011) Establishment and maintenance of alternative chromatin states at a multicopy gene locus. Cell 145:543–554

62. Zentner GE, Saiakhova A, Manaenkov P, Adams MD, Scacheri PC (2011) Integrative genomic analysis of human ribosomal DNA. Nucleic Acids Res 39:4949–4960

63. Herdman C, Mars J-C, Stefanovsky VY, Tremblay MG, Sabourin-Felix M, Lindsay H, Robinson MD, Moss T (2017) A unique enhancer boundary complex on the mouse ribosomal RNA genes persists after loss of Rrn3 or UBF and the inactivation of RNA polymerase I transcription. PLoS Genet 13:e1006899

64. Mars J-C, Sabourin-Felix M, Tremblay MG, Moss T (2018) A deconvolution protocol for ChIP-Seq reveals analogous enhancer structures on the mouse and human ribosomal RNA genes. G3 (Bethesda) 8:303–314

65. Stros M, Launholt D, Grasser KD (2007) The HMG-box: a versatile protein domain occurring in a wide variety of DNA-binding proteins. Cell Mol Life Sci 64:2590–2606

66. Sanij E, Hannan RD (2009) The role of UBF in regulating the structure and dynamics of transcriptionally active rDNA chromatin. Epigenetics 4:374–382

67. Wright JE, Mais C, Prieto J-L, McStay B (2006) A role for upstream binding factor in organizing ribosomal gene chromatin. Biochem Soc Symp 73:77–84

68. Bell SP, Learned RM, Jantzen HM, Tjian R (1988) Functional cooperativity between transcription factors UBF1 and SL1 mediates human ribosomal RNA synthesis. Science 241:1192–1197

69. Pikaard CS, McStay B, Schultz MC, Bell SP, Reeder RH (1989) The Xenopus ribosomal gene enhancers bind an essential polymerase I transcription factor, xUBF. Genes Dev 3:1779–1788

70. Pikaard CS, Smith SD, Reeder RH, Rothblum L (1990) rUBF, an RNA polymerase I transcription factor from rats, produces DNase I footprints identical to those produced by xUBF, its homolog from frogs. Mol Cell Biol 10:3810–3812

71. Moss T, Stefanovsky VY, Pelletier G (1998) The structural and architectural role of upstream binding factor, UBF. In: Paule MR (ed) Transcription of ribosomal RNA genes by eukaryotic RNA polymerase I. Springer, Berlin, pp 75–94

72. Bazett-Jones DP, Leblanc B, Herfort M, Moss T (1994) Short-range DNA looping by the Xenopus HMG-box transcription factor, xUBF. Science 264:1134–1137

73. Hamdane N, Stefanovsky VY, Tremblay MG, Németh A, Paquet E, Lessard F, Sanij E, Hannan R, Moss T (2014) Conditional inactivation of Upstream Binding Factor reveals its epigenetic functions and the existence of a somatic nucleolar precursor body. PLoS Genet 10:e1004505

74. O'Sullivan AC, Sullivan GJ, McStay B (2002) UBF binding in vivo is not restricted to regulatory sequences within the vertebrate ribosomal DNA repeat. Mol Cell Biol 22:657–668

75. Roussel P, André C, Masson C, Géraud G, Hernandez-Verdun D (1993) Localization of the RNA polymerase I transcription factor hUBF during the cell cycle. J Cell Sci 104 (Pt 2):327–337

76. Jordan P, Mannervik M, Tora L, Carmo-Fonseca M (1996) In vivo evidence that TATA-binding protein/SL1 colocalizes with UBF and RNA polymerase I when rRNA synthesis is either active or inactive. J Cell Biol 133:225–234

77. Roussel P, André C, Comai L, Hernandez-Verdun D (1996) The rDNA transcription machinery is assembled during mitosis in active NORs and absent in inactive NORs. J Cell Biol 133:235–246

78. Zatsepina OV, Schöfer C, Weipoltshammer K, Mosgoeller W, Almeder M, Stefanova VN, Jordan EG, Wachtler F (1996) The RNA polymerase I transcription factor UBF and rDNA are located at the same major sites in both interphase and mitotic pig embryonic kidney (PK) cells. Cytogenet Cell Genet 73:274–278

79. Heitz E (1931) Die Ursache der gesetzmässigen Zahl, Lage, Form und Grösse pflanzlicher Nukleolen. Planta 12:775–844

80. Heliot L, Kaplan H, Lucas L, Klein C, Beorchia A, Doco-Fenzy M, Menager M, Thiry M, O'Donohue MF, Ploton D (1997) Electron tomography of metaphase nucleolar organizer regions: evidence for a twisted-loop organization. Mol Biol Cell 8:2199–2216

81. McClintock B (1934) The relation of a particular chromosomal element to the development of the nucleoli in Zea mays. Z Für Zellforsch Mikrosk Anat 21:294–326

82. Albert B, Colleran C, Léger-Silvestre I, Berger AB, Dez C, Normand C, Perez-Fernandez J, McStay B, Gadal O (2013) Structure-function analysis of Hmo1 unveils an ancestral organization of HMG-Box factors involved in ribosomal DNA transcription from yeast to human. Nucleic Acids Res 41:10135–10149

83. Gadal O, Labarre S, Boschiero C, Thuriaux P (2002) Hmo1, an HMG-box protein, belongs to the yeast ribosomal DNA transcription system. EMBO J 21:5498–5507

84. Berger AB, Decourty L, Badis G, Nehrbass U, Jacquier A, Gadal O (2007) Hmo1 is required for TOR-dependent regulation of ribosomal protein gene transcription. Mol Cell Biol 27:8015–8026

85. Hall DB, Wade JT, Struhl K (2006) An HMG protein, Hmo1, associates with promoters of many ribosomal protein genes and throughout the rRNA gene locus in Saccharomyces cerevisiae. Mol Cell Biol 26:3672–3679

86. Kasahara K, Ohtsuki K, Ki S, Aoyama K, Takahashi H, Kobayashi T, Shirahige K, Kokubo T (2007) Assembly of regulatory factors on rRNA and ribosomal protein genes in Saccharomyces cerevisiae. Mol Cell Biol 27: 6686–6705

87. Kermekchiev M, Workman JL, Pikaard CS (1997) Nucleosome binding by the polymerase I transactivator upstream binding factor displaces linker histone H1. Mol Cell Biol 17:5833–5842

88. McCauley MJ, Huo R, Becker N, Holte MN, Muthurajan UM, Rouzina I, Luger K, Maher LJ, Israeloff NE, Williams MC (2019) Single and double box HMGB proteins differentially destabilize nucleosomes. Nucleic Acids Res 47:666–678

89. Murugesapillai D, McCauley MJ, Huo R, Nelson Holte MH, Stepanyants A, Maher LJ, Israeloff NE, Williams MC (2014) DNA bridging and looping by HMO1 provides a mechanism for stabilizing nucleosome-free chromatin. Nucleic Acids Res 42:8996–9004

90. Hu CH, McStay B, Jeong SW, Reeder RH (1994) xUBF, an RNA polymerase I transcription factor, binds crossover DNA with low sequence specificity. Mol Cell Biol 14: 2871–2882

91. Kamau E, Bauerle KT, Grove A (2004) The Saccharomyces cerevisiae high mobility group box protein HMO1 contains two functional DNA binding domains. J Biol Chem 279: 55234–55240

92. Leblanc B, Read C, Moss T (1993) Recognition of the Xenopus ribosomal core promoter by the transcription factor xUBF involves multiple HMG box domains and leads to an xUBF interdomain interaction. EMBO J 12: 513–525

93. Sanij E, Diesch J, Lesmana A, Poortinga G, Hein N, Lidgerwood G, Cameron DP, Ellul J, Goodall GJ, Wong LH, Dhillon AS, Hamdane N, Rothblum LI, Pearson RB, Haviv I, Moss T, Hannan RD (2015) A novel role for the Pol I transcription factor UBTF in maintaining genome stability through the regulation of highly transcribed Pol II genes. Genome Res 25:201–212

94. Achar YJ, Adhil M, Choudhary R, Gilbert N, Foiani M (2020) Negative supercoil at gene boundaries modulates gene topology. Nature 577:701–705

95. Mais C, Wright JE, Prieto J-L, Raggett SL, McStay B (2005) UBF-binding site arrays form pseudo-NORs and sequester the RNA polymerase I transcription machinery. Genes Dev 19:50–64

96. Prieto J-L, McStay B (2008) Pseudo-NORs: a novel model for studying nucleoli. Biochim Biophys Acta 1783:2116–2123

97. Prieto J-L, McStay B (2007) Recruitment of factors linking transcription and processing of pre-rRNA to NOR chromatin is UBF-dependent and occurs independent of transcription in human cells. Genes Dev 21: 2041–2054

98. Lucchini R, Sogo JM (1995) Replication of transcriptionally active chromatin. Nature 374:276–280

99. Scott RS, Truong KY, Vos JM (1997) Replication initiation and elongation fork rates within a differentially expressed human multicopy locus in early S phase. Nucleic Acids Res 25:4505–4512

100. Sandmeier JJ, French S, Osheim Y, Cheung WL, Gallo CM, Beyer AL, Smith JS (2002) RPD3 is required for the inactivation of yeast ribosomal DNA genes in stationary phase. EMBO J 21:4959–4968

101. Fahy D, Conconi A, Smerdon MJ (2005) Rapid changes in transcription and chromatin structure of ribosomal genes in yeast during growth phase transitions. Exp Cell Res 305: 365–373

102. Tremblay M, Charton R, Wittner M, Levasseur G, Griesenbeck J, Conconi A (2014) UV light-induced DNA lesions cause dissociation of yeast RNA polymerases-I and establishment of a specialized chromatin structure at rRNA genes. Nucleic Acids Res 42:380–395

103. Conconi A, Paquette M, Fahy D, Bespalov VA, Smerdon MJ (2005) Repair-independent chromatin assembly onto active ribosomal genes in yeast after UV irradiation. Mol Cell Biol 25:9773–9783

104. Sanij E, Poortinga G, Sharkey K, Hung S, Holloway TP, Quin J, Robb E, Wong LH, Thomas WG, Stefanovsky V, Moss T, Rothblum L, Hannan KM, McArthur GA, Pearson RB, Hannan RD (2008) UBF levels determine the number of active ribosomal RNA genes in mammals. J Cell Biol 183: 1259–1274

105. Birch JL, Tan BC-M, Panov KI, Panova TB, Andersen JS, Owen-Hughes TA, Russell J, Lee S-C, Zomerdijk JCBM (2009) FACT facilitates chromatin transcription by RNA polymerases I and III. EMBO J 28:854–865

106. Cutler S, Lee LJ, Tsukiyama T (2018) Chromatin remodeling factors Isw2 and Ino80 regulate chromatin, replication, and copy number of the Saccharomyces cerevisiae ribosomal DNA locus. Genetics 210:1543–1556

107. Hamperl S, Brown CR, Garea AV, Perez-Fernandez J, Bruckmann A, Huber K, Wittner M, Babl V, Stoeckl U, Deutzmann R, Boeger H, Tschochner H, Milkereit P, Griesenbeck J (2014) Compositional and structural analysis of selected chromosomal domains from Saccharomyces cerevisiae. Nucleic Acids Res 42:e2

108. Zhang Y, Anderson SJ, French SL, Sikes ML, Viktorovskaya OV, Huband J, Holcomb K, Hartman JL, Beyer AL, Schneider DA (2013) The SWI/SNF chromatin remodeling complex influences transcription by RNA polymerase I in Saccharomyces cerevisiae. PloS One 8:e56793

109. Anderson SJ, Sikes ML, Zhang Y, French SL, Salgia S, Beyer AL, Nomura M, Schneider DA (2011) The transcription elongation factor Spt5 influences transcription by RNA polymerase I positively and negatively. J Biol Chem 286:18816–18824

110. Engel KL, French SL, Viktorovskaya OV, Beyer AL, Schneider DA (2015) Spt6 is essential for rRNA synthesis by RNA polymerase I. Mol Cell Biol 35:2321–2331

111. Iben S, Tschochner H, Bier M, Hoogstraten D, Hozák P, Egly JM, Grummt I (2002) TFIIH plays an essential role in RNA polymerase I transcription. Cell 109:297–306

112. Schneider DA, French SL, Osheim YN, Bailey AO, Vu L, Dodd J, Yates JR, Beyer AL, Nomura M (2006) RNA polymerase II elongation factors Spt4p and Spt5p play roles in transcription elongation by RNA polymerase I and rRNA processing. Proc Natl Acad Sci U S A 103:12707–12712

113. Zhang Y, Sikes ML, Beyer AL, Schneider DA (2009) The Paf1 complex is required for efficient transcription elongation by RNA polymerase I. Proc Natl Acad Sci U S A 106:2153–2158

114. Zhang Y, French SL, Beyer AL, Schneider DA (2016) The transcription factor THO promotes transcription initiation and elongation by RNA polymerase I. J Biol Chem 291:3010–3018

115. Gallagher JEG, Dunbar DA, Granneman S, Mitchell BM, Osheim Y, Beyer AL, Baserga SJ (2004) RNA polymerase I transcription and pre-rRNA processing are linked by specific SSU processome components. Genes Dev 18:2506–2517

116. Merkl PE, Pilsl M, Fremter T, Schwank K, Engel C, Längst G, Milkereit P, Griesenbeck J, Tschochner H (2020) RNA polymerase I (Pol I) passage through nucleosomes depends on Pol I subunits binding its lobe structure. J Biol Chem 295:4782–4795

117. Hermans N, Huisman JJ, Brouwer TB, Schächner C, van Heusden GPH, Griesenbeck J, van Noort J (2017) Toehold-enhanced LNA probes for selective pull down and single-molecule analysis of native chromatin. Sci Rep 7:16721

# Chapter 3

# Analysis of Yeast RNAP I Transcription of Nucleosomal Templates In Vitro

## Philipp E. Merkl, Christopher Schächner, Michael Pilsl, Katrin Schwank, Kristin Hergert, Gernot Längst, Philipp Milkereit, Joachim Griesenbeck, and Herbert Tschochner

## Abstract

Nuclear eukaryotic RNA polymerases (RNAPs) transcribe a chromatin template in vivo. Since the basic unit of chromatin, the nucleosome, renders the DNA largely inaccessible, RNAPs have to overcome the nucleosomal barrier for efficient RNA synthesis. Gaining mechanistical insights in the transcription of chromatin templates will be essential to understand the complex process of eukaryotic gene expression. In this article we describe the use of defined in vitro transcription systems for comparative analysis of highly purified RNAPs I–III from *S. cerevisiae* (hereafter called yeast) transcribing in vitro reconstituted nucleosomal templates. We also provide a protocol to study promoter-dependent RNAP I transcription of purified native 35S ribosomal RNA (rRNA) gene chromatin.

**Key words** Transcription, Chromatin, Nucleosomes, Histones, RNA polymerase I, RNA polymerase II, RNA polymerase III, Ribosomal RNA gene chromatin, Rrn3, Core factor, Net1, In vitro assays, *Saccharomyces cerevisiae*, Yeast

## 1 Introduction

In all eukaryotes there are at least three different nuclear multi-subunit RNAPs (RNA polymerases) termed I–III (reviewed in [1], see also short reviews from Merkl et al., and Pilsl et al. in this issue). The enzymes share common subunits and a similar core structure but clearly differ in their composition and function (reviewed in [1], see also short reviews from Merkl et al., and Pilsl et al. in this issue). The template transcribed by RNAPs I–III in vivo is chromatin. In chromatin, approximately 146 bp of DNA are wrapped around an octameric core of histone proteins forming a basic repeating unit called the nucleosome (reviewed in [2–4]). This

---

Philipp E. Merkl and Christopher Schächner contributed equally with all other contributors.

Karl-Dieter Entian (ed.), *Ribosome Biogenesis: Methods and Protocols*, Methods in Molecular Biology, vol. 2533,
https://doi.org/10.1007/978-1-0716-2501-9_3, © The Author(s) 2022

leads to compaction and impairs access to the genetic information. Therefore, chromatin structure must be transiently altered allowing transcription at defined genomic loci. Accordingly, characteristic chromatin transitions have been observed in vivo, when genes switch from an transcriptionally inactive to an actively transcribed state (reviewed in [5, 6]). There is evidence that RNAPs I–III deal differently with the chromatin template ([7], see also short reviews from Merkl et al. and Schächner et al. in this issue).

Defined in vitro systems including purified components contributed substantially to our current understanding of mechanisms of eukaryotic transcription (reviewed in [8]). The possibility to use in vitro reconstituted nucleosomal templates provided a minimal model system for transcription in the context of chromatin (reviewed in [9]). Here, we describe a protocol for comparative analyses of yeast RNAPs I–III in promoter-independent transcription of in vitro reconstituted chromatin templates. To this end, we developed a purification procedure for affinity purification of the three enzymes under identical conditions [10, 11]. The purified enzymes were devoid of cross-contamination with other RNAPs or transcription factors. For promoter-independent transcription, tailed DNA templates containing a 3′ overhang can be employed (Fig. 1a) [12]. From 3′ overhangs all RNAPs can initiate transcription without additional transcription factors. These templates in combination with the strong 601 nucleosome positioning sequence (601 templates) [13] were used for nucleosome assembly at defined positions (Fig. 1b). To determine the transcription efficiency through an assembled nucleosome, radioactively labeled RNA synthesized by the different RNAPs from the nucleosomal 601 templates are detected and quantified (Fig. 1c, d). Each transcription reaction contains another nucleosome-free reference template of different size, which serves as an internal control for the transcriptional activity of the respective RNAP. Additionally, transcription reactions are performed containing the naked 601 templates and the reference template (Fig. 1c). The transcription efficiency through a nucleosome is then calculated by dividing the quotient of transcripts from nucleosomal 601 template to reference template by the quotient of transcripts from naked 601 template to reference template. These analyses revealed marked differences between transcription of nucleosomal templates by RNAPs I–III ((Fig. 1d), and [7]). Whereas RNAPs I and III could readily transcribe through an in vitro assembled nucleosome RNAP II transcription was strongly impaired.

Nucleosomal templates obtained after salt dialysis have the advantage that they are fully defined. However, it is unclear in how far they reflect endogenous chromatin, the native template of nuclear transcription. Thus, we established a technique allowing the excision of a genomic region of interest in its native chromatin context by site-specific recombination in specifically engineered

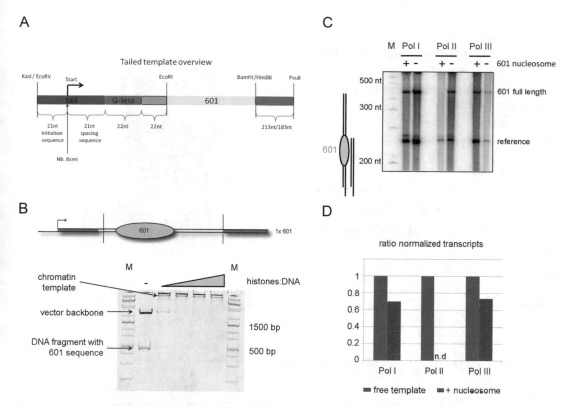

**Fig. 1** Promoter-independent transcription of in vitro assembled nucleosomal templates by RNAPs I–III. (**a**) Schematic representation of the template for nucleosome assembly containing a 601 nucleosome positioning sequence (601 template). The reference template lacks the nucleosome positioning sequence but is otherwise identical. Restriction sites used to release the templates from plasmids K1253 and K1573 are indicated. (**b**) Electrophoretic mobility shift assay after nucleosome assembly. Purified core histones H2A, H2B, H3, and H4 from chicken erythrocytes were assembled on the 601 template shown in (**a**) by salt gradient dialysis. Assembly reactions with different histone to DNA ratios (Table 7) were analyzed in a native polyacrylamide gel as described in Subheading 3.2. The position of the nucleosome-free template and the K1253 vector backbone and the chromatin template after assembly are indicated on the left. Sizes of selected DNA fragments in DNA markers (M) are indicated on the right. (**c, d**) Purified RNAPs I–III transcribe through a nucleosome on tailed templates with different efficiencies. (**c**) Transcription reactions were performed in the presence of a reference template and the 601 template before (−) or after (+) nucleosome assembly. The cartoon on the left indicates the length of the transcripts derived from the different templates. In vitro transcription assays were performed using 7.5 nM of purified RNAPs, identical buffer conditions and 10 nM of each of the different templates. Radiolabeled transcripts were separated on a denaturing polyacrylamide gel and visualized as described in Subheading 3.5.2. Sizes of selected RNA fragments in an RNA marker (M) are indicated on the left. (**d**) Quantification of the experiments shown in (**c**) was performed as described in Subheading 3.5.3

yeast strains (Fig. 2a) [17–19]. To assist affinity purification of the released chromatin domain, the genomic region of interest contains a cluster of DNA binding sites for the bacterial LexA protein. In the yeast strains used for recombination, recombinant LexA C-terminally fused to a tandem affinity purification (TAP) tag is constitutively expressed. The protein binds to its binding sites

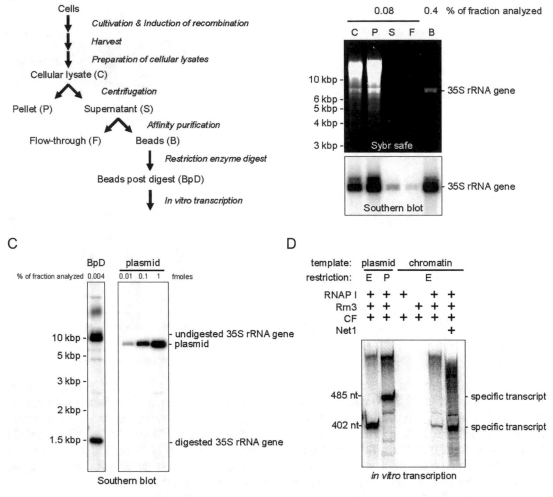

**Fig. 2** Promoter-dependent transcription of purified native rRNA gene chromatin by RNAP I. (**a**) Schematic representation of purification and restriction enzyme digest of yeast native 35S rRNA gene chromatin. (**b**) DNA analysis of samples withdrawn during the purification procedure (shown in **a**, and described in Subheadings 3.3.1 and 3.3.2). DNA of the indicated fraction of individual samples depicted on the top was isolated as described in Subheading 3.3.4, linearized with SacII and separated by electrophoresis in a 1% agarose gel. An image of the agarose gel stained with SYBR safe is shown on the top. The same gel was subjected to the Southern blot procedure with a radioactively labeled probe described in Subheading 2.3. The autoradiogram of the blot is shown at the bottom. The positions and respective length of DNA marker fragments (NEB 1 kb ladder, not shown) are depicted on the left of the gel picture. The position of the rDNA fragment derived from the 35S rRNA gene chromatin domain in the gel and on the blot is depicted on the right. (**c**) Quantitative Southern blot analysis of the "beads post EcoRV digest" sample (BpD) together with a titration from 0.1 to 1 fmol of plasmid K375. The isolated DNA was digested with PflmI prior to electrophoresis in a 1.5% agarose gel which was subjected to the Southern blot procedure. The positions and respective length of DNA marker fragments (NEB 1 kb ladder, not shown) are depicted on the left of the autoradiogram. The positions of PflmI fragments derived from the EcoRV digested or undigested 35S rRNA gene chromatin domain, as well as from the PflmI/EcoRV digested plasmid K375 are depicted on the right of the autoradiogram. (**d**) Promoter-dependent in vitro transcription of native rRNA gene chromatin. Promoter-dependent in in vitro transcription was performed as described in [14] using either 10 nM of EcoRV (E) or PvuII (P) linearized plasmid K375 or

within the chromatin domain and serves as bait for subsequent affinity purification of the genomic target region (Fig. 2b). The isolated native chromatin domains are suitable substrates for compositional analysis by mass spectrometry, structural analysis by electron microscopy or biophysical molecular tweezer analysis [20–23]. Furthermore, they can be used in functional assays to study transcription factor binding, chromatin remodeling, or transcription on native templates in vitro [18, 24, 25]. Here, we show that purified native 35S rRNA gene chromatin can be used as template for promoter-dependent RNAP I transcription. To this end, the chromatin domain bound to the affinity matrix is linearized by restriction enzyme digest to produce transcripts of a defined length (Fig. 2c). Promoter-dependent transcription of the purified chromatin domain requires at least purified RNAP I, as well as two components of the RNAP I transcription machinery, the three-subunit core factor (CF) and the initiation factor Rrn3 (Fig. 2d). We find that the Net1 protein, which has previously been characterized as an activator of RNAP I transcription in vitro and in vivo [15, 26], leads to a robust stimulation of RNAP I dependent native chromatin transcription (Fig. 2d).

In summary, combining analyses involving strictly defined in vitro assembled nucleosomal templates and ex vivo purified native chromatin will likely help to gain further insights in mechanisms of nuclear transcription by eukaryotic RNAPs.

## 2 Materials

### 2.1 Preparation of Tailed Templates

Details about construction of plasmids K1253 (pUC19 tail g—601) and K1573 (pUC19 tail g—w/o BS) can be found elsewhere [10, 11]. Plasmids and related sequence information are available upon request.

1. Plasmid K1253 for nucleosome reconstitution, and reference plasmid K1573.

2. Nb. BsmI, KasI, PvuII, and respective buffers (NEB).

3. RNase-free water.

4. Competitor oligo o2207, with the same sequence

---

**Fig. 2** (continued) 10 nM of EcoRV linearized rRNA gene chromatin as template. Note that only 20% of the chromatin template were properly digested by EcoRV and produce transcripts with a defined length. Individual transcription reactions were performed in the presence or absence of RNAP I (5 nM), CF (20 nM), Rrn3 (70 nM), and the RNAP I transcription activator Net1 (20 nM) [15, 16], as indicated on top. Radiolabeled transcripts were separated on a denaturing polyacrylamide gel and visualized as described in Subheading 3.5.2. The positions and respective lengths of RNAs synthesized from PvuII or EcoRV digested plasmid K375 or chromatin templates are indicated on the left and the right of the autoradiogram

**Table 1**
**Buffers for chromatin assembly**

| Buffer | Ingredients | Concentration/percentage |
|---|---|---|
| High salt buffer | Tris pH 7.6<br>NaCl<br>EDTA<br>NP40<br>2-mercaptoethanol | 10 mM<br>2 M<br>1 mM<br>0.05%<br>1 mM |
| 20× low salt buffer | Tris pH 7.6<br>NaCl<br>EDTA<br>NP40<br>2-mercaptoethanol | 200 mM<br>1 M<br>20 mM<br>1%<br>20 mM |
| 6× loading buffer | Glycerol<br>Orange G | 60% |

(5′- CGAGTAAGTATAGGGTAAGGTGAT -3′) as the 24 nt overhang generated by Nb.BsmI/KasI digest of plasmid K1253 or K1573.

5. Thermocycler.

6. NanoDrop spectrophotometer (Thermo Fisher Scientific).

**2.2  In Vitro Nucleosome Assembly**

1. Purified core histones H2A, H2B, H3 and H4 from chicken erythrocytes (prepared as described in [27]).

2. Bovine serum albumin (10 mg/mL), RNase free.

3. DNA template (*see* Subheading 3.1).

4. Siliconized micro tubes (Eppendorf).

5. Buffers *see* Table 1.

6. Polyacrylamide gel for electrophoretic mobility shift assay (EMSA) (Table 2).

7. 6× EMSA buffer (60% glycerol, Orange G).

8. FLA3000 (Fuji) Imager or equivalent imaging system for Ethidium bromide staining.

9. Gel dryer (Drystar).

10. Whatman filter paper (Macherey-Nagel, MN 827 B).

**2.3  Purification and Restriction Enzyme Digest of Native Yeast Chromatin**

Materials for strain construction, cell growth and harvesting (preparation of yeast cell "spaghetti"), as well as for coupling of rabbit immunoglobulin G (IgG) to epoxy-activated magnetic beads, and protein analysis have been described elsewhere [19, 20]. Strain y2381 used for the purification of a 35S rRNA gene chromatin domain and plasmid K375 which contains an entire rDNA repeat were used in the experiments shown in Fig. 2 and have been

**Table 2**
**Composition of native polyacrylamide gel for EMSA**

| Component | Volume [mL] |
|---|---|
| Rotiphorese Gel 30 AA/Bis-AA solution (37.5:1) (Roth) | 2 |
| 5× TBE | 0.8 |
| Water | 7.2 |
| APS (10% w/v) | 0.08 |
| TEMED | 0.008 |

described earlier [20, 28]. The template to obtain the radioactively labeled probe in the Southern blots shown in Fig. 2b, c was obtained by PCR from plasmid K358 (pM49.2) [17] with primers o597 (5'-GAAACAGCTATGACCATG-3') and o598 (5'-GCCTGACTGCAGAAC GTACTACTGTACATATAAC-3'). Strains, plasmids as well as related sequence information are available upon request.

*2.3.1 Preparation of Cellular Lysates*

1. Coffee grinder (Tefal Prep'Line).
2. PARAFILM® M.
3. Proteinase inhibitors (100× PIs): benzamidine (33 mg/mL), PMSF (17 mg/mL) in ethanol p.a., stored at −20 °C.
4. Dry ice pellets (150 g per purification).
5. Frozen yeast cell "spaghetti" (3 g per purification).
6. Magnetic bead buffer (MB100): 20 mM Tris-HCl pH 8.0, 100 mM KCl, 5 mM MgAc, 0.5% Triton X-100 (w/v), 0.1% Tween 20 (w/v). Buffer MB (without additives) can be stored at room temperature and should be cooled to 4 °C prior to use. 2-Mercaptoethanol (final concentration 1.5 mM) and proteinase inhibitors (final concentration 1× PIs) should only be added prior to use.
7. Bio-Rad Protein Assay Dye Reagent Concentrate.

*2.3.2 Affinity Chromatography of Native Chromatin Domains*

1. IgG coupled to magnetic beads, prepared as previously described [19].
2. BcMag Separator (Bioclone Inc., MS-04).
3. Rotating wheel or alternative rotation device.
4. Magnetic bead Buffer (MB100), as described in Subheading 3.3.1.

*2.3.3 Restriction Enzyme Digest of Purified Native Chromatin Domains*

1. Restriction enzymes and respective buffer (NEB).
2. Thermomixer® Dry Block Heating Shaker (Eppendorf).

| | |
|---|---|
| *2.3.4  DNA Analysis* | 1. Buffer IRN: 50 mM Tris-HCl, pH 8.0, 20 mM EDTA, 0.5 M NaCl. |

1. Buffer IRN: 50 mM Tris-HCl, pH 8.0, 20 mM EDTA, 0.5 M NaCl.

2. Buffer TE: 10 mM Tris-HCl, pH 7.5, 1 mM EDTA.

3. RNase A (20 mg/mL) (Invitrogen).

4. Proteinase K (20 mg/mL) (Sigma), dissolved in 50 mM Tris-HCl pH 8.0, 1 mM $CaCl_2$ and stored in aliquots at $-20$ °C.

5. Yeast tRNA (10 mg/mL) (Sigma), dissolved in nuclease-free water.

6. Roti® phenol–chloroform–isoamyl alcohol (25:24:1) (Roth), stored at 4 °C in the dark.

7. Ethanol p.a., stored at room temperature.

8. Restriction enzymes and respective buffer (NEB).

**2.4  Purification of RNAPs I, II, and III from S. cerevisiae**

1. Vibrax-VXR (IKA), rotary shaker.

2. IgG coupled to magnetic beads, and BcMag Separator, rotating wheel as described in Subheading 3.3.2.

3. Thermomixer® Dry Block Heating Shaker (Eppendorf).

4. Glass beads (ø 0.75–1 mm) (Roth).

5. YPD medium: 2% (w/v) Bacto™ Peptone, 1% (w/v) Bacto™ Yeast Extract, 2% (w/v) Glucose.

6. Proteinase inhibitors (100×), as described in Subheading 3.3.1.

7. Purified recombinant 6× His-tagged Tobacco Etch Virus (TEV) protease produced in *E. coli*.

8. Yeast strains (Table 3).

9. Buffers (Table 4).

**Table 3**
**Yeast strains used for RNA polymerase purification**

| # | Name | Genotype | Reference |
|---|---|---|---|
| y2423 | BY4741 A135-TEV-ProtA | MATa, his3-Δ1 leu2-Δ0 met15-Δ0 ura3-Δ0 rpa135:: RPA135-TEV-ProtA-kanMX6 | [10] |
| y2424 | BY4741 Rpb2-TEV-ProtA | MATa, his3-Δ1 leu2-Δ0 met15-Δ0 ura3-Δ0 rpb2::RPB2-TEV-ProtA-kanMX6 | [10] |
| y2425 | BY4741 C128-TEV-ProtA | MATa, his3-Δ1 leu2-Δ0 met15-Δ0 ura3-Δ0 c128::C128-TEV-ProtA-kanMX6 | [10] |

**Table 4**
**Buffers for RNA polymerase purification**

| Buffer | Ingredients | Concentration/percentage |
|---|---|---|
| P1 KOAc | KOAc<br>Hepes pH 7.8<br>$MgCl_2$<br>Glycerol<br>PIs | 200 mM<br>20 mM<br>1 mM<br>20%<br>1× |
| P2 KOAc | KOAc<br>Hepes pH 7.8<br>$MgCl_2$<br>Glycerol<br>NP40<br>(PIs) | 200 mM<br>20 mM<br>1 mM<br>20%<br>0.1%<br>(1×) |
| P1 KCl | KCl<br>Tris/HCl pH 8<br>MgAc<br>Glycerol<br>PIs | 200 mM<br>20 mM<br>5 mM<br>20%<br>1× |
| P2 KCl | KCl<br>Tris/HCl pH 8<br>MgAc<br>Glycerol<br>NP40<br>(PIs) | 200 mM<br>20 mM<br>5 mM<br>20%<br>0.1%<br>(1×) |

*2.5 In Vitro Transcription of Chromatin Templates*

1. Buffers for in vitro transcription (Table 5).
2. Buffers for denaturing polyacrylamide gel electrophoresis (Table 6).
3. GelSave (Applichem).

# 3 Methods

*3.1 Preparation of Tailed Templates*

1. Fragments for tailed template preparation are released from 10 μg plasmid K1253 or the reference plasmid K1573 using restriction enzymes PvuII and KasI for 1.5 h at 37 °C in a total volume of 100 μL, followed by heat inactivation of these enzymes at the appropriate temperature as indicated by the manufacturer.

2. DNA is precipitated by the addition of 0.1 volume of 3 M sodium acetate and 2.5 volumes of 100% EtOH and incubation at −20 °C for at least 30 min. The template DNA is pelleted by centrifugation at $16,000 \times g$ for 20 min at 4 °C, washed with 70% EtOH and resuspended in RNase-free water to result in a final concentration of 2 mg/mL.

**Table 5**
**Buffers for in vitro transcription experiments**

| Buffer | Ingredients | Concentration/percentage |
|---|---|---|
| 10× new transcription buffer (NTB) | Hepes pH 8 | 200 mM |
| | $MgCl_2$ | 100 mM |
| | EDTA | 50 mM |
| | EGTA | 0.5 mM |
| | DTT | 25 mM |
| Proteinase K storage buffer | Tris–HCl pH 7.5 | 20 mM |
| | $CaCl_2$ | 1 mM |
| | Glycerol | 50% |
| Proteinase K buffer | NaCl | 300 mM |
| | Tris/HCl pH 7.5 | 10 mM |
| | EDTA | 5 mM |
| | SDS | 0.6% |
| Proteinase K mix (20 reactions) | Proteinase K (20 mg/mL) | 110 μL |
| | Proteinase K buffer | 4.7 mL |
| TBE | Tris | 50 mM |
| | Boric acid | 50 mM |
| | EDTA | 1 mM |
| Denaturing RNA loading buffer | Formamide deionized | 80% |
| | TBE | 0.5× |
| | Bromophenol blue | Spatula tip |
| | Xylene cyanole | Spatula tip |

**Table 6**
**Composition of denaturing polyacrylamide gel for RNA electrophoresis**

| Component | Volume/weight |
|---|---|
| Rotiphorese gel 30 AA/Bis-AA solution (37.5:1) (Roth) | 3.3 mL |
| 5× TBE | 2 mL |
| $H_2O$ | 8 mL |
| Urea | 6.4 g |
| TEMED | 20 μL |
| 20% APS | 100 μL |

3. The template DNA is incubated with the sequence-specific nicking endonuclease Nb.BsmI at 65 °C for 1.5 h in the buffer recommended by the manufacturer.

4. Nb.BsmI is heat-inactivated by incubation at 80 °C for 20 min in a thermocycler.

**Table 7**
**Assembly reaction setup**

| Ratio: Histones: DNA | 0.4: 1 | 0.6: 1 | 0.8: 1 | 1: 1 |
|---|---|---|---|---|
| High salt buffer | 44 µL | 42.75 µL | 41.5 µL | 40.25 µL |
| BSA (10 mg/mL) | 1 µL | | | |
| DNA template (2 µg/µL) | 2.5 µL | | | |
| Chicken histones (0.8 mg/mL) | 2.5 µL | 3.75 µL | 5 µL | 6.25 µL |
| Total volume | 50 µL | | | |

5. 10 min after starting the heat inactivation, competitor oligo o2207 is added in molar excess to anneal with the 5′ single strand DNA fragment which is released upon the nicking reaction.

6. After incubation at 80 °C for 10 min, the sample is slowly cooled down to room temperature using a shallow gradient from −1 °C/min in a thermocycler.

7. EtOH precipitation is performed as described above and DNA concentration is adjusted to 2 mg/mL.

### 3.2 In Vitro Nucleosome Assembly

Nucleosomes are reconstituted on tailed templates which contain one or multiple 601 positioning sequences [13]. The 601 sequence directs precise nucleosome positioning upon assembly, which is a prerequisite to obtain homogeneous chromatin templates.

1. For in vitro transcription, only fully assembled template DNA is used. To determine optimal assembly conditions, several assembly reactions with different histone to DNA ratios are prepared (Table 7).

2. Dialysis chambers are prepared by removing the conical tip of siliconized 1.4 mL micro tubes (Eppendorf) and perforation of the cap with a hot metal rod (approximately 0.5 mm in diameter).

3. Dialysis membrane (molecular weight cutoff 6–8 kDa) is equilibrated in high salt buffer. The equilibrated dialysis membrane is fixed between tube and cap to build a dialysis chamber.

4. Dialysis chambers are placed in a floater in a 5 L beaker containing 300 mL high salt buffer and air bubbles at the bottom of the dialysis chambers are removed with a Pasteur pipette that was bent in the flame of a Bunsen burner.

5. The assembly reactions (**step 1**) are transferred into the dialysis chambers. The volume in the mini-dialysis chamber should not be below 40 µL and the DNA concentration should be above 100 ng/µL to obtain reproducible assembly reactions.

6. Using a peristaltic pump 3 L of low salt buffer containing 1 mM 2-mercaptoethanol are transferred at 200 mL/h into the 5 L beaker with the dialysis chambers overnight at 4 °C (or at room temperature). This results in a slow reduction of the salt concentration from 2 M NaCl to 0.23 M NaCl.

7. The floater is transferred to a 500 mL beaker with 300 mL of low salt buffer containing 1 mM 2-mercaptoethanol. Air bubbles at the bottom of the dialysis chambers are removed with the Pasteur pipette and the assembly reactions are dialyzed for an additional hour.

8. The assembly reactions are transferred to a siliconized microtube and stored at 4 °C. Nucleosomes are stable for at least 6 months in the fridge and should not be frozen.

9. To verify successful nucleosome reconstitution, 5 μL of the assembly reaction (about 0.2 μg template) is supplemented with 1 μL 6× EMSA buffer and analyzed on a native TBE gel.

10. After electrophoresis the gel is stained for 15 min in 0.4× TBE containing 0.5 μg/mL ethidium bromide at room temperature and fluorescence is visualized using a FLA3000 imaging system (or equivalent). The fraction where the free DNA band has just vanished is then further used in in vitro transcription experiments.

### 3.3 Purification and Restriction Enzyme Digest of Native Yeast Chromatin

Details on strain construction, cell growth and harvesting (preparation of yeast cell "spaghetti,") as well as instructions for coupling of rabbit IgGs to epoxy-activated magnetic beads analyses, and protein analysis can be found elsewhere [19, 20]. Subheadings 3.3.1, 3.3.2, and 3.3.4 have been adapted from [19] with modifications.

#### 3.3.1 Preparation of Cellular Lysates

Unless noted otherwise all manipulations are carried out at 4 °C.

1. A commercial coffee grinder (Tefal, Prep'Line) is precooled by grinding 30–50 g of dry ice pellets under strong shaking two times for approximately 30 s. The resulting dry ice powder is used for cell lysis (see Note 1).

2. 3 g of cells are added to roughly 50 g of the dry ice powder in the coffee mill (see Note 2).

3. The junctions between lid and coffee mill are sealed with PARAFILM to prevent leaking of the yeast/dry ice powder during grinding.

4. Yeast cells are ground for 3 × 1 min under strong shaking with 1 min interruptions to prevent heating of the coffee mill (see Note 3).

5. The resulting fine powder can be stored at −80 °C prior to use or is transferred directly to a 25–50 mL plastic beaker with a stir bar. Gentle stirring of the powder using a magnetic stirrer accelerates evaporation of the dry ice (see Note 4).

6. After evaporation of most of the dry ice 1 mL of cold buffer MB100 supplemented with 1.5 mM 2-mercaptoethanol and 1× proteinase inhibitors per 1 g of ground yeast cells are added to the frozen yeast cell powder.

7. The cellular lysate is stirred for another 5–15 min.

8. The cellular lysate is transferred to a 15 mL conical tube. The beaker is rinsed once with 0.5 mL of MB100 to recover residual crude extract which is added to the 15 mL conical tube.

9. Samples for DNA and protein analysis are withdrawn from the cellular lysate (sample "C," 20 and 10 μL, respectively). Samples can be stored at −20 °C prior to analysis (*see* **Note 5**).

10. The cellular lysate is transferred into several 2 mL micro tubes and cellular debris is sedimented by centrifugation (30 min, 16,000 × *g* at 4 °C).

11. The clear supernatant is transferred to a 15 mL conical tube.

12. The protein concentration in the supernatant is determined using Bio-Rad Protein Assay Dye Reagent Concentrate, according to the manufacturer's instructions (*see* **Note 6**).

13. Samples for DNA and protein analysis are taken from the supernatant (sample "S," 20 and 10 μL, respectively).

14. Cellular debris in the pellet remaining in the 2 mL tubes after centrifugation is suspended in the same volume, which has been removed as supernatant.

15. Samples for DNA and protein analysis are withdrawn from the pellet suspension (sample "P," 20 and 10 μL, respectively).

*3.3.2 Affinity Chromatography*

Unless noted otherwise all manipulations are carried out at 4 °C.

1. Magnetic beads coupled with IgGs (around $6.8 × 10^8$ beads, 200 μL of the magnetic bead slurry when prepared as previously described [19]) are transferred in a fresh 1.5 mL reaction tube.

2. The tube is placed in the BcMag separator until all the beads are captured at the side of the magnet. The clear supernatant is removed.

3. The beads are washed two times by suspension in 0.5 mL MB100. After each washing step the supernatant is removed as described in **step 2**.

4. The beads are equilibrated in 0.5 mL MB100 for 30 min on a rotating wheel. After equilibration the supernatant is removed as described in **step 2**.

5. The beads are suspended in 0.5 mL of the supernatant defined in Subheading 3.3.1, **step 11** and transferred to the rest of the supernatant in the 15 mL conical tube.

6. Magnetic beads and supernatant are incubated on a rotating wheel for at least 1 h.

7. After affinity purification, the flow-through is collected in a fresh 15 mL tube.

8. Samples for DNA and protein analysis are withdrawn from the flow-through (sample "F," 20 and 10 μL, respectively).

9. The beads containing the purified chromatin domains are suspended in 0.5 mL of MB100 supplemented with 1.5 mM 2-mercaptoethanol and transferred into a 1.5 mL micro tube. The supernatant is removed as described in **step 2**.

10. The beads are washed five times by suspension in 0.5 mL MB100 and incubation for 10 min on a rotating wheel. After each washing step the supernatant is removed as described in **step 2**.

11. The beads are suspended in 0.5 mL of the 1× NEB buffer suggested for the respective restriction enzyme.

12. Samples for DNA and protein analysis are withdrawn from the bead suspension (sample "B," 20 and 10 μL, respectively).

*3.3.3 Restriction Enzyme Digest of Purified Native Chromatin Domains*

1. The 1× NEB buffer is removed from beads as described in Subheading 3.3.2, **step 2**.

2. The beads are suspended 100 μL of fresh 1× NEB buffer.

3. The respective restriction enzyme is added to the bead suspension to a final concentration of 0.2 u/μL.

4. The bead suspension is incubated under shaking with 1000 rpm in a Thermomixer at 37 °C for 30 min. After incubation the supernatant is removed as described in Subheading 3.3.2, **step 2**.

5. The beads are washed twice with 0.5 mL of MB100. After each washing step the supernatant is removed as described in Subheading 3.3.2, **step 2**.

6. The beads are suspended in 0.5 mL MB100.

7. Samples for DNA and protein analysis are withdrawn from the bead suspension (sample beads post digest "BpD," 20 and 10 μL).

8. The beads are stored at 4 °C until use in in vitro transcription (*see* **Note 7**).

*3.3.4 DNA Analysis*

1. Samples are adjusted to a total volume of 100 μL using TE buffer, followed by the addition of 100 μL of IRN buffer.

2. Samples are supplemented with 10 μL of 10% SDS and 2 μL of Proteinase K (20 mg/mL), mixed and incubated for 1 h at 56 °C.

3. Nucleic acids are extracted by the addition of 150 μL of cold phenol-chloroform-isoamyl alcohol.

4. Samples are thoroughly mixed on a VORTEX mixer for 10 s and are centrifuged (5 min, 16,000 × $g$ at room temperature).

5. Aqueous phase is removed carefully and is added to 2.5 volumes (500 μL) of ethanol p.a.

6. Samples are supplemented with 1 μL of yeast tRNAs (10 mg/mL), mixed and nucleic acids are precipitated at −20 °C for at least 20 min (*see* **Note 8**).

7. Nucleic acids are sedimented by centrifugation (20 min, 16,000 × $g$ at 4 °C).

8. The supernatant is removed and the nucleic acid pellet is washed once with 150 μL of 70% ethanol p.a.

9. Nucleic acids are sedimented by centrifugation (20 min, 16,000 × $g$ at 4 °C).

10. The supernatant is removed, and the nucleic acid pellet is air-dried for 15 min at room temperature.

11. Nucleic acids are suspended in 50 μL TE containing 50 μg/mL RNase A.

12. The samples are incubated under shaking in a Thermomixer at 37 °C for 30 min.

13. Before analysis, the DNA samples are digested with appropriate restriction enzymes.

14. The amount of the specific DNA region within the purified native chromatin domain can be quantified by Southern blot analysis or quantitative PCR (*see* **Note 9**).

15. Standard methods for nucleic acid separation in native agarose gel, capillary transfer, and hybridization with radioactively labeled probes are employed for Southern blot analysis [29–31].

**3.4  Purification of RNAPs I, II, and III from S. cerevisiae**

Wild-type RNAPs I, II, and III are purified from yeast strains y2423 (RNAP I), y2424 (RNAP II), and y2425 (RNAP III) (Table 3) via IgG-protein A affinity purification [10, 11]. In each strain, the second largest subunit of the respective RNAP is expressed as a C-terminal fusion protein with protein A tag. A recognition site for TEV protease located between the C-terminus of the RNAP subunit and the protein A tag enables efficient elution of the different RNAPs (see below).

1. A 20 mL YPD culture is grown to stationary phase at 30 °C. From this culture, 2 L of YPD are inoculated to an OD600 such that it results in an OD600 of 1.5 after overnight cultivation at 30 °C.

2. At OD600 1.5, the cells are harvested (4000 × $g$, 6 min, room temperature) and washed in 200 mL ice cold water. Cells are split in aliquots representing 400 mL culture volume and again sedimented (4000 × $g$, 6 min, 4 °C). The supernatant is discarded, and the cell aliquots are frozen in liquid nitrogen and stored at −20 °C.

3. All subsequent steps are carried out in a cold room or refrigerated centrifuges at 4 °C unless stated otherwise.

4. RNAP purification is performed with 1–4 cell aliquots.

5. Cells are thawed on ice, washed in 5 mL P1 + protease inhibitors (PIs) and sedimented (4000 × $g$, 6 min).

6. The supernatant is discarded, the pellet is weighed and suspended in 1.5 mL of the respective P1 + PIs per gram.

7. 0.7 mL of this solution are added to 2 mL reaction tubes containing 1.4 g glass beads. Cells are lysed on an IKA Vibrax VXR basic shaker at maximum speed for 15 min, followed by 5 min cooling of the samples on ice. This procedure is repeated four times.

8. To collect the cell lysates, the bottom and cap of microtubes are pierced with a hot (syringe) needle and placed in a 15-mL tube. After centrifugation (130 × $g$, 1 min) the glass beads remain in the microtubes and are discarded. The crude cell lysates, which are collected in the 15-mL tubes, are transferred into new 1.5-mL microtubes.

9. Cell debris is removed by centrifugation at 16,000 × $g$ for 30 min. The protein concentration in the supernatant is determined with the Bradford assay, and should be between 20 and 50 mg/mL.

10. The lysate is supplemented with NP40 to a concentration of 0.5% and 100× PIs are added to achieve a final concentration of 1×.

11. Equal protein amounts (usually 1 mL cell extract, 30–40 mg) are incubated with 200 μL of IgG coupled magnetic beads slurry for 1 h on a rotating wheel.

12. The beads are washed three times with 700 μL of P2 + PIs and then washed three times with 700 μL P2 (KOAc).

13. For elution, the beads are suspended in 25 μL P2 (KOAc) supplemented with 10 μg of TEV protease. Cleavage is performed for 2 h at 16 °C in a Thermomixer at 1000 rpm. The supernatant is collected, the beads are washed with 25 μL P2 (KOAc) and both fractions combined.

14. This elution fraction containing either RNAP I, II, or III is split in 10 μL aliquots, frozen in liquid nitrogen and stored at −80 °C. RNAP concentration is usually between 100 and 200 nM.

**Table 8**
**Composition of a standard in vitro transcription reaction**

| Substance | Final concentration/quantity |
|---|---|
| Template DNA | ~200 fmol (30–100 ng) |
| $\alpha$-$^{32}$P]-CTP (400 Ci/mmol, 10 µCi/µL, Hartmann Analytic) | 1.25 µM (1 µL) |
| Cold CTP (100 µM) | 24 µM (4.8 µL) |
| Mix of cold ATP, UTP, and GTP (10 mM each) | 0.5 mM each (1 µL) |
| 2.5 M KOAc | 50 mM/150 mM (0.4 µL/1.2 µL) |
| 10× new transcription buffer (NTB) | 1× (2 µL) |
| RNasin | 10–20 U (0.5 µL) |
| RNA polymerase (100–150 nM) | 1 µL |
| RNase-free $H_2O$ | to 20 µL |

**3.5 In Vitro Transcription of Chromatin Templates**

Transcription from tailed templates containing a 3′ overhang starts precisely at the nucleotide where the DNA becomes double stranded again. RNAP I promoter dependent transcription starts within the core element (CE I) [32].

*3.5.1 Reaction Setup and RNA Extraction*

All components are kept on ice until the start of the reaction. Filter tips are used for pipetting.

1. Transcriptions reactions are assembled as detailed in Table 8. If multiple reactions are carried out, prepare a master mix from the constituents except chromatin and RNAPs.

2. The transcription reaction is started by adding the RNAP (final concentration 5–10 nM), thorough mixing, and incubation for 30 min at 30 °C.

3. The transcription reaction is stopped by adding 200 µL Proteinase K mix and incubation at 37 °C for 15 min.

4. To precipitate RNA, 22 µL of 3 M NaOAc, 2 µL glycogen solution (5 mg/mL, Ambion), and 750 µL ethanol p.a. are added and samples are incubated −20 °C overnight.

5. RNA is sedimented at $16,000 \times g$ for 20 min at 4 °C.

6. The supernatant is discarded. Pellets are washed with 50 µL 70% EtOH, centrifuged at $16,000 \times g$ for 20 min at 4 °C.

7. The supernatant is discarded, and pellets are dried at 90 °C for 15 s.

8. RNA is dissolved in 9 µL of loading buffer, by heating the sample at 70 °C for 10 min.

9. Samples are kept at 4 °C until analysis or stored at −20 °C.

*3.5.2 Denaturing Gel Electrophoresis and Visualization of Radiolabeled Transcripts*

Transcripts are separated in a denaturing polyacrylamide gel (20 cm × 0.3 cm × 17 cm).

1. Before pouring the gel, glass plates, spacers and the comb were treated with 0.1% SDS to remove RNases, and SDS is washed away with RNase free water and 70% ethanol.

2. One plate is silanized with GelSave. This allows for smooth removal of the gel from the plates after electrophoresis.

3. After assembly of plates and spacers in an appropriate casting device a denaturing polyacrylamide gel solution is prepared (Table 6) and rapidly transferred between the glass plates.

4. The gel is prerun gel at 25 W for 1 h, until the temperature at the surface of the glass plates is above 40 °C.

5. After loading the samples RNAs are separated at 25 W for approx. 30 min, until the bromophenol blue dye has left the gel and the xylene cyanole dye migrates within the lower third of the gel.

6. The gel is transferred to Whatman filter paper and dried at 80 °C for 45 min.

7. The gel is exposed to an imaging plate. Phosphorescence from the imaging plate is recorded by a FLA3000 imaging system (or equivalent).

*3.5.3 Transcript Quantification*

1. To determine the efficiency of chromatin transcription each transcription reaction contains equal molar amounts of the 601 template of interest and a reference template of different size (e.g., template generated from plasmids K1253 and K1573, respectively) in every reaction for normalization. This results in two radioactively labeled transcript populations per lane.

2. The relative radioactive signal intensity of a single band is background corrected and divided by the signal area.

3. Relative signal intensities of transcripts derived from 601 templates with and without assembled nucleosome are divided by the signal intensities of transcripts derived from the reference template. This yields the normalized transcript levels derived from nucleosomal and nucleosome-free 601 templates. The quotient of the normalized transcript levels derived from the nucleosomal 601 template and derived from the nucleosome-free 601 template is taken as measure for the efficiency of transcription through a nucleosome.

# 4  Notes

1. Strong shaking of the coffee mill prevents sticking of the dry ice powder to the inside wall of the grinder. (Cryo-)gloves should be used to protect the hands during grinding.

2. The amount of dry ice needed for a grinding cycle depends on the coffee grinder and should be determined in pilot experiments. Dry ice evaporates during the procedure, and at least 10 g of dry ice/yeast powder should remain in the coffee-grinder at the end of the grinding cycle. If tested before, the grinding procedure may be performed at the laboratory bench at room temperature, which can be more convenient.

3. Grinding of yeast cells with dry ice in a coffee mill is a relatively mild lysis procedure. Shearing forces on genomic DNA are significantly lower than in the glass-bead mediated cell disruption described in Subheading 3.4. This reduces the amount of contaminating chromosomal chromatin fragments in the supernatant after centrifugation of the crude lysate.

4. This step critically depends on the performance of the magnetic stirrer since the dry ice/yeast powder may be spilled if the stir bar rotation is not properly adjusted.

5. Protein analysis by the Western blot procedure is described elsewhere [33, 34]. The Western blot analysis is performed to detect the TAP-tagged LexA bait protein, which binds to its recognition sites within the recombined chromatin domain of interest. Good retention of chromatin domains is only guaranteed if the LexA-TAP protein is largely depleted in the flow-through obtained after affinity purification. LexA-TAP can be either detected via an antibody directed against the calmodulin binding peptide (CBP) [19], or peroxidase–anti-peroxidase soluble complex (Sigma-Aldrich, Inc., P 1291) which interacts with protein A. CBP and protein A are components of the TAP-tag [35].

6. Using the ratio of cells to buffer indicated in Subheading 3.3.1, **step 6**, a protein concentration of 15–20 mg/mL is routinely obtained. If protein concentrations are significantly lower the grinding procedure needs to be optimized.

7. Restriction enzyme digestion of the native chromatin bound to the beads is usually incomplete, since the respective restriction site may occasionally be protected by nucleosomes (*see* Fig. 2c, undigested 35S rRNA gene).

8. Yeast tRNAs act as a carrier molecule upon ethanol precipitation and are required for quantitative recovery of nucleic acids from the "B" and "BpD" samples.

9. For absolute quantitation of the linearized DNA region within the purified native chromatin domains, a titration series of distinct amounts of an isolated DNA fragment containing the DNA region of interest (e.g., from plasmid DNA, or a purified PCR product) should be included in the analyses (*see* Fig. 2c). Note that only the digested 35S rRNA gene chromatin will produce a transcript of the expected size.

## Acknowledgments

We thank the members of the Department of Biochemistry III for constant support and discussion. This work was funded by the Deutsche Forschungsgemeinschaft (DFG) in the context of the SFB960. P. E. M. was partly supported by a fellowship of the German National Academic Foundation.

## References

1. Vannini A, Cramer P (2012) Conservation between the RNA polymerase I, II, and III transcription initiation machineries. Mol Cell 45:439–446

2. Kornberg RD, Lorch Y (1999) Twenty-five years of the nucleosome, fundamental particle of the eukaryote chromosome. Cell 98: 285–294

3. Olins DE, Olins AL (2003) Chromatin history: our view from the bridge. Nat Rev Mol Cell Biol 4:809–814

4. Andrews AJ, Luger K (2011) Nucleosome structure(s) and stability: variations on a theme. Annu Rev Biophys 40:99–117

5. Lai WKM, Pugh BF (2017) Understanding nucleosome dynamics and their links to gene expression and DNA replication. Nat Rev Mol Cell Biol 18:548–562

6. Rando OJ, Winston F (2012) Chromatin and transcription in yeast. Genetics 190:351–387

7. Merkl PE, Pilsl M, Fremter T, Schwank K, Engel C, Längst G, Milkereit P, Griesenbeck J, Tschochner H (2020) RNA polymerase I (Pol I) passage through nucleosomes depends on Pol I subunits binding its lobe structure. J Biol Chem 295:4782–4795

8. Kornberg RD (2007) The molecular basis of eukaryotic transcription. Proc Natl Acad Sci U S A 104:12955–12961

9. Lusser A, Kadonaga JT (2004) Strategies for the reconstitution of chromatin. Nat Methods 1:19–26

10. Merkl P, Perez-Fernandez J, Pilsl M, Reiter A, Williams L, Gerber J, Böhm M, Deutzmann R, Griesenbeck J, Milkereit P, Tschochner H (2014) Binding of the termination factor Nsi1 to its cognate DNA site is sufficient to terminate RNA polymerase I transcription in vitro and to induce termination in vivo. Mol Cell Biol 34:3817–3827

11. Merkl P (2014) Comparative studies on elongation and termination of the three RNA polymerases from S. cerevisiae in vitro. PhD thesis. Universität Regensburg, Regensburg

12. Kadesch TR, Chamberlin MJ (1982) Studies of in vitro transcription by calf thymus RNA polymerase II using a novel duplex DNA template. J Biol Chem 257:5286–5295

13. Lowary PT, Widom J (1998) New DNA sequence rules for high affinity binding to histone octamer and sequence-directed nucleosome positioning. J Mol Biol 276:19–42

14. Pilsl M, Merkl PE, Milkereit P, Griesenbeck J, Tschochner H (2016) Analysis of S. cerevisiae RNA polymerase I transcription in vitro. Methods Mol Biol Clifton NJ 1455:99–108

15. Shou W, Sakamoto KM, Keener J, Morimoto KW, Traverso EE, Azzam R, Hoppe GJ, Feldman RM, DeModena J, Moazed D, Charbonneau H, Nomura M, Deshaies RJ (2001) Net1 stimulates RNA polymerase I transcription and regulates nucleolar structure independently of controlling mitotic exit. Mol Cell 8:45–55

16. Hannig K (2016) Net1 - ein modular aufgebautes und multifunktionales Protein im Nukleolus der Hefe Saccharomyces cerevisiae. PhD thesis. Universität Regensburg, Regensburg

17. Griesenbeck J, Boeger H, Strattan JS, Kornberg RD (2004) Purification of defined chromosomal domains. Methods Enzymol 375: 170–178

18. Griesenbeck J, Boeger H, Strattan JS, Kornberg RD (2003) Affinity purification of specific chromatin segments from chromosomal loci in yeast. Mol Cell Biol 23:9275–9282

19. Hamperl S, Brown CR, Perez-Fernandez J, Huber K, Wittner M, Babl V, Stöckl U, Boeger H, Tschochner H, Milkereit P, Griesenbeck J (2014) Purification of specific chromatin domains from single-copy gene loci in Saccharomyces cerevisiae. Methods Mol Biol Clifton NJ 1094:329–341

20. Hamperl S, Brown CR, Garea AV, Perez-Fernandez J, Bruckmann A, Huber K, Wittner M, Babl V, Stoeckl U, Deutzmann R, Boeger H, Tschochner H, Milkereit P, Griesenbeck J (2014) Compositional and structural

analysis of selected chromosomal domains from Saccharomyces cerevisiae. Nucleic Acids Res 42:e2

21. Hermans N, Huisman JJ, Brouwer TB, Schächner C, van Heusden GPH, Griesenbeck J, van Noort J (2017) Toehold-enhanced LNA probes for selective pull down and single-molecule analysis of native chromatin. Sci Rep 7:16721

22. Brown CR, Eskin JA, Hamperl S, Griesenbeck J, Jurica MS, Boeger H (2015) Chromatin structure analysis of single gene molecules by psoralen cross-linking and electron microscopy. Methods Mol Biol Clifton NJ 1228:93–121

23. Brown CR, Mao C, Falkovskaia E, Jurica MS, Boeger H (2013) Linking stochastic fluctuations in chromatin structure and gene expression. PLoS Biol 11:e1001621

24. Lorch Y, Griesenbeck J, Boeger H, Maier-Davis B, Kornberg RD (2011) Selective removal of promoter nucleosomes by the RSC chromatin-remodeling complex. Nat Struct Mol Biol 18:881–885

25. Nagai S, Davis RE, Mattei PJ, Eagen KP, Kornberg RD (2017) Chromatin potentiates transcription. Proc Natl Acad Sci U S A 114:1536–1541

26. Hannig K, Babl V, Hergert K, Maier A, Pilsl M, Schächner C, Stöckl U, Milkereit P, Tschochner H, Seufert W, Griesenbeck J (2019) The C-terminal region of Net1 is an activator of RNA polymerase I transcription with conserved features from yeast to human. PLoS Genet 15:e1008006

27. Neelin JM, Butler GC (1959) The fractionation of the histones of calf thymus and chicken erythrocytes by cation-exchange chromatography with sodium salts. Can J Biochem Physiol 37:843–859

28. Reiter A, Hamperl S, Seitz H, Merkl P, Perez-Fernandez J, Williams L, Gerber J, Németh A,

Léger I, Gadal O, Milkereit P, Griesenbeck J, Tschochner H (2012) The Reb1-homologue Ydr026c/Nsi1 is required for efficient RNA polymerase I termination in yeast. EMBO J 31:3480–3493

29. Merz K, Hondele M, Goetze H, Gmelch K, Stoeckl U, Griesenbeck J (2008) Actively transcribed rRNA genes in S. cerevisiae are organized in a specialized chromatin associated with the high-mobility group protein Hmo1 and are largely devoid of histone molecules. Genes Dev 22:1190–1204

30. Allefs JJ, Salentijn EM, Krens FA, Rouwendal GJ (1990) Optimization of non-radioactive Southern blot hybridization: single copy detection and reuse of blots. Nucleic Acids Res 18:3099–3100

31. Green MR, Sambrook J (2012) Molecular cloning: a laboratory manual (Fourth Edition): three-volume set, 4th edn. Cold Spring Harbor Laboratory Press, Cold Spring Harbor

32. Keener J, Josaitis CA, Dodd JA, Nomura M (1998) Reconstitution of yeast RNA polymerase I transcription in vitro from purified components. TATA-binding protein is not required for basal transcription. J Biol Chem 273:33795–33802

33. Towbin H, Staehelin T, Gordon J (1979) Electrophoretic transfer of proteins from polyacrylamide gels to nitrocellulose sheets: procedure and some applications. Proc Natl Acad Sci U S A 76:4350–4354

34. Laemmli UK (1970) Cleavage of structural proteins during the assembly of the head of bacteriophage T4. Nature 227:680–685

35. Rigaut G, Shevchenko A, Rutz B, Wilm M, Mann M, Séraphin B (1999) A generic protein purification method for protein complex characterization and proteome exploration. Nat Biotechnol 17:1030–1032

# Part III

**RNA Polymerases**

# Chapter 4

## Specialization of RNA Polymerase I in Comparison to Other Nuclear RNA Polymerases of *Saccharomyces cerevisiae*

**Philipp E. Merkl, Christopher Schächner, Michael Pilsl, Katrin Schwank, Catharina Schmid, Gernot Längst, Philipp Milkereit, Joachim Griesenbeck, and Herbert Tschochner**

## Abstract

In archaea and bacteria the major classes of RNAs are synthesized by one DNA-dependent RNA polymerase (RNAP). In contrast, most eukaryotes have three highly specialized RNAPs to transcribe the nuclear genome. RNAP I synthesizes almost exclusively ribosomal (r)RNA, RNAP II synthesizes mRNA as well as many noncoding RNAs involved in RNA processing or RNA silencing pathways and RNAP III synthesizes mainly tRNA and 5S rRNA. This review discusses functional differences of the three nuclear core RNAPs in the yeast *S. cerevisiae* with a particular focus on RNAP I transcription of nucleolar ribosomal (r)DNA chromatin.

**Key words** RNA polymerase I, RNA polymerase II, RNA polymerase III, Transcription, Chromatin, Nucleosomes, Ribosomal RNA genes, Transcription factors, Gene expression, Yeast, *Saccharomyces cerevisiae*

---

## 1 RNA Polymerase I Has Only One Essential Genomic Target

Nuclear yeast RNAPs are protein complexes consisting of 12 (RNAP II), 14 (RNAP I) and 17 (RNAP III) subunits. They all share a conserved architecture of the RNAP core, which catalyzes the highly accurate polymerization of RNA from single NTP molecules [1–3] (see review by Pilsl and Engel in this issue). Based on structural analyses and on functional in vitro assays, on the one hand the molecular mechanisms driving the RNA polymerization appear to be similar in all RNAPs. On the other hand, all three enzymes have special features, supporting their specific in vivo tasks [1, 2]. Thus, RNAP II has to transcribe thousands of different genes and produces transcripts from a few hundred to several thousand of bases in length. To account for dynamic changes in cellular gene expression RNAP II has (a) to recognize many

Karl-Dieter Entian (ed.), *Ribosome Biogenesis: Methods and Protocols*, Methods in Molecular Biology, vol. 2533,
https://doi.org/10.1007/978-1-0716-2501-9_4, © The Author(s) 2022

promoters, (b) to access differently modified chromatin templates, which probably requires to adjust its elongation and termination properties. To fulfill these multiple tasks, RNAP II interacts with many different factors at each step of the transcription process [4, 5]. In contrast, RNAP III recognizes only three distinct classes of promoters and has probably a distinct transcription termination mechanism [6]. RNAP III synthesizes mainly short noncoding RNAs (typically <200 bp) with high efficiency in rapidly growing cells. Accordingly, the RNAP III transcription machinery is rather well defined [7–10]. Finally, the yeast RNAP I transcription machinery has only one known genomic target, the multicopy 9.1 kb 35S rRNA genes [11]. The rRNA genes are transcribed at very high rates accounting for up to 60% of RNA synthesis upon cellular growth [12]. Accordingly, electron micrographs of chromatin spreads show an extremely high density of RNAP I molecules at rRNA genes, whereas most RNAP II-dependent genes are only sparsely covered with polymerases [13–15]. Furthermore, RNAP I and RNAP III-dependent genes are constitutively transcribed in actively dividing cells and—as opposed to the majority of RNAP II transcribed genes—apparently devoid of nucleosomes (see as review [16–18] and Schächner et al., within this issue).

## 2    RNA Polymerase I Contains Additional Subunits Resembling Transcription Factors of RNAP II

RNAPs I, II, and III contain ten conserved subunits which form the catalytic core. In addition, all three enzymes contain a 2-subunit stalk structure, which is distantly related and consists of subunits A14/A43, Rpb4/Rpb7 and C17/C25 in RNAPs I, II and III, respectively. In RNAP III an additional heterotrimer C82/C34/C3 connects the stalk with the RNAP III clamp, which probably helps to open the DNA duplex [19]. The overall architecture of the three RNAPs differs mainly in vicinity of the lobe structure, which is formed by the second largest subunits Rpa135, Rpb2 and Rpc128, respectively. Only one subunit—Rpb9—is bound to the RNAP II lobe, whereas the heterodimer A34.5/49 and subunit A12.2 bind to the lobe of RNAP I, and the homologous C17/C25 and C11 subunits to the lobe of RNAP III. RNAP I subunits A34.5 and A49 consist of three subdomains: a dimerization module formed by A34.5 and the N-terminal part of A49 (full length A34.5 and aa 1–110 of A49); the A49 linker (aa 105–187 of A49); and the C-terminal part of A49 (aa 187–415). The dimerization module binds to the "lobe" and "external" domains of the second largest Pol I subunit A135 on the core module side [20–22]. In contrast, the C-terminal part of A49 which contains a tandem winged helix can be detected at the upstream face of the clamp core in several states of transcriptional active RNAP I molecules and seems to be flexible attached [20, 21, 23–31]. Bio-chemical and cell biological experiments showed that A34.5/A49 support transcription initiation, enhance RNAP I elongation and stimulate the intrinsic RNAP I RNA cleavage activity [26, 28, 32–36]. RNA cleavage activity depends on the dimerization module which is located in close proximity to A12.2 whose C-terminal part is also important for efficient RNA cleavage [26]. Deletion of A12.2 results in growth inhibition at elevated temperature, sensitivity to nucleotide-reducing drugs, and inefficient transcription termination; hampers the assembly of the RNAP I enzyme; and leads to incorporation of wrong NTPs [37–40]. The lack of A12.2 may also lead to the loss of A34.5/A49, and might influence the intrinsic stability of elongation and termination complexes [40, 41].

Based on amino acid sequence similarities, position on the enzyme and function, the heterodimer formed by A34.5 and the N-terminus of A49 was suggested to be homologous to the RNAP II transcription factor TFIIF [26, 33]. TFIIF is predominantly found at promoter-proximal regions suggesting a crucial role in transcription initiation [42, 43]. On the other hand, TFIIF was suggested to leave the promoter—at least transiently—in complex with RNAP II, likely supporting early elongation [42–45]. A role of TFIIF in RNAP II elongation is further corroborated by in vitro studies, where it increases transcription rates by suppressing RNAP II pausing [46–48]. Several studies propose that TFIIF promotes transcription elongation in concert with the RNA cleavage supporting factor TFIIS, which structurally resembles the C-terminus of the RNAP I subunit A12.2 (reviewed in [3, 48–51]. In the RNAP II system, TFIIF and TFIIS are independently capable to release arrested RNAP II to resume productive elongation. However, these factors may synergistically enhance resumption of RNAP II transcription especially in conditions when the paused enzyme has additionally backtracked on the template [49]. Backtracked RNAP I requires the C-terminal, RNA cleavage activating part of A12.2 to resume elongation [52]. It is, however, unknown if the heterodimer A34.5/A49 participates in this process.

Finally, the C-terminus of A49 structurally and functionally resembles the tandem winged helix of TFIIE [33]. As TFIIE in RNAP II transcription, the C-terminal domain of A49 binds DNA and supports promoter-dependent transcription initiation in vitro [28] and RNAP I promoter recruitment in vivo [32]. In contrast to TFIIE, the A49 subunit stays associated with the enzyme after promoter clearance in vivo [32], and supports elongation of RNA from a DNA/RNA scaffold in vitro [33]. Recent studies suggest a more dynamic association of the heterodimer A34.5/A49 to the RNAP I lobe, since the heterodimer was absent from the core enzyme and A12.2 C-terminus was rearranged when RNAP I elongation was artificially blocked by addition of a nonhydrolyzable nucleotide [53].

A specific challenge for all elongating RNAPs is the transcription of chromatin templates. Since RNAP I and III transcribe nucleosome-depleted chromatin templates ( [13–15] see short review of Schächner et al. this issue). This indicates that nucleosomes are displaced from the chromatin template in the initial round of transcription, and it is possible that the lobe associated subunits of RNAP I and III may be involved in the process of nucleosome depletion.

## 3   Nuclear RNAPs Transcribe Chromatin Templates

In eukaryotic cells, nuclear DNA is assembled into repeated units called nucleosomes consisting of 146 bp of DNA wrapped around an octameric complex of histone proteins [54]. Nucleosomes generally provide a strong barrier for elongating RNAP II in vitro [46, 55, 56]. DNA attached to nucleosomes recoils on the octamer, locking the enzyme in an arrested state [57] thereby providing four major superhelical pausing sites [58]. Additional factors are required for passage of RNAP II through this barrier (see below). The mechanism how purified RNAP II complexes passes nucleosomes in vitro was thoroughly studied [59, 60]. Whether assembled nucleosomes stay associated or are evicted during RNAP II transcription depends on the formation of a small intranucleosomal DNA loop and on the transcription efficiency (rate) [61]. Accordingly, various RNAP II complexes can remodel chromatin to a different extent [59, 60].

It was suggested, that RNAP II can only pass nucleosomes if uncoiling of the DNA from the surface of the octamer is facilitated and if transcription elongation factors keep the polymerase in a transcriptionally competent state [62]. TFIIF and TFIIS may prevent the release of RNAP II at nucleosomal barriers and thereby support transcription through a nucleosome in a synergistic manner [63]. Passage of purified RNAP II through in vitro assembled nucleosomes was also supported by elongation factor Spt4/Spt5 [64] and in the presence of TFIIS together with Spt4/5 and elongation factor Elf1 [65]. Insights in the molecular mechanism how Spt4/5 together with Elf1 facilitate progression of RNAP II through a nucleosome were recently obtained using high resolution structures by cryo-EM of different stalled elongation complexes [65]. Other factors that were reported to partially disassemble nucleosomes similar to Spt4/Spt5 are the histone chaperone FACT and Paf1c [66–68].

Much less is known about how RNAP I and RNAP III interact with nucleosomes in vitro. However, in vivo there is ample evidence that RNAP I and RNAP III genes are largely devoid of nucleosomes (reviewed in [16–18], see short review of Schächner et al. in this issue). It is an open question how RNAP I and RNAP III deal with nucleosomal genes in the initial round of transcription. In contrast to RNAP II which has only subunit Rpb9 associated to the lobe structure, yeast RNAP I and RNAP III have the TFIIF- and TFIIS-homologous subunits A34.5/A49, A12.2 (RNAP I), and C37/C53, C11 (RNAP III) tightly associated to the lobe. Similar to TFIIF and TFIIS in RNAP II transcription, the homologous Pol I subunits A34.5/A49 and A12.2 facilitate RNAP I passage through nucleosomes [35]. Depletion of either the heterodimeric subunits A34.5/A49 or the cleavage supporting activity of A12.2 resulted in both reduced Pol I processivity and impaired passage though nucleosomes [35]. It is tempting to speculate that the homologous RNAP III subunits could play a similar role in RNAP III chromatin transcription. Furthermore, additional factors like FACT, Spt4/Spt5, or Paf1c have all been suggested to support RNAP I elongation [69–72]. Appropriate in vitro transcription system using highly purified factors and defined nucleosome templates will be the key to elucidate details of the molecular mechanisms of RNAP I and RNAP III transcription in the context of chromatin (see chapter by Merkl et al. in this issue).

## Acknowledgments

We thank all the members of the department of Biochemistry III for constant support and discussion. This work was funded by the Deutsche Forschungsgemeinschaft (DFG) in the context of the SFB960. P. E. M. was partly supported by a fellowship of the German National Academic Foundation.

## References

1. Engel C, Neyer S, Cramer P (2018) Distinct mechanisms of transcription initiation by RNA polymerases I and II. Annu Rev Biophys 47:425–446

2. Khatter H, Vorländer MK, Müller CW (2017) RNA polymerase I and III: similar yet unique. Curr Opin Struct Biol 47:88–94

3. Vannini A, Cramer P (2012) Conservation between the RNA polymerase I, II, and III transcription initiation machineries. Mol Cell 45:439–446

4. Chen FX, Smith ER, Shilatifard A (2018) Born to run: control of transcription elongation by RNA polymerase II. Nat Rev Mol Cell Biol 19:464–478

5. Haberle V, Stark A (2018) Eukaryotic core promoters and the functional basis of transcription initiation. Nat Rev Mol Cell Biol 19:621–637

6. Arimbasseri AG, Rijal K, Maraia RJ (2013) Transcription termination by the eukaryotic RNA polymerase III. Biochim Biophys Acta 1829:318–330

7. Arimbasseri AG, Rijal K, Maraia RJ (2014) Comparative overview of RNA polymerase II and III transcription cycles, with focus on RNA polymerase III termination and reinitiation. Transcription 5:e27639

8. Graczyk D, Cieśla M, Boguta M (2018) Regulation of tRNA synthesis by the general transcription factors of RNA polymerase III - TFIIIB and TFIIIC, and by the MAF1 protein. Biochim Biophys Acta Gene Regul Mech 1861:320–329

9. Moir RD, Willis IM (2013) Regulation of pol III transcription by nutrient and stress signaling pathways. Biochim Biophys Acta 1829:361–375

10. Willis IM, Moir RD (2018) Signaling to and from the RNA polymerase III transcription and processing machinery. Annu Rev Biochem 87: 75–100

11. Nogi Y, Yano R, Nomura M (1991) Synthesis of large rRNAs by RNA polymerase II in mutants of *Saccharomyces cerevisiae* defective in RNA polymerase I. Proc Natl Acad Sci U S A 88:3962–3966

12. Warner JR (1999) The economics of ribosome biosynthesis in yeast. Trends Biochem Sci 24: 437–440

13. French SL, Osheim YN, Cioci F, Nomura M, Beyer AL (2003) In exponentially growing *Saccharomyces cerevisiae* cells, rRNA synthesis is determined by the summed RNA polymerase I loading rate rather than by the number of active genes. Mol Cell Biol 23:1558–1568

14. French SL, Osheim YN, Schneider DA, Sikes ML, Fernandez CF, Copela LA, Misra VA, Nomura M, Wolin SL, Beyer AL (2008) Visual analysis of the yeast 5S rRNA gene transcriptome: regulation and role of La protein. Mol Cell Biol 28:4576–4587

15. Laird CD, Chooi WY (1976) Morphology of transcription units in Drosophila melanogaster. Chromosoma 58:193–218

16. Hamperl S, Wittner M, Babl V, Perez-Fernandez J, Tschochner H, Griesenbeck J (2013) Chromatin states at ribosomal DNA loci. Biochim Biophys Acta 1829:405–417

17. Morse RH, Roth SY, Simpson RT (1992) A transcriptionally active tRNA gene interferes with nucleosome positioning in vivo. Mol Cell Biol 12:4015–4025

18. Moss T, Mars J-C, Tremblay MG, Sabourin-Felix M (2019) The chromatin landscape of the ribosomal RNA genes in mouse and human. Chromosome Res 27(1-2):31–40. https://doi.org/10.1007/s10577-018-09603-9

19. Hoffmann NA, Jakobi AJ, Moreno-Morcillo-M, Glatt S, Kosinski J, Hagen WJH, Sachse C, Müller CW (2015) Molecular structures of unbound and transcribing RNA polymerase III. Nature 528:231–236

20. Engel C, Sainsbury S, Cheung AC, Kostrewa D, Cramer P (2013) RNA polymerase I structure and transcription regulation. Nature 502:650–655

21. Fernández-Tornero C, Moreno-Morcillo M, Rashid UJ, Taylor NMI, Ruiz FM, Gruene T, Legrand P, Steuerwald U, Müller CW (2013) Crystal structure of the 14-subunit RNA polymerase I. Nature 502:644–649

22. Jennebach S, Herzog F, Aebersold R, Cramer P (2012) Crosslinking-MS analysis reveals RNA polymerase I domain architecture and basis of rRNA cleavage. Nucleic Acids Res 40: 5591–5601

23. Engel C, Gubbey T, Neyer S, Sainsbury S, Oberthuer C, Baejen C, Bernecky C, Cramer P (2017) Structural basis of RNA polymerase I transcription initiation. Cell 169:120–131.e22

24. Han Y, Yan C, Nguyen THD, Jackobel AJ, Ivanov I, Knutson BA, He Y (2017) Structural mechanism of ATP-independent transcription initiation by RNA polymerase I. elife 6:e27414

25. Kostrewa D, Kuhn C-D, Engel C, Cramer P (2015) An alternative RNA polymerase I structure reveals a dimer hinge. Acta Crystallogr D Biol Crystallogr 71:1850–1855

26. Kuhn C-D, Geiger SR, Baumli S, Gartmann M, Gerber J, Jennebach S, Mielke T, Tschochner H, Beckmann R, Cramer P (2007) Functional architecture of RNA polymerase I. Cell 131:1260–1272

27. Neyer S, Kunz M, Geiss C, Hantsche M, Hodirnau V-V, Seybert A, Engel C, Scheffer MP, Cramer P, Frangakis AS (2016) Structure of RNA polymerase I transcribing ribosomal DNA genes. Nature 540(7634):607–610. https://doi.org/10.1038/nature20561

28. Pilsl M, Crucifix C, Papai G, Krupp F, Steinbauer R, Griesenbeck J, Milkereit P, Tschochner H, Schultz P (2016) Structure of the initiation-competent RNA polymerase I and its implication for transcription. Nat Commun 7:12126

29. Sadian Y, Tafur L, Kosinski J, Jakobi AJ, Wetzel R, Buczak K, Hagen WJ, Beck M, Sachse C, Müller CW (2017) Structural insights into transcription initiation by yeast RNA polymerase I. EMBO J 36:2698–2709

30. Sanz-Murillo M, Xu J, Belogurov GA, Calvo O, Gil-Carton D, Moreno-Morcillo M, Wang D, Fernández-Tornero C (2018) Structural basis of RNA polymerase I stalling at UV light-induced DNA damage. Proc Natl Acad Sci U S A 115:8972–8977

31. Tafur L, Sadian Y, Hoffmann NA, Jakobi AJ, Wetzel R, Hagen WJH, Sachse C, Müller CW (2016) Molecular structures of transcribing RNA polymerase I. Mol Cell 64:1135–1143

32. Beckouet F, Labarre-Mariotte S, Albert B, Imazawa Y, Werner M, Gadal O, Nogi Y, Thuriaux P (2008) Two RNA polymerase I subunits control the binding and release of Rrn3 during transcription. Mol Cell Biol 28:1596–1605

33. Geiger SR, Lorenzen K, Schreieck A, Hanecker P, Kostrewa D, Heck AJR, Cramer P (2010) RNA polymerase I contains a TFIIF-related DNA-binding subcomplex. Mol Cell 39:583–594

34. Liljelund P, Mariotte S, Buhler JM, Sentenac A (1992) Characterization and mutagenesis of the gene encoding the A49 subunit of RNA polymerase A in Saccharomyces cerevisiae. Proc Natl Acad Sci U S A 89:9302–9305

35. Merkl PE, Pilsl M, Fremter T, Schwank K, Engel C, Längst G, Milkereit P, Griesenbeck J, Tschochner H (2020) RNA polymerase I (Pol I) passage through nucleosomes depends on Pol I subunits binding its lobe structure. J Biol Chem 295:4782–4795

36. Knutson BA, McNamar R, Rothblum LI (2020) Dynamics of the RNA polymerase I TFIIF/TFIIE-like subcomplex: a mini-review. Biochem Soc Trans 48:1917–1927

37. Gout J-F, Li W, Fritsch C, Li A, Haroon S, Singh L, Hua D, Fazelinia H, Smith Z, Seeholzer S, Thomas K, Lynch M, Vermulst M (2017) The landscape of transcription errors in eukaryotic cells. Sci Adv 3:e1701484

38. Nogi Y, Yano R, Dodd J, Carles C, Nomura M (1993) Gene RRN4 in Saccharomyces cerevisiae encodes the A12.2 subunit of RNA polymerase I and is essential only at high temperatures. Mol Cell Biol 13:114–122

39. Prescott EM, Osheim YN, Jones HS, Alen CM, Roan JG, Reeder RH, Beyer AL, Proudfoot NJ (2004) Transcriptional termination by RNA polymerase I requires the small subunit Rpa12p. Proc Natl Acad Sci U S A 101:6068–6073

40. Van Mullem V, Landrieux E, Vandenhaute J, Thuriaux P (2002) Rpa12p, a conserved RNA polymerase I subunit with two functional domains. Mol Microbiol 43:1105–1113

41. Appling FD, Scull CE, Lucius AL, Schneider DA (2018) The A12.2 subunit is an intrinsic destabilizer of the RNA polymerase I elongation complex. Biophys J 114:2507–2515

42. Krogan NJ, Kim M, Ahn SH, Zhong G, Kobor MS, Cagney G, Emili A, Shilatifard A, Buratowski S, Greenblatt JF (2002) RNA polymerase II elongation factors of Saccharomyces cerevisiae: a targeted proteomics approach. Mol Cell Biol 22:6979–6992

43. Mayer A, Lidschreiber M, Siebert M, Leike K, Söding J, Cramer P (2010) Uniform transitions of the general RNA polymerase II transcription complex. Nat Struct Mol Biol 17:1272–1278

44. Cojocaru M, Jeronimo C, Forget D, Bouchard A, Bergeron D, Côte P, Poirier GG, Greenblatt J, Coulombe B (2008) Genomic location of the human RNA polymerase II general machinery: evidence for a role of TFIIF and Rpb7 at both early and late stages of transcription. Biochem J 409:139–147

45. Rani PG, Ranish JA, Hahn S (2004) RNA polymerase II (Pol II)-TFIIF and Pol II-mediator complexes: the major stable Pol II complexes and their activity in transcription initiation and reinitiation. Mol Cell Biol 24:1709–1720

46. Izban MG, Luse DS (1992) Factor-stimulated RNA polymerase II transcribes at physiological elongation rates on naked DNA but very poorly on chromatin templates. J Biol Chem 267:13647–13655

47. Renner DB, Yamaguchi Y, Wada T, Handa H, Price DH (2001) A highly purified RNA polymerase II elongation control system. J Biol Chem 276:42601–42609

48. Zhang C, Yan H, Burton ZF (2003) Combinatorial control of human RNA polymerase II (RNAP II) pausing and transcript cleavage by transcription factor IIF, hepatitis delta antigen, and stimulatory factor II. J Biol Chem 278:50101–50111

49. Schweikhard V, Meng C, Murakami K, Kaplan CD, Kornberg RD, Block SM (2014) Transcription factors TFIIF and TFIIS promote transcript elongation by RNA polymerase II by synergistic and independent mechanisms. Proc Natl Acad Sci U S A 111:6642–6647

50. Zhang C, Burton ZF (2004) Transcription factors IIF and IIS and nucleoside triphosphate substrates as dynamic probes of the human RNA polymerase II mechanism. J Mol Biol 342:1085–1099

51. Zhang C, Zobeck KL, Burton ZF (2005) Human RNA polymerase II elongation in slow motion: role of the TFIIF RAP74 alpha1 helix in nucleoside triphosphate-driven translocation. Mol Cell Biol 25:3583–3595

52. Lisica A, Engel C, Jahnel M, Roldán É, Galburt EA, Cramer P, Grill SW (2016) Mechanisms of backtrack recovery by RNA polymerases I and II. Proc Natl Acad Sci U S A 113:2946–2951

53. Tafur L, Sadian Y, Hanske J, Wetzel R, Weis F, Müller CW (2019) The cryo-EM structure of a 12-subunit variant of RNA polymerase I reveals dissociation of the A49-A34.5 heterodimer and rearrangement of subunit A12.2. eLife 8:e43204

54. Kornberg RD (1974) Chromatin structure: a repeating unit of histones and DNA. Science 184:868–871

55. Chang CH, Luse DS (1997) The H3/H4 tetramer blocks transcript elongation by RNA polymerase II in vitro. J Biol Chem 272:23427–23434

56. Izban MG, Luse DS (1991) Transcription on nucleosomal templates by RNA polymerase II in vitro: inhibition of elongation with

enhancement of sequence-specific pausing. Genes Dev 5:683–696

57. Gaykalova DA, Kulaeva OI, Volokh O, Shaytan AK, Hsieh F-K, Kirpichnikov MP, Sokolova OS, Studitsky VM (2015) Structural analysis of nucleosomal barrier to transcription. Proc Natl Acad Sci U S A 112:E5787–E5795

58. Kujirai T, Ehara H, Fujino Y, Shirouzu M, Sekine S-I, Kurumizaka H (2018) Structural basis of the nucleosome transition during RNA polymerase II passage. Science 362: 595–598

59. Dangkulwanich M, Ishibashi T, Bintu L, Bustamante C (2014) Molecular mechanisms of transcription through single-molecule experiments. Chem Rev 114:3203–3223

60. Kulaeva OI, Hsieh F-K, Chang H-W, Luse DS, Studitsky VM (2013) Mechanism of transcription through a nucleosome by RNA polymerase II. Biochim Biophys Acta 1829:76–83

61. Bintu L, Kopaczynska M, Hodges C, Lubkowska L, Kashlev M, Bustamante C (2011) The elongation rate of RNA polymerase determines the fate of transcribed nucleosomes. Nat Struct Mol Biol 18:1394–1399

62. Luse DS, Studitsky VM (2011) The mechanism of nucleosome traversal by RNA polymerase II: roles for template uncoiling and transcript elongation factors. RNA Biol 8: 581–585

63. Luse DS, Spangler LC, Újvári A (2011) Efficient and rapid nucleosome traversal by RNA polymerase II depends on a combination of transcript elongation factors. J Biol Chem 286:6040–6048

64. Crickard JB, Lee J, Lee T-H, Reese JC (2017) The elongation factor Spt4/5 regulates RNA polymerase II transcription through the nucleosome. Nucleic Acids Res 45:6362–6374

65. Ehara H, Kujirai T, Fujino Y, Shirouzu M, Kurumizaka H, Sekine S-I (2019) Structural insight into nucleosome transcription by RNA

polymerase II with elongation factors. Science 363:744–747

66. Belotserkovskaya R, Oh S, Bondarenko VA, Orphanides G, Studitsky VM, Reinberg D (2003) FACT facilitates transcription-dependent nucleosome alteration. Science 301:1090–1093

67. Hsieh F-K, Kulaeva OI, Patel SS, Dyer PN, Luger K, Reinberg D, Studitsky VM (2013) Histone chaperone FACT action during transcription through chromatin by RNA polymerase II. Proc Natl Acad Sci U S A 110: 7654–7659

68. Kim J, Guermah M, Roeder RG (2010) The human PAF1 complex acts in chromatin transcription elongation both independently and cooperatively with SII/TFIIS. Cell 140: 491–503

69. Birch JL, Tan BC-M, Panov KI, Panova TB, Andersen JS, Owen-Hughes TA, Russell J, Lee S-C, Zomerdijk JCBM (2009) FACT facilitates chromatin transcription by RNA polymerases I and III. EMBO J 28:854–865

70. Schneider DA, French SL, Osheim YN, Bailey AO, Vu L, Dodd J, Yates JR, Beyer AL, Nomura M (2006) RNA polymerase II elongation factors Spt4p and Spt5p play roles in transcription elongation by RNA polymerase I and rRNA processing. Proc Natl Acad Sci U S A 103:12707–12712

71. Zhang Y, Sikes ML, Beyer AL, Schneider DA (2009) The Paf1 complex is required for efficient transcription elongation by RNA polymerase I. Proc Natl Acad Sci U S A 106: 2153–2158

72. Zhang Y, Smith AD, Renfrow MB, Schneider DA (2010) The RNA polymerase-associated factor 1 complex (Paf1C) directly increases the elongation rate of RNA polymerase I and is required for efficient regulation of rRNA synthesis. J Biol Chem 285:14152–14159

# Chapter 5

# Structural Studies of Eukaryotic RNA Polymerase I Using Cryo-Electron Microscopy

## Michael Pilsl and Christoph Engel

## Abstract

Technical advances have pushed the resolution limit of single-particle cryo-electron microscopy (cryo-EM) throughout the past decade and made the technique accessible to a wide range of samples. Among them, multisubunit DNA-dependent RNA polymerases (Pols) are a prominent example. This review aims at briefly summarizing the architecture and structural adaptations of Pol I, highlighting the importance of cryo-electron microscopy in determining the structures of transcription complexes.

**Key words** RNA polymerase I, Cryo-electron microscopy, Pre-rRNA transcription

## 1 Cryo-Electron Microscopy: The New Standard in Transcription Research

The visualization of macromolecular complexes is essential to our understanding of their function. This is especially true for eukaryotic RNA polymerases (Pol) I, II, and III. These enzymes play a pivotal role within the central dogma of molecular biology by synthesizing the 35S ribosomal RNA precursor (Pol I), messenger and many noncoding RNAs (Pol II), and tRNAs, 5S rRNA, U6 snRNA as well as other small, structured RNAs (Pol III).

Almost 20 years ago, advances in cryo-crystallography allowed solving the structure of RNA polymerase II, first in its 10-subunit form [1], later comprising all 12 subunits [2], providing insights into the function of this molecular machine at an unprecedented level of detail. This gave rise to a number of follow-up studies, resulting in structures of an actively elongating Pol II form [3, 4] and elongation [5, 6] or initiation [7, 8] factor–bound Pol II. Thereby, the molecular mechanisms of transcription, as well as regulatory and catalytic functions of transcription factors, could be deciphered.

However, X-ray diffraction analysis relies on the availability and quality of the analyzed crystals. It is therefore not surprising that a

Karl-Dieter Entian (ed.), *Ribosome Biogenesis: Methods and Protocols*, Methods in Molecular Biology, vol. 2533, https://doi.org/10.1007/978-1-0716-2501-9_5, © The Author(s) 2022

number of transcription factors could never be successfully studied in complex with their respective polymerase by crystallography. This includes the general Pol II initiation factors TFIIF and TFIIE, which are involved in initiation complex formation and promoter DNA melting [9]. A crystal structure of Pol I was solved 10 years after Pol II in an inactive conformation [10, 11], a Pol III crystal structure is still lacking to date. Crystallization depends on high amounts of purified material. Whereas conformational heterogeneity usually is problematic for crystal formation, cryo-EM allows for visualization of different functional states of proteins in vitrified ice, therefore capturing close-to-native states. Technical improvements such as the development of direct electron detectors [10], highly stable microscopes and improved processing software [11, 12] pushed previous limitations of the technique and led to the often quoted "resolution revolution" in cryo-EM [13]. Within this book, we describe protocols for a sample preparation and single-particle cryo-EM screening workflow, adapted to RNA polymerase complexes (Chapter 6 ).

Here, we aim to briefly outline the benefits and limitations of single-particle cryo-EM for the analysis of transcription complexes at the example of RNA polymerase I in the context of functional characterization reviewed by Merkl et al. in the same issue.

## 2   Pol I Specific Subunits Resemble Built-in Transcription Factors

Yeast Pol I has a molecular weight of 590 kDa and consists of 14 protein subunits. A core of ten subunits includes the large subunits A190 and A135, the subcomplex AC40/AC19 (shared with Pol III), the common subunits Rpb5, Rpb6, Rpb8, Rpb10, and Rpb12 (also included in Pol II and Pol III) and the subunit A12.2. Pol I also contains the specific subunit complex A14/A43 forming the "stalk" and the specific heterodimer subcomplex A49/A34.5. In Fig. 1, we present a "hybrid model" of Pol I, constructed using the software package COOT [14]. The model combines structural information obtained from cryo-EM reconstructions of elongation and initiation complexes and the dimer crystal structure (see below). The Pol I subunit complex A49/A34.5 structurally and functionally resembles a built-in version of subunits Tfg1/2 constituting the Pol II initiation factor TFIIF [15] and is involved in open complex stabilization as well as promoter escape. Nevertheless, subcomplex A49/A34.5 may also contribute to transcript cleavage activity [16] and may play a role in elongation [17], as reviewed by Merkl et al. in this book. The Pol I subunit A12.2 displays features of the Pol II subunit Rpb9, as well as the Pol II elongation/cleavage factor TFIIS, explaining the intrinsic ability of Pol I for transcript cleavage [18] and efficient recovery from deep backtracks [19].

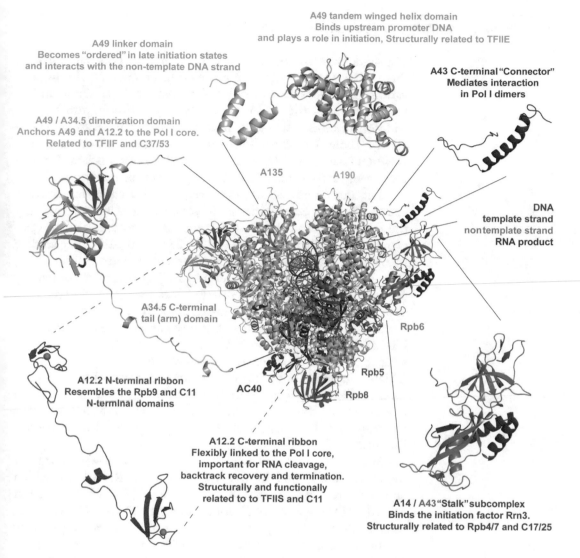

**A49 tandem winged helix domain**
Binds upstream promoter DNA
and plays a role in initiation, Structurally related to TFIIE

**A49 linker domain**
Becomes "ordered" in late initiation states
and interacts with the non-template DNA strand

**A43 C-terminal "Connector"**
Mediates interaction
in Pol I dimers

**A49 / A34.5 dimerization domain**
Anchors A49 and A12.2 to the Pol I core.
Related to TFIIF and C37/53

A135

A190

**DNA
template strand
nontemplate strand
RNA product**

**A34.5 C-terminal
tail (arm) domain**

Rpb6

Rpb5

**A12.2 N-terminal ribbon**
Resembles the Rpb9 and C11
N-terminal domains

AC40

Rpb8

**A12.2 C-terminal ribbon**
Flexibly linked to the Pol I core,
important for RNA cleavage,
backtrack recovery and termination.
Structurally and functionally
related to to TFIIS and C11

**A14 / A43 "Stalk" subcomplex**
Binds the initiation factor Rrn3.
Structurally related to Rpb4/7 and C17/25

**Fig. 1** Ribbon model of RNA polymerase I highlighting specific subunits and –domains. Hybrid model constructed using COOT [14] for demonstration purposes. The structure of the Pol I elongation complex (PDB 5M3F) was extended by adding (a) a model of the C-terminal domain of subunit A12.2, (b) the "connector" domain of subunit A43 from the crystal structure (both from PDB 4C2M) and (c) the linker and tandem-winged helix domains [15] from an ITC reconstruction (PDB 5 W66). The "front view" looks along the incoming ("downstream") DNA. Subunits not visible in the front view but present in the model are AC19, Rpb10, and Rpb12. Cyan spheres depict coordinated zinc atoms

The constitutive association of subunits A12.2 and A49/A34.5 may be a symptom of the enzyme's adaptation to transcribing one specific, extraordinarily long gene. A differential regulation of Pol I transcription similar to the conditional, gene-specific regulation of Pols II and III is most likely not required. Instead, a binary activity switch can be achieved by posttranslational modification of the polymerase or its initiation factors [20–23].

## 3 The Pol I Transcription Cycle Visualized In Vitro

Throughout transcription of a DNA template, Pols pass through three main phases, which are more or less conserved throughout various organisms. First, the Pol is recruited to the template sequence, melts the DNA duplex with or without the help of additional factors and begins the synthesis of an RNA strand (initiation). Thereafter, the initial RNA is extended according to the DNA template strand (elongation). Finally, Pol dissociates from its DNA template and releases its RNA product (termination) [24].

The Pol I transcription cycle requires few basic transcription factors [25, 26]. Basal initiation in yeast can be achieved with only the factor Rrn3 and the Core Factor (CF) complex, consisting of proteins Rrn6, Rrn7, and Rrn11 [27, 28]. Elongation may involve regulatory factors in vivo, but can commence in vitro without them [25, 26]. Termination finally requires a Myb-domain containing protein, Nsi1 in yeast [29, 30]. Pol I can adopt a dimeric state specific to this enzyme, [31], in which both molecules are inactivated [32] and prevented from binding initiation factors Rrn3 and CF [33–35]. Dimerization is reversible [33] and may play a role in storage of Pol I molecules during starvation [36, 37]. Using cryo-EM in many variations, our understanding of the Pol I transcription cycle has been significantly improved in recent years. A structural description of the Pol I transcription cycle allowed a detailed structure–function analysis and the comparison to other transcription systems [38–41].

Specifically, single-particle cryo-EM analyses showed how Pol I monomers are bound by the initiation factor Rrn3 [42], which allows for recruitment of CF subunit Rrn7 [37, 43, 44] that is related to the general Pol II initiation factor TFIIB [45, 46]. The interaction with Rrn3 prevents the formation of transcriptionally inactive Pol I dimers. In baker's yeast (*Saccharomyces cerevisiae*) Pol I dimerization depends on the specialized, nonconserved "connector" domain of subunit A43, suggesting that this mode of regulation is specific to *S. cerevisiae* [37]. However, recent cryo-EM studies of Pol I from fission yeast (*Schizosaccharomyces pombe*) demonstrated that inactive dimers can form independent of the connector domain utilizing divergent structure elements [47]. It is therefore possible that different organisms evolved different dimer interfaces, but use the same strategy of Pol I hibernation by dimerization during periods of starvation.

Monomeric Pol I bound to Rrn3 can be recruited by promoter-engaged CF. Whereas the structure of CF was determined by X-ray crystallography [48], its interaction with the Pol I–Rrn3 complex was apparently too flexible for this method to succeed. Instead, three independent studies used cryo-EM to visualize a reconstituted initially transcribing complex (ITC) that relies on an artificially stabilized, mismatched transcription bubble with a short initial product RNA [48–50]. Comparison of these studies shows that seemingly similar experimental cryo-EM approaches may yield different, though highly complementary results. This demonstrates the influence of sample preparation and experimental conditions on the outcome of a cryo-EM experiment and the strength of single-particle cryo-EM to elucidate dynamic processes. Specifically, some complexes exist in conformations that fail to bind Rrn3 [49], which is required essential to the initiation process and dissociates after promoter escape [42, 51, 52]. These complexes may represent later initiation intermediates. In another structure, the RNA primer is lost and the C-terminal domain of subunit A12.2 is inserted into the funnel domain of Pol I, as would be expected during RNA cleavage events [50]. A third reconstruction showed local resolution differences suggesting high flexibility in distal CF regions [48]. More recently, consolidating structures of close-to-native preinitiation complexes were reported [53, 54]. A closed and an open complex could be reconstructed from a small fraction of recorded particles but yielded important information about the roles of a flexible loop in Rrn3 in CF engagement, and the role of the linker/tWH domain of subunit A49 in template DNA melting, open bubble stabilization, and Rrn3 dissociation [53].

Following initiation, Pol I adopts an actively elongating conformation. This conformation was never successfully crystallized but was reconstructed by single-particle cryo-EM [55, 56]. It is still under debate, whether dissociation/transient association of the A49/A34.5 heterodimer and formation of a 12-subunit polymerase has a physiological function under some circumstances. Chromatin immunoprecipitation (ChIP) data does not suggest subunit depletion along the 35S gene body in vivo [57], although a lack of density in cryo-EM reconstructions of *S. cerevisiae* and *S. pombe* Pol I ECs suggests that subdomain relocation can take place [47, 58]. Upon initiation, the central DNA-binding cleft contracts and tightly binds downstream DNA and the DNA–RNA hybrid region, thus facilitating processive elongation. Contraction upon activation is apparently common to Pol I regulation in different organisms [47] but differs from Pol II [3] and III [59]. The various Pol I EC reconstructions demonstrated the versatile nature of the specific subunits A12.2, A49, and A34.5 [47, 55, 56, 58], and the importance of a Pol I-specific arginine residue in the "bridge-helix" in stalling at DNA lesions caused by UV radiation [60]. Furthermore, the physiological relevance of a contracted Pol I state was confirmed by the 3D-reconstruction of the enzyme from ex vivo purified, actively transcribing Pol I using electron cryo-tomography [55]. Interestingly enough, the underlying preparation technique has been used to describe Pol I functionality since the 1960s [61].

Structural information on transient and highly dynamic states of the Pol I transcription cycle, such as termination, are still lacking to date.

# 4   Outlook

Continuing investigation of the Pol I transcription system currently aims at defining the structural basis of promoter recruitment in the context of TATA-binding protein [62] and yeast upstream activating factor (UAF) which are important to achieve full initiation levels under physiological conditions [27, 63]. The structural investigations of these complexes and their interplay with the Pol I enzyme will be the key to understand this initiation systems in comparison with Pol II [64, 65] and Pol III [66, 67]. Ultimately, such comparative structure–function analyses will enable us to understand the particular adaptation of the Pol I transcription system to pre-rRNA transcription.

Cryo-EM has now firmly established itself as the method of choice to analyze the structure of such mega-Dalton sized, dynamic, macromolecular complexes. However, the method has also proven to be prone to certain errors. Especially the lack of tools for intrinsic validation of density interpretation may be an issue for initial sequence assignment at resolutions worse than 4 Å. Continuing method development at the experimental and the computational level continues and may soon overcome issues of flexibility and density assignment. For the time being, however, the interpretation of cryo-EM reconstructions should be carefully evaluated and supported by functional data or mutational analysis. Results can also be strengthened by crystallization or small angle X-ray scattering analysis of flexible domains [68], native mass spectrometry [15], hydrogen–deuterium exchange mass-spectrometry evaluation [69], or single-molecule FRET analysis [70]. Especially distance restrains obtained from protein crosslinking coupled to mass spectrometry provides architectural information and may assist low-resolution density assignment [71, 72].

# Acknowledgements

The authors thank all members of the Structural Biochemistry group and Biochemistry I/III departments of the University of Regensburg for help and discussions. This work was supported by the Emmy-Noether-Programme (DFG grant no. EN 1204/1-1 to CE) and SFB 960 TP-A8.

## References

1. Cramer P, Bushnell DA, Kornberg RD (2001) Structural basis of transcription: RNA polymerase II at 2.8 angstrom resolution. Science 292: 1863–1876. https://doi.org/10.1126/science.1059493

2. Armache J-K, Mitterweger S, Meinhart A, Cramer P (2004) Structures of complete RNA polymerase II and its subcomplex, Rpb4/7. J Biol Chem 280(8):7131–7134. https://doi.org/10.1074/jbc.M413038200

3. Gnatt AL, Cramer P, Fu J, Bushnell DA, Kornberg RD (2001) Structural basis of transcription: an RNA polymerase II elongation complex at 3.3 Å resolution. Science 292:1876–1882. https://doi.org/10.1126/science.1059495

4. Kettenberger H, Armache K-J, Cramer P (2004) Complete RNA polymerase II elongation complex structure and its interactions with NTP and TFIIS. Mol Cell 16:955–965. https://doi.org/10.1016/j.molcel.2004.11.040

5. Kettenberger H, Armache K-J, Cramer P (2003) Architecture of the RNA polymerase II-TFIIS complex and implications for mRNA cleavage. Cell 114:347–357. https://doi.org/10.1016/S0092-8674(03)00598-1

6. Wang D, Bushnell DA, Huang X, Westover KD, Levitt M, Kornberg RD (2009) Structural basis of transcription: Backtracked RNA polymerase II at 3.4 Å resolution. Science 324:1203–1206. https://doi.org/10.1126/science.1168729

7. Liu X, Bushnell DA, Wang D, Calero G, Kornberg RD (2010) Structure of an RNA polymerase II–TFIIB complex and the transcription initiation mechanism. Science 327:206. https://doi.org/10.1126/science.1182015

8. Sainsbury S, Niesser J, Cramer P (2013) Structure and function of the initially transcribing RNA polymerase II-TFIIB complex. Nature 493:437–440. https://doi.org/10.1038/nature11715

9. Sainsbury S, Bernecky C, Cramer P (2015) Structural basis of transcription initiation by RNA polymerase II. Nat Rev Mol Cell Biol 16:129–143. https://doi.org/10.1038/nrm3952

10. McMullan G, Faruqi AR, Henderson R (2016) Direct electron detectors. Methods Enzymol 579:1–17. https://doi.org/10.1016/bs.mie.2016.05.056

11. Scheres SHW (2012) A Bayesian view on cryo-EM structure determination. J Mol Biol 415:406–418. https://doi.org/10.1016/j.jmb.2011.11.010

12. Zivanov J, Nakane T, Forsberg B, Kimanius D, Hagen WJH, Lindahl E, Scheres SHW (2018) RELION-3: new tools for automated high-resolution cryo-EM structure determination. bioRxiv. https://doi.org/10.1101/421123

13. Kühlbrandt W (2014) Biochemistry. The resolution revolution. Science 343:1443–1444. https://doi.org/10.1126/science.1251652

14. Emsley P, Cowtan K (2004) Coot: model-building tools for molecular graphics. Acta Crystallogr D Biol Crystallogr 60:2126–2132. https://doi.org/10.1107/S0907444904019158

15. Geiger SR, Lorenzen K, Schreieck A, Hanecker P, Kostrewa D, Heck AJR, Cramer P (2010) RNA polymerase I contains a TFIIF-related DNA-binding subcomplex. Mol Cell 39:583–594. https://doi.org/10.1016/j.molcel.2010.07.028

16. Kuhn C-D, Geiger SR, Baumli S, Gartmann M, Gerber J, Jennebach S, Mielke T, Tschochner H, Beckmann R, Cramer P (2007) Functional architecture of RNA polymerase I. Cell 131:1260–1272. https://doi.org/10.1016/j.cell.2007.10.051

17. Merkl PE, Pilsl M, Fremter T, Schwank K, Engel C, Längst G, Milkereit P, Griesenbeck J, Tschochner H (2020) RNA polymerase I (Pol I) passage through nucleosomes depends on Pol I subunits binding its lobe structure. J Biol Chem 295:4782–4795. https://doi.org/10.1074/jbc.RA119.011827

18. Jennebach S, Herzog F, Aebersold R, Cramer P (2012) Crosslinking-MS analysis reveals RNA polymerase I domain architecture and basis of rRNA cleavage. Nucleic Acids Res 40:5591–5601. https://doi.org/10.1093/nar/gks220

19. Lisica A, Engel C, Jahnel M, Roldán É, Galburt EA, Cramer P, Grill SW (2016) Mechanisms of backtrack recovery by RNA polymerases I and II. Proc Natl Acad Sci U S A 113:2946–2951. https://doi.org/10.1073/pnas.1517011113

20. Fath S, Kobor MS, Philippi A, Greenblatt J, Tschochner H (2004) Dephosphorylation of RNA polymerase I by Fcp1p is required for efficient rRNA synthesis. J Biol Chem 279:25251–25259. https://doi.org/10.1074/jbc.M401867200

21. Clemente-Blanco A, Mayán-Santos M, Schneider DA, Machín F, Jarmuz A, Tschochner H, Aragón L (2009) Cdc14 inhibits transcription by RNA polymerase I during anaphase. Nature 458:219–222. https://doi.org/10.1038/nature07652

22. Mayer C, Zhao J, Yuan X, Grummt I (2004) mTOR-dependent activation of the transcription factor TIF-IA links rRNA synthesis to nutrient availability. Genes Dev 18:423–434. https://doi.org/10.1101/gad.285504

23. Hannan KM, Brandenburger Y, Jenkins A, Sharkey K, Cavanaugh A, Rothblum L, Moss T, Poortinga G, McArthur GA, Pearson RB, Hannan RD (2003) mTOR-dependent regulation of ribosomal gene transcription requires S6K1 and is mediated by phosphorylation of the carboxy-terminal activation domain of the nucleolar transcription factor UBF. Mol Cell Biol 23:8862–8877. https://

doi.org/10.1128/mcb.23.23.8862-8877. 2003

24. Cheung ACM, Cramer P (2012) A movie of RNA polymerase II transcription. Cell 149: 1431–1437. https://doi.org/10.1016/j.cell. 2012.06.006

25. Moss T, Langlois F, Gagnon-Kugler T, Stefanovsky V (2007) A housekeeper with power of attorney: the rRNA genes in ribosome biogenesis. Cell Mol Life Sci 64:29–49. https://doi. org/10.1007/s00018-006-6278-1

26. Goodfellow SJ, Zomerdijk JCBM (2013) Basic mechanisms in RNA polymerase I transcription of the ribosomal RNA genes. Subcell Biochem 61:211–236. https://doi.org/10.1007/978-94-007-4525-4_10

27. Keener J, Josaitis CA, Dodd JA, Nomura M (1998) Reconstitution of yeast RNA polymerase I transcription in vitro from purified components. TATA-binding protein is not required for basal transcription. J Biol Chem 273: 33795–33802

28. Milkereit P, Tschochner H (1998) A specialized form of RNA polymerase I, essential for initiation and growth-dependent regulation of rRNA synthesis, is disrupted during transcription. EMBO J 17:3692–3703. https:// doi.org/10.1093/emboj/17.13.3692

29. Reiter A, Hamperl S, Seitz H, Merkl P, Perez-Fernandez J, Williams L, Gerber J, Németh A, Léger I, Gadal O, Milkereit P, Griesenbeck J, Tschochner H (2012) The Reb1-homologue Ydr026c/Nsi1 is required for efficient RNA polymerase I termination in yeast. EMBO J 31:3480–3493. https://doi.org/10.1038/emboj.2012.185

30. Merkl P, Perez-Fernandez J, Pilsl M, Reiter A, Williams L, Gerber J, Böhm M, Deutzmann R, Griesenbeck J, Milkereit P, Tschochner H (2014) Binding of the termination factor Nsi1 to its cognate DNA site is sufficient to terminate RNA polymerase I transcription in vitro and to induce termination in vivo. Mol Cell Biol 34:3817–3827. https://doi.org/10. 1128/MCB.00395-14

31. Bischler N, Brino L, Carles C, Riva M, Tschochner H, Mallouh V, Schultz P (2002) Localization of the yeast RNA polymerase I-specific subunits. EMBO J 21:4136–4144. https://doi.org/10.1093/emboj/cdf392

32. Milkereit P, Schultz P, Tschochner H (1997) Resolution of RNA polymerase I into dimers and monomers and their function in transcription. Biol Chem 378:1433–1443

33. Engel C, Sainsbury S, Cheung AC, Kostrewa D, Cramer P (2013) RNA polymerase I structure and transcription regulation. Nature 502:650–655. https://doi.org/10. 1038/nature12712

34. Fernández-Tornero C, Moreno-Morcillo M, Rashid UJ, Taylor NMI, Ruiz FM, Gruene T, Legrand P, Steuerwald U, Müller CW (2013) Crystal structure of the 14-subunit RNA polymerase I. Nature 502:644–649. https://doi. org/10.1038/nature12636

35. Kostrewa D, Kuhn C-D, Engel C, Cramer P (2015) An alternative RNA polymerase I structure reveals a dimer hinge. Acta Crystallogr D Biol Crystallogr 71:1850–1855. https://doi. org/10.1107/S1399004715012651

36. Fernández-Tornero C (2018) RNA polymerase I activation and hibernation: unique mechanisms for unique genes. Transcription 9:248–254. https://doi.org/10.1080/21541264.2017.1416267

37. Torreira E, Louro JA, Pazos I, González-Polo N, Gil-Carton D, Duran AG, Tosi S, Gallego O, Calvo O, Fernández-Tornero C (2017) The dynamic assembly of distinct RNA polymerase I complexes modulates rDNA transcription. elife 6:e20832. https:// doi.org/10.7554/eLife.20832

38. Hanske J, Sadian Y, Müller CW (2018) The cryo-EM resolution revolution and transcription complexes. Curr Opin Struct Biol 52:8–15. https://doi.org/10.1016/j.sbi.2018. 07.002

39. Engel C, Neyer S, Cramer P (2018) Distinct mechanisms of transcription initiation by RNA polymerases I and II. Annu Rev Biophys 47: 425–446. https://doi.org/10.1146/annurev-biophys-070317-033058

40. Jochem L, Ramsay EP, Vannini A (2017) RNA polymerase I, bending the rules? EMBO J 36: 2664–2666. https://doi.org/10.15252/embj.201797924

41. Jackobel AJ, Han Y, He Y, Knutson BA (2018) Breaking the mold: structures of the RNA polymerase I transcription complex reveal a new path for initiation. Transcription 9:255–261. https://doi.org/10.1080/21541264. 2017.1416268

42. Blattner C, Jennebach S, Herzog F, Mayer A, Cheung ACM, Witte G, Lorenzen K, Hopfner K-P, Heck AJR, Aebersold R, Cramer P (2011) Molecular basis of Rrn3-regulated RNA polymerase I initiation and cell growth. Genes Dev 25:2093–2105. https://doi.org/10.1101/gad.17363311

43. Engel C, Plitzko J, Cramer P (2016) RNA polymerase I-Rrn3 complex at 4.8 Å resolution. Nat Commun 7:12129. https://doi. org/10.1038/ncomms12129

44. Pilsl M, Crucifix C, Papai G, Krupp F, Steinbauer R, Griesenbeck J, Milkereit P, Tschochner H, Schultz P (2016) Structure of the initiation-competent RNA polymerase I and its implication for transcription. Nat Commun 7:12126. https://doi.org/10.1038/ncomms12126

45. Knutson BA, Hahn S (2011) Yeast Rrn7 and human TAF1B are TFIIB-related RNA polymerase I general transcription factors. Science 333:1637–1640. https://doi.org/10.1126/science.1207699

46. Naidu S, Friedrich JK, Russell J, Zomerdijk JCBM (2011) TAF1B is a TFIIB-like component of the basal transcription machinery for RNA polymerase I. Science 333:1640–1642. https://doi.org/10.1126/science.1207656

47. Heiss FB, Daiß JL, Becker P, Engel C (2021) Conserved strategies of RNA polymerase I hibernation and activation. Nat Commun 12:758. https://doi.org/10.1038/s41467-021-21031-8

48. Engel C, Gubbey T, Neyer S, Sainsbury S, Oberthuer C, Baejen C, Bernecky C, Cramer P (2017) Structural basis of RNA polymerase I transcription initiation. Cell 169:120–131. e22. https://doi.org/10.1016/j.cell.2017.03.003

49. Han Y, Yan C, Nguyen THD, Jackobel AJ, Ivanov I, Knutson BA, He Y (2017) Structural mechanism of ATP-independent transcription initiation by RNA polymerase I. elife 6: e27414. https://doi.org/10.7554/eLife.27414

50. Sadian Y, Tafur L, Kosinski J, Jakobi AJ, Wetzel R, Buczak K, Hagen WJ, Beck M, Sachse C, Müller CW (2017) Structural insights into transcription initiation by yeast RNA polymerase I. EMBO J 36:2698–2709. https://doi.org/10.15252/embj.201796958

51. Bier M, Fath S, Tschochner H (2004) The composition of the RNA polymerase I transcription machinery switches from initiation to elongation mode. FEBS Lett 564:41–46. https://doi.org/10.1016/S0014-5793(04)00311-4

52. Herdman C, Mars J-C, Stefanovsky VY, Tremblay MG, Sabourin-Felix M, Lindsay H, Robinson MD, Moss T (2017) A unique enhancer boundary complex on the mouse ribosomal RNA genes persists after loss of Rrn3 or UBF and the inactivation of RNA polymerase I transcription. PLoS Genet 13: e1006899. https://doi.org/10.1371/journal.pgen.1006899

53. Sadian Y, Baudin F, Tafur L, Murciano B, Wetzel R, Weis F, Müller CW (2019) Molecular insight into RNA polymerase I promoter recognition and promoter melting. Nat Commun 10:5543. https://doi.org/10.1038/s41467-019-13510-w

54. Pilsl M, Engel C (2020) Structural basis of RNA polymerase I pre-initiation complex formation and promoter melting. Nat Commun 11:1206. https://doi.org/10.1038/s41467-020-15052-y

55. Neyer S, Kunz M, Geiss C, Hantsche M, Hodirnau V-V, Seybert A, Engel C, Scheffer MP, Cramer P, Frangakis AS (2016) Structure of RNA polymerase I transcribing ribosomal DNA genes. Nature 540(7634):607–610. https://doi.org/10.1038/nature20561

56. Tafur L, Sadian Y, Hoffmann NA, Jakobi AJ, Wetzel R, Hagen WJH, Sachse C, Müller CW (2016) Molecular structures of transcribing RNA polymerase I. Mol Cell 64:1135–1143. https://doi.org/10.1016/j.molcel.2016.11.013

57. Beckouet F, Labarre-Mariotte S, Albert B, Imazawa Y, Werner M, Gadal O, Nogi Y, Thuriaux P (2008) Two RNA polymerase I subunits control the binding and release of Rrn3 during transcription. Mol Cell Biol 28:1596–1605. https://doi.org/10.1128/MCB.01464-07

58. Tafur L, Sadian Y, Hanske J, Wetzel R, Weis F, Müller CW (2019) The cryo-EM structure of a 12-subunit variant of RNA polymerase I reveals dissociation of the A49-A34.5 heterodimer and rearrangement of subunit A12.2. elife 8: e43204. https://doi.org/10.7554/eLife.43204

59. Hoffmann NA, Jakobi AJ, Moreno-Morcillo M, Glatt S, Kosinski J, Hagen WJH, Sachse C, Müller CW (2015) Molecular structures of unbound and transcribing RNA polymerase III. Nature 528:231–236. https://doi.org/10.1038/nature16143

60. Sanz-Murillo M, Xu J, Belogurov GA, Calvo O, Gil-Carton D, Moreno-Morcillo M, Wang D, Fernández-Tornero C (2018) Structural basis of RNA polymerase I stalling at UV light-induced DNA damage. Proc Natl Acad Sci U S A 115:8972–8977. https://doi.org/10.1073/pnas.1802626115

61. Miller OL, Beatty BR (1969) Visualization of nucleolar genes. Science 164:955–957. https://doi.org/10.1126/science.164.3882.955

62. Kramm K, Engel C, Grohmann D (2019) Transcription initiation factor TBP: old friend new questions. Biochem Soc Trans 47:411–423. https://doi.org/10.1042/BST20180623

63. Bedwell GJ, Appling FD, Anderson SJ, Schneider DA (2012) Efficient transcription by RNA

polymerase I using recombinant core factor. Gene 492:94–99. https://doi.org/10.1016/j.gene.2011.10.049

64. Schilbach S, Hantsche M, Tegunov D, Dienemann C, Wigge C, Urlaub H, Cramer P (2017) Structures of transcription pre-initiation complex with TFIIH and mediator. Nature 551:204–209. https://doi.org/10.1038/nature24282

65. He Y, Yan C, Fang J, Inouye C, Tjian R, Ivanov I, Nogales E (2016) Near-atomic resolution visualization of human transcription promoter opening. Nature 533:359–365. https://doi.org/10.1038/nature17970

66. Abascal-Palacios G, Ramsay EP, Beuron F, Morris E, Vannini A (2018) Structural basis of RNA polymerase III transcription initiation. Nature 553:301–306. https://doi.org/10.1038/nature25441

67. Vorländer MK, Khatter H, Wetzel R, Hagen WJH, Müller CW (2018) Molecular mechanism of promoter opening by RNA polymerase III. Nature 553:295–300. https://doi.org/10.1038/nature25440

68. Ramsay EP, Abascal-Palacios G, Daiß JL, King H, Gouge J, Pilsl M, Beuron F, Morris E, Gunkel P, Engel C, Vannini A (2020) Structure of human RNA polymerase III. Nat Commun 11:6409. https://doi.org/10.1038/s41467-020-20262-5

69. Shukla AK, Westfield GH, Xiao K, Reis RI, Huang L-Y, Tripathi-Shukla P, Qian J, Li S, Blanc A, Oleskie AN, Dosey AM, Su M, Liang C-R, Gu L-L, Shan J-M, Chen X, Hanna R, Choi M, Yao XJ, Klink BU, Kahsai AW, Sidhu SS, Koide S, Penczek PA, Kossiakoff AA, Woods VL, Kobilka BK, Skiniotis G, Lefkowitz RJ (2014) Visualization of arrestin recruitment by a G-protein-coupled receptor. Nature 512:218–222. https://doi.org/10.1038/nature13430

70. Kramm K, Schröder T, Gouge J, Vera AM, Gupta K, Heiss FB, Liedl T, Engel C, Berger I, Vannini A, Tinnefeld P, Grohmann D (2020) DNA origami-based single-molecule force spectroscopy elucidates RNA polymerase III pre-initiation complex stability. Nat Commun 11:2828. https://doi.org/10.1038/s41467-020-16702-x

71. Leitner A, Faini M, Stengel F, Aebersold R (2016) Crosslinking and mass spectrometry: an integrated technology to understand the structure and function of molecular machines. Trends Biochem Sci 41:20–32. https://doi.org/10.1016/j.tibs.2015.10.008

72. Schmidt C, Urlaub H (2017) Combining cryo-electron microscopy (cryo-EM) and cross-linking mass spectrometry (CX-MS) for structural elucidation of large protein assemblies. Curr Opin Struct Biol 46:157–168. https://doi.org/10.1016/j.sbi.2017.10.005

# Chapter 6

## Preparation of RNA Polymerase Complexes for Their Analysis by Single-Particle Cryo-Electron Microscopy

Michael Pilsl, Florian B. Heiss, Gisela Pöll, Mona Höcherl, Philipp Milkereit, and Christoph Engel

### Abstract

Recent technological progress revealed new prospects of high-resolution structure determination of macromolecular complexes using cryo-electron microscopy (cryo-EM). In the field of RNA polymerase (Pol) I research, a number of cryo-EM studies contributed to understanding the highly specialized mechanisms underlying the transcription of ribosomal RNA genes. Despite a broad applicability of the cryo-EM method itself, preparation of samples for high-resolution data collection can be challenging. Here, we describe strategies for the purification and stabilization of Pol I complexes, exemplarily considering advantages and disadvantages of the methodology. We further provide an easy-to-implement protocol for the coating of EM-grids with self-made carbon support films. In sum, we present an efficient workflow for cryo-grid preparation and optimization, including early stage cryo-EM screening that can be adapted to a wide range of soluble samples for high-resolution structure determination.

**Key words** RNA polymerase I, Preparation of transcription complexes, Single-particle cryo-electron microscopy, Grid preparation, Plunge freezing, Negative staining

---

## 1 Introduction

During the past years, development of more sophisticated microscopes, new direct electron detectors, and advances in computational image processing caused a "resolution revolution" [1] in the field of cryo-electron microscopy (cryo-EM). This culminated in the award of the Nobel Prize in Chemistry to three scientists driving these developments: Joachim Frank, Richard Henderson, and Jacques Dubochet in 2017. Recent developments have been summarized in detail [2–8]. With its increasing popularity, the technique is now more easily accessible and widely used in many areas of structural biology research, such as the analysis of transcription complexes [9]. Among many others, cryo-EM studies on RNA polymerase (Pol) I complexes became possible and advanced our understanding of the molecular mechanisms employed by this

Karl-Dieter Entian (ed.), *Ribosome Biogenesis: Methods and Protocols*, Methods in Molecular Biology, vol. 2533,
https://doi.org/10.1007/978-1-0716-2501-9_6, © The Author(s) 2022

highly specialized enzyme [10–19]. Here, we describe the work-flow of biochemical purification and sample preparation of Pol I complexes and the optimization of cryo-grid preparation containing frozen, hydrated single particle specimens with the goal of acquiring high resolution images for structure determination. We focus on grid preparation, quality control, and EM screening in an iterative manner. We also emphasize the steps necessary for establishment of a customized workflow that can be tailored to the needs of any sample suitable for single-particle analysis.

The success of structure determination by single-particle cryo-EM depends on high-quality biochemical preparation and characterization of the molecule(s) of interest. Buffer optimization and stabilization of complexes should be done in the initial phase of a project, strategies are described in detail [20]. We previously presented protocols for the purification of 14-subunit, 590 kDa Pol I complexes and their characterization in vitro [21, 22]. Starting from this, we detail the specimen features which are important for successful structure determination using single-particle cryo-EM and suggest approaches for their optimization. For this purpose, we compare complex preparation- and assembly strategies using endogenously purified Pol I and recombinant transcription factors on nucleic acid templates. Transcription factor complexes can be (a) assembled on a biotinylated DNA, enriched using the interaction with bead-coupled streptavidin and eluted with restriction enzymes [23]. Alternatively (b), size exclusion chromatography (SEC) may yield homogenous and stable complexes that are well-suited for cryo-grid preparation. Large macromolecules can also be enriched using density gradient centrifugation protocols (c). As such, the gradient-fixation (GraFix)-method relies on a sedimentation step coupled with an intra- and intermolecular cross-linking step combining purification and complex stabilization [24, 25]. Following GraFix, a buffer exchange is required to remove sucrose or glycerol that would otherwise interfere with the subsequent freezing process and may increase background noise in cryo-EM images. Generally, cross-linking of protein-protein or protein-nucleic acid complexes can improve their stability during the grid preparation process. This cross-linking can be coupled to a purification step (as in GraFix), or performed directly before grid-plunging (d). These preparation techniques can also be combined, for example, carrying out an SEC run after batch cross-linking. Such a strategy combines the advantages of sample stabilization and purification while directly including the transition to a suitable buffer system but requires larger quantities of sample.

In addition to sample preparation and stabilization, we discuss the use of different grid types and support materials. General cryo-EM sample preparation techniques applicable to a wide range of samples were described in detail [26, 27]. Adsorption of particles to a thin support film can aid sample concentration, alter bias in orientation distribution, or protect fragile particles from denaturation on air–water interfaces [28]. To this end, grids covered with thin carbon layer substrates are commonly used. Additionally, graphene oxide or hydrogenated graphene were reported to be well-suited support materials as they are almost transparent to electrons [29–31]. While holey carbon grids covered with ultrathin support layers are commercially available (*see* Subheading 2), many support types can be manually prepared more economically at similar or higher quality. We also describe a technical gadget to float an ultrathin carbon film on holey carbon grids. This is similar to other floatation techniques [32], but allows for sample adsorption on precoated grids directly prior to plunging and may thus be helpful to some users. This device is based on [33] and is commercially available in a modified form (SKU 10840; LADD Research Industries, Williston, VT, USA).

In addition to sample optimization and the choice of grid type, various physical parameters influence the preparation of cryo-EM grids. Glow discharge settings, grid type variation, buffer choice, and the mechanics of the blotting device should be carefully considered for each individual sample.

In general, we recommend initial optimization using negative staining EM, followed by two stages of cryo-EM screening (Fig. 1). The first cryo-screening stage aims at an evaluation of grid types, support films, or blotting conditions and gives information on sample behavior in ice. In a second phase of cryo-screening, intermediate-resolution single-particle maps may be reconstructed. Phase I cryo-screening results yield insights into sample behavior, whereas results of the second cryo-screening phase indicate whether the sample is suitable for high-resolution data collection by identifying flexibilities within the macromolecular complex and bias in orientation distribution.

For screening, we recommend the acquisition of low-magnification grid maps for navigation and evaluation of overall ice distribution. Low dose acquisition strategies to avoid beam-induced particle damage are used. This workflow includes focusing and exposure-dose measurement at higher magnifications on grid areas adjacent to the foil-hole of interest using image/beam shift functions, as for the acquisition of high-resolution images. Overviews of sample preparation, the use of cryo-holders and imaging strategies have been described [34–37]. For automated data collection, the SerialEM software includes many more features that have been recently summarized [38]. The open-source software is freely available and can be adapted to a wide range of microscopes and camera systems. Recent developments include the implementation of "on-the-fly" data processing and evaluation strategies into the software packages RELION, Warp, cryoSPARC, and SPHIRE, that may be useful in sample evaluation [39–42]. Here, we focus on the sample and grid preparation, as well as phase I cryo-EM screening approaches for multisubunit RNA polymerases.

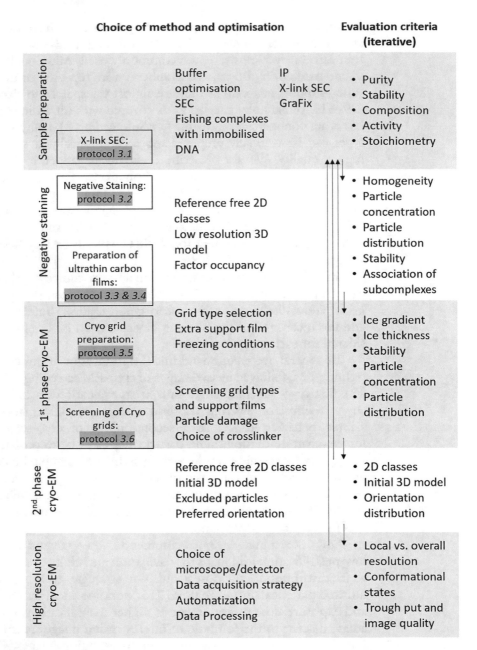

**Fig. 1** Overview of a workflow for (cryo-)EM sample screening and grid optimization. We suggest five phases, starting with sample preparation and iterative evaluation of screening results. Detailed protocols for individual steps are referenced and listed in Subheadings 3.1–3.6

# 2 Materials

## 2.1 Assembly of Pol I Complexes

### 2.1.1 Materials

1. Amicon Ultra Concentrators 100 kDa MWCO (Millipore).
2. Superose 6 Increase 3.2/300 column (GE Healthcare).
3. Microvolume FPLC system (e.g., Ettan LC or Aekta Micro; GE Healthcare).
4. Bis(sulfosuccinimidyl)suberate (BS3) crosslinker (Thermo Fisher Scientific).

### 2.1.2 Buffers

1. Quenching buffer: 2 M ammonium hydrogen carbonate.
2. H0 buffer: 20 mM HEPES–KOH pH 7.8, 5 mM DTT.
3. SEC buffer: 20 mM HEPES–KOH pH 7.8, 150 mM potassium acetate, 1 mM magnesium chloride, 10 µM zinc chloride, 5 mM DTT.

## 2.2 Negative Staining

### 2.2.1 Materials

1. Parafilm M (Bemis Flexible Packaging).
2. Uranyl Formate (powder; Science Services).
3. Bidest. water (unfiltered).
4. Filter paper grade 1 (Whatman).
5. Carbon coated EM grid (e.g., Plano S160 or homemade on 300 mesh copper grids).
6. Glow discharge device (Harrick: Plasma Cleaner/Sterilizer PDC-3xG, or Pelco 'EasiGlow' plasma cleaner (Ted Pella), or similar).

## 2.3 Preparation of Ultrathin Carbon Film Coated Grids

1. Cressington 208 carbon coater (Cressington) or similar.
2. Self-made Floatation device (acrylic glass chamber, foldback binder clip, metal support mesh) (see Fig. 2).
3. Carbon rods (6.15 × 305 mm; Elektronen-Optik-Service GmbH).
4. Freshly cleaved mica (Glimmer "V3" 75 × 25 mm; PLANO GmbH).
5. Glass slide (for light microscopy; Menzel-Gläser or similar).
6. Filter paper grade 1 (Whatman).
7. Reverse forceps ('N5'; Dumont).
8. Petri dish (glass; ~90 mm diameter).
9. EM grids (Quantifoil R 2/1 or 2/2).
10. Bidest. water.
11. Glow discharge device, (Harrick: Plasma Cleaner/Sterilizer PDC-3xG).

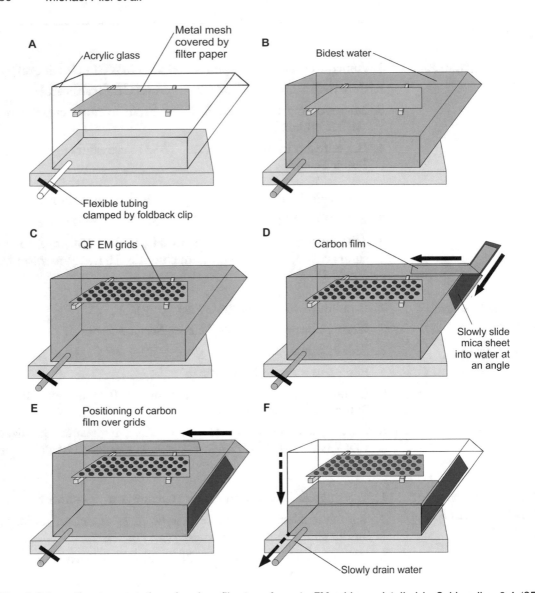

**Fig. 2** Schematic representation of carbon film transfer onto EM grids as detailed in Subheading 3.4 (QF: Quantifoil, EM: Electron Microscopy)

**2.4 Cryo-Grid Preparation**

1. Liquid nitrogen.

2. Ethane (3.5, Linde).

3. EM grids: "R 1.2/1.3" (Quantifoil); "R 2/1" (Quantifoil); "R 2/1 + 2 nm Carbon" (Quantifoil); homemade ultrathin carbon film floated on "R 2/1" (Quantifoil).

4. Cryo grid storage boxes (Plano).

5. Pelco "EasiGlow" plasma cleaner (Ted Pella), or similar.

6. Vitrobot Mark IV (Thermo Fisher Scientific).

**2.5 Cryo-Electron Microscopy**

1. JEM 2100F (JEOL) operating at 200 kV equipped with a 4 k × 4 k CMOS camera (TemCam-F416, TVIPS GmbH) or similar.

2. Liquid Nitrogen.

3. Gatan 626 Cryo Transfer Holder (Gatan), or similar.

4. Clip Ring (Gatan).

5. Clip Ring Tool (Gatan).

6. SerialEM software package [43].

# 3 Methods

**3.1 Assembly of Pol I Complexes**

1. Equilibrate Superose 6 Increase 3.2/300 column with two column volumes (CVs) SEC buffer on micro-volume SEC system.

2. Mix proteins and nucleic acids (stoichiometry, assembly and incubation conditions subject of optimization). We typically load ~100 µg protein to the SEC column for non–cross-linked samples and start with ~200 µg if the complex will be cross-linked before the SEC run.

3. Adjust salt concentration of the assembly reaction with buffer H0 to 150 mM potassium acetate (SEC buffer).

4. Incubate for 30 min at 4 °C (up to 25 °C).

5. Add BS3-crosslinker to a final concentration of 1 mM and incubate for 30 min at 30 °C (*see* **Note 1**).

6. Quench cross-linking reaction with ammonium hydrogen carbonate at a final concentration of 100 mM for 15 min at 30 °C (*see* **Note 2**).

7. Concentrate the sample to a final volume of 20–50 µl using the Amicon Ultra Concentrators 100 kDa MWCO (Millipore) if necessary.

8. Centrifuge sample 5 min at $15,000 \times g$ to remove large aggregates. Transfer supernatant to fresh tube.

9. Load sample onto the equilibrated Superose 6 Increase 3.2/300 column and collect 50 µl fractions.

10. Evaluate 260 and 280 nm UV spectra for comigration of nucleic acids, pool peak fractions (*see* **Note 3**).

**3.2 Negative Staining**

1. Prepare saturated uranyl formate solution: Add ~10–20 mg of uranyl formate in 1.5 ml tube, add 400 µl bidest water, vigorously vortex for 2 min and centrifuge for >10 min at $15,000 \times g$ (*see* **Note 4**).

2. Glow discharge EM grid(s) for 30 s.

3. Prepare a drop of 500 µl bidest. Water on a clean surface (Parafilm).

4. Apply 5 µl sample to a freshly glow-discharged, carbon-coated EM grid and adsorb for 30 s (*see* **Note 5**).

5. Wash the grid for 20 s in the droplet of bidest. Water.

6. Add 5 µl of uranyl formate, incubate for 20 s and blot liquid from the edge of the grid (Whatman filter paper). Repeat this step two more times (three staining steps in total) (*see* **Note 6**).

7. Dry grid for >5 min before storage. Grids can be directly imaged or long-term stored in a dry place but must be protected from dust.

8. We evaluate the negative stain image for homogeneity, complex stability, and concentration. Collection of small datasets comprising at least 10,000 negatively stained particles (20–100 images should be sufficient at magnifications of 30,000–50,000×) can be used to calculate initial low-resolution 2D and 3D classes (*see* **Note 7**).

### 3.3 Preparation of Ultrathin Carbon Film

1. Fix freshly cleaved mica halves on glass slide using small strips of tape on both ends. Slide a piece of filter paper under mica (*see* **Note 8**).

2. Vent and open the carbon coater and place glass slide with mica on stage.

3. Check carbon rods: left rod should have a smooth tip, right rod should have a plain face, both rods have to be in physical contact.

4. Close the recipient chamber. Turn on Cressington carbon coater device and wait for the vacuum to be under $4 \times 10^{-5}$ mbar.

5. Degas carbon rods: Slowly turn up voltage to 2 V, hold until carbon rod glows red. Wait for vacuum to recover and repeat two more times.

6. Switch on the thickness monitor and evaporate carbon at 3.6 V for 10 s. Do not remove shield to ensure indirect evaporation. Wait at least 30 s before reading the carbon film thickness from the monitor, the film should be ~2 nm. Repeat evaporation if necessary (*see* **Note 9**).

7. Vent the recipient chamber, wait at least 5 min before opening it (evaporation source will become hot during evaporation). Store carbon films on mica carrier for >3 days (ideally >10 days) in a petri dish before use (*see* **Note 10**).

### 3.4 Carbon Film Transfer onto EM Grids

1. Construct a floatation chamber well in advance (compare Fig. 2). The design was described in [33] and should be adaptable in a scientific workshop. A commercial version (SKU

10840) of a similar apparatus is available from LADD Research Industries (Williston, VT, USA). We also use this flotation chamber to transfer surface assembled graphene oxide [44] onto EM grids.

2. Prepare a sheet of filter paper that is slightly bigger than the carbon film produced in "Preparation of ultrathin carbon film" and mark the rough outline of the carbon film on this filter paper with a pencil.

3. Place metal support mesh on beams in floatation chamber and place marked filter paper on top of metal mesh. Close the flexible outlet tube at the chamber bottom using a clip or connect to peristaltic pump.

4. Fill the chamber with bidest. Water to about 0.5 cm above the filter paper.

5. Carefully place freshly glow-discharged EM grids (30 s on setting "low") on the filter paper (*see* **Note 11**).

6. Pick up the carbon-covered mica sheet (see above) with forceps at a position previously covered by tape (no carbon film).

7. Slowly slide the mica sheet into the water with the carbon film facing upward and monitor carbon film detachment on the surface. Slowly and continuously slide the mica into the water until fully submerged (*see* Fig. 2).

8. Carefully position the floating carbon film on top of the grids using the forceps.

9. Slowly drain the water by opening the clip on the outlet tube and continue to guide the carbon film over the grids.

10. Place the filter paper (with the wet, now coated grids on top) in a petri dish containing an additional filter paper at the bottom. Cover and allow to dry over-night.

11. Check carbon film under binocular reflection microscope: Are holey Quantifoil film and the carbon support on the same side? Only one layer of untorn support must be visible on a grid (this can also be checked in a transmission electron microscope) (*see* **Note 12**).

**3.5 Cryo-Grid Preparation**

1. Prepare the Vitrobot Mark IV plunge freezer according to manufacturer's instruction (Thermo Fisher): Fill water reservoir of the humidifier with 60 ml water, place new filter papers and cool down humidity chamber of the Vitrobot to 4° for ~45 min. Set humidity to 100% after 30 min and enable the humidifier, to moisten the filter paper (*see* **Note 13**).

2. Check Vitrobot settings and perform a test run without grid or forceps. Vitrobot settings: 4 °C, 100%, Blotting settings: wait 0 s, blot 5 s, drain 0 s, Blot force 12 (*see* **Note 14**).

3. Cool the cryogen container with liquid nitrogen for 5 min.

4. Condense ethane (handle with caution under fume hood, wear eye and skin protection) (*see* **Note 15**).

5. Wait until solid ethane precipitates at the edges of the cryogen container, remove cooling "spider" apparatus and transfer the cryogen-containing assembly to the Vitrobot (*see* **Note 16**).

6. Glow discharge EM grids (carbon side up, if applicable), for holey carbon grids: 2 × 100 s, 15 mA, 0.4 mbar; for grids coated with ultrathin carbon film: 30 s, 15 mA, 0.4 mbar.

7. Label and place grid storage boxes in cavities inside the cooling container.

8. Pick up a freshly glow-discharged grid with the Vitrobot tweezers, be sure you only touch the rim of the grid and mount the tweezers with the grid on the Vitrobot plunging rod.

9. Click "continue" to lift the forceps into the humidity chamber and the Styrofoam nitrogen cup with the cryogen container.

10. Apply 3–5 µl of sample and start the blotting and plunging process (*see* **Note 17**).

11. Once the grid was plunged into the ethane container and automatically retracted from the humidity chamber, carefully slide the tweezer from the plunging rod. Make sure to keep the grid covered with liquid ethane while removing the Styrofoam container from its holder in the Vitrobot (*see* **Note 18**).

12. Transfer the grid from liquid ethane to liquid nitrogen and into the storage box. Close full storage boxes and store in nitrogen at the bottom of the Styrofoam container until transfer to a storage container (*see* **Note 19**).

13. Store grid boxes in a liquid nitrogen tank (*see* **Note 20**).

### 3.6 Cryo-Electron Microscopy

1. Place Gatan 626 cryo holder in transfer station and fill the transfer station with liquid nitrogen. Fill the holder Dewar (which will keep the specimen cold during the transfer and microscopy process) with liquid nitrogen directly afterward (*see* **Note 21**).

2. Wait for ~15 min until station is equilibrated (nitrogen stops boiling). Optional: Connect the temperature control unit to the holder and confirm stable temperature is around $-180\,^{\circ}\mathrm{C}$.

3. Precool all tweezers and other tools used from here on in liquid nitrogen to avoid heating of the vitreous sample.

4. Transfer EM grid to the slot at the tip of the holder and fix it with the clip ring (*see* **Note 22**).

5. Close the shield over the sample by sliding the lever on the back for the holder Dewar to protect it during grid transfer to the microscope.

*Optional*: Prepare electron microscope by tilting the stage 30° to avoid spilling liquid nitrogen during holder insertion.

6. Insert holder into the microscope and evacuate the lock. Wait until vacuum recovers.

7. Start SerialEM software [43] and check microscope alignment, low-dose mode settings and imaging states and determine the eucentric height of the specimen (*see* **Note 23**).

8. Create a map of the entire grid at low magnification (80–100×). If using the FEI Vitrobot for plunging, a gradient in ice thickness should be visible. Ice in some regions may be too thick for electrons to pass through and appear black, while regions on the opposite side of the grid may be almost dry.

9. Start the Serial-EM "Navigator" function. Create a map from the atlas and select grid squares with different ice appearance to be screened at higher magnifications. Using the 'add points' feature of the navigator to save coordinates may be helpful.

10. Acquire images at intermediate magnification (2000×) to correlate overall ice appearance with local distribution. Eventually make maps at this intermediate magnification, this could help navigating on the grid-square and is useful, if some more micrographs should be collected.

11. Image areas with distinct ice thickness and distribution. We acquire images at 40,000× magnification (2.7 Å/pixel) using the low dose mode setup in SerialEM, taking focus images at the carbon support foil. Ensure the illuminated area for the focus does not overlap with the area to be imaged. Relying on the calibration of our electron beam we acquire images at 20–50 $e^-/A^2$.

12. We evaluate the grid atlas based on ice distribution, to eventually adjust blotting or glow discharge parameters. Higher magnification images are evaluated on sample heterogeneity, stability, behavior of the sample in thinner and thicker ice, and particle concentration and distribution.

# 4    Notes

1. Optimal concentration of crosslinker can be determined with a titration experiment, depending on temperature and time we suggest 0.1–5 mM for BS3.

2. A short prior quenching with lysine, aspartate or a mixture of amino acids will modify surface properties and could influence orientation distribution.

3. For quality control, we compare cross-linked/non–cross-linked SEC fractions using negative stain EM and SDS-PAGE (silver stain).

4. Solution should have a dark yellow color with precipitation at the bottom of the tube. Optional addition of NaOH drops could improve staining, but also lead to more precipitation.

5. Longer absorption times will increase the particle density, but may lead to evaporation effects (precipitation of salts on grid).

6. Do not blot completely dry, leave a thin film of staining solution on surface of the grid between the staining steps. Particles should be embedded into the heavy metal stain, complete blotting of the stain may introduce artifacts such as positive staining of the particles.

7. Although the resolution will be limited by the stain, one may obtain important information about factor occupancy and particle damage. However, the heavy metal staining at low pH values may introduce artifacts. Therefore, this serves only as a first insight into the quality of your sample.

8. The filter paper serves as internal control whether the coating has worked and also as optical thickness comparison with other batches.

9. The carbon film is not as transparent as alternatives described above, introduces some background signal and might be problematic to use with smaller particles with low intrinsic signal to noise ratio. However, the carbon support works well for Pol I complexes, which have molecular masses of >600 kDa.

10. Carbon films on mica sheets can be stored in petri dishes over years. 2 nm films are used for cryo-grid preparations, thicker films (5–8 nm) can be used for negative staining.

11. Take care that they do not turn; the holey film should face upward. Grids must not overlap.

12. Holy film and carbon will appear shiny, rainbow-like colored; backside should not have this appearance.

13. During the cryo-grid preparation process, surface effects play an important role. The behavior of protein complexes at air–water and grid support–water interfaces can hardly be predicted. Evaporation effects may lead to increasing salt concentrations and surface saturation resulting in protein aggregation [26]. We recommend using low temperatures at 100% humidity as described.

14. We initially used apo ferritin and Pol I [45, 46] to find starting conditions on our Vitrobot. Adaptation of blot force (−20 to +20), wait time (<2 min), sample volumes of 2–8 μl, blotting times from 1 to 10 s, and glow discharge conditions may be worth screening. For our machine and sample types, 5 s blotting at blot force 12 without wait or drain time for a 3 μl sample seem to work well as starting conditions.

15. We hold the tip of the ethane outlet to the lower bottom edge of the ethane container and slowly lift it near the surface of liquid ethane in the pot. A slurping sound will ensure the right flowrate of ethane gas.

16. Liquid ethane is the mostly used cryogen for cryo-grid freezing. The temperature of the cryogen is critical for the vitrification process. At temperatures higher than 133 K ($-140$ °C), vitreous water will be transformed into cubic or hexagonal ice, the grid is no longer usable. Ethane should be used close to its melting point (90.4 K; $-182.8$ °C) but is still liquid at higher temperatures (boiling point ethane: 184.6 K; $-88.4$ °C) not suitable for sample vitrification [47]. To achieve this, we wait until we observe some freezing ethane on edges of the ethane container. However, too much solid ethane can damage grids or forceps. Addition of 10% propane will lower the melting temperature and the cryogen will stay liquid. Alternatively, the use of a cryostat system to control the ethane/cryogen temperature can be an option and applied to most plunge freezing systems [48]. [Boiling point nitrogen: 77.4 K ($-195.8$ °C), Melting point ethane: 90.4 K ($-182.8$ °C), Boiling point ethane: 184.6 K ($-88.4$ °C)].

17. For Cryo-EM grid preparation, only little sample amounts are required. If the sample is adsorbed to a thin carbon film, concentrations as low as 50 ng/µl of sample concentration are sufficient. Even lover amounts can be used in customized humidity chambers if adsorption times are significantly increased [19]. Negative stain quality control is recommended to monitor particle homogeneity and distribution. For preparation of unsupported holey carbon grids, the required sample concentration is 2–5× higher to yield similar particles densities.

18. Use of a face mask may help to prevent surface ice contamination, as nitrogen atmosphere will not be disturbed. Avoid contact of ice-covered tools with liquid nitrogen or ethane to prevent sample contamination.

19. Even though the procedure is not fully reproducible in our hands, the blotting procedure introduces a gradient and the method is robust enough to generate vitrified ice of different quality. Depending on grid types, high-resolution data collection usually requires no more than 20 squares with suitable ice.

20. Visible ethane contamination on the grid surface will sublimate within one or two days of storage in liquid nitrogen tank. During storage, ice flakes in the liquid nitrogen may start contaminating your grids. Thus, we use cryo-grids no longer than 3 months following plunging.

21. Measures to reduce ice contamination may be helpful: Work should be carried out in a low-humidity environment. A protective mask can be worn. Dewars should be covered with lids while equilibrating. Start filling of liquid nitrogen at the tip of the holder, then the Dewar, to avoid ice formation at the specimen tip. Each tool used should be heated and dried after use in nitrogen.

22. First-time users may practice at room temperature and with empty grids first.

23. Our screening workflow is highly compatible with the SerialEM software package. We recommend setup of the low-dose mode to avoid exposure-induced damage by unnecessary illumination of the sample. The software is freely available, constantly updated and can be adapted to most microscopes and cameras.

## Acknowledgments

We thank Herbert Tschochner and Joachim Griesenbeck for discussions, Lena Heuschneider for technical assistance, and Reinhard Rachel for practical advice. We acknowledge funding by SFB960 of the DFG (TP-A8 to CE and TP-B1 to PM) and by the "Emmy-Noether-Programme" (DFG grant no. EN 1204/1-1 to CE).

## References

1. Kühlbrandt W (2014) Biochemistry. The resolution revolution. Science 343:1443–1444. https://doi.org/10.1126/science.1251652

2. Callaway E (2015) The revolution will not be crystallized: a new method sweeps through structural biology. Nature 525:172–174. https://doi.org/10.1038/525172a

3. Vinothkumar KR, Henderson R (2016) Single particle electron cryomicroscopy: trends, issues and future perspective. Q Rev Biophys 49:e13. https://doi.org/10.1017/S0033583516000068

4. Fernandez-Leiro R, Scheres SHW (2016) Unravelling biological macromolecules with cryo-electron microscopy. Nature 537:339–346. https://doi.org/10.1038/nature19948

5. Frank J (2017) Advances in the field of single-particle cryo-electron microscopy over the last decade. Nat Protoc 12:209–212. https://doi.org/10.1038/nprot.2017.004

6. Lyumkis D (2019) Challenges and opportunities in cryo-EM single-particle analysis. J Biol Chem 294:5181–5197. https://doi.org/10.1074/jbc.REV118.005602

7. Nogales E (2016) The development of cryo-EM into a mainstream structural biology technique. Nat Methods 13:24–27

8. Glaeser RM (2019) How good can single-particle cryo-EM become? What remains before it approaches its physical limits? Annu Rev Biophys 48:45–61. https://doi.org/10.1146/annurev-biophys-070317-032828

9. Hanske J, Sadian Y, Müller CW (2018) The cryo-EM resolution revolution and transcription complexes. Curr Opin Struct Biol 52:8–15. https://doi.org/10.1016/j.sbi.2018.07.002

10. Pilsl M, Crucifix C, Papai G, Krupp F, Steinbauer R, Griesenbeck J, Milkereit P, Tschochner H, Schultz P (2016) Structure of the initiation-competent RNA polymerase I and its implication for transcription. Nat Commun 7:12126. https://doi.org/10.1038/ncomms12126

11. Engel C, Plitzko J, Cramer P (2016) RNA polymerase I–Rrn3 complex at 4.8 Å resolution. Nat Commun 7:12129. https://doi.org/10.1038/ncomms12129

12. Engel C, Gubbey T, Neyer S, Sainsbury S, Oberthuer C, Baejen C, Bernecky C, Cramer P (2017) Structural basis of RNA polymerase I transcription initiation. Cell 169:120–131. e22. https://doi.org/10.1016/j.cell.2017. 03.003

13. Tafur L, Sadian Y, Hoffmann NA, Jakobi AJ, Wetzel R, Hagen WJH, Sachse C, Müller CW (2016) Molecular structures of transcribing RNA polymerase I. Mol Cell 64:1135–1143. https://doi.org/10.1016/j.molcel.2016. 11.013

14. Neyer S, Kunz M, Geiss C, Hantsche M, Hodirnau V-V, Seybert A, Engel C, Scheffer MP, Cramer P, Frangakis AS (2016) Structure of RNA polymerase I transcribing ribosomal DNA genes. Nature 540:607–610. https:// doi.org/10.1038/nature20561

15. Heiss FB, Daiß JL, Becker P, Engel C (2021) Conserved strategies of RNA polymerase I hibernation and activation. Nat Commun 12: 758. https://doi.org/10.1038/s41467-021-21031-8

16. Pilsl M, Engel C (2020) Structural basis of RNA polymerase I pre-initiation complex formation and promoter melting. Nat Commun 11:1206. https://doi.org/10.1038/s41467-020-15052-y

17. Torreira E, Louro JA, Pazos I, González-Polo N, Gil-Carton D, Duran AG, Tosi S, Gallego O, Calvo O, Fernández-Tornero C (2017) The dynamic assembly of distinct RNA polymerase I complexes modulates rDNA transcription. elife 6:e20832. https://doi.org/10.7554/eLife.20832

18. Sanz-Murillo M, Xu J, Belogurov GA, Calvo O, Gil-Carton D, Moreno-Morcillo M, Wang D, Fernández-Tornero C (2018) Structural basis of RNA polymerase I stalling at UV light-induced DNA damage. Proc Natl Acad Sci U S A 115:8972–8977. https://doi.org/10.1073/pnas.1802626115

19. Han Y, Yan C, Nguyen THD, Jackobel AJ, Ivanov I, Knutson BA, He Y (2017) Structural mechanism of ATP-independent transcription initiation by RNA polymerase I. elife 6: e27414. https://doi.org/10.7554/eLife. 27414

20. Stark H, Chari A (2016) Sample preparation of biological macromolecular assemblies for the determination of high-resolution structures by cryo-electron microscopy. Microscopy (Oxf) 65:23–34. https://doi.org/10.1093/jmicro/dfv367

21. Engel C (2016) Purification of crystallization-grade RNA polymerase I from S. cerevisiae. Methods Mol Biol 1455:85–97. https://doi.org/10.1007/978-1-4939-3792-9_7

22. Pilsl M, Merkl PE, Milkereit P, Griesenbeck J, Tschochner H (2016) Analysis of S. cerevisiae RNA polymerase I transcription in vitro. Methods Mol Biol 1455:99–108. https://doi.org/10.1007/978-1-4939-3792-9_8

23. He Y, Fang J, Taatjes DJ, Nogales E (2013) Structural visualization of key steps in human transcription initiation. Nature 495:481–486. https://doi.org/10.1038/nature11991

24. Kastner B, Fischer N, Golas MM, Sander B, Dube P, Boehringer D, Hartmuth K, Deckert J, Hauer F, Wolf E, Uchtenhagen H, Urlaub H, Herzog F, Peters JM, Poerschke D, Lührmann R, Stark H (2008) GraFix: sample preparation for single-particle electron cryomicroscopy. Nat Methods 5:53–55. https://doi.org/10.1038/nmeth1139

25. Stark H (2010) GraFix: stabilization of fragile macromolecular complexes for single particle cryo-EM. Methods Enzymol 481:109–126

26. Passmore LA, Russo CJ (2016) Specimen preparation for high-resolution Cryo-EM. Methods Enzymol 579:51–86. https://doi.org/10.1016/bs.mie.2016. 04.011

27. Thompson RF, Walker M, Siebert CA, Muench SP, Ranson NA (2016) An introduction to sample preparation and imaging by cryo-electron microscopy for structural biology. Methods 100:3–15. https://doi.org/10. 1016/j.ymeth.2016.02.017

28. D'Imprima E, Floris D, Joppe M, Sánchez R, Grininger M, Kühlbrandt W (2019) Protein denaturation at the air-water interface and how to prevent it. elife 8:e42747. https://doi.org/10.7554/eLife.42747

29. Pantelic RS, Meyer JC, Kaiser U, Baumeister W, Plitzko JM (2010) Graphene oxide: a substrate for optimizing preparations of frozen-hydrated samples. J Struct Biol 170: 152–156. https://doi.org/10.1016/j.jsb. 2009.12.020

30. Pantelic RS, Suk JW, Magnuson CW, Meyer JC, Wachsmuth P, Kaiser U, Ruoff RS, Stahlberg H (2011) Graphene: substrate preparation and introduction. J Struct Biol 174:234–238. https://doi.org/10.1016/j.jsb.2010. 10.002

31. Russo CJ, Passmore LA (2014) Controlling protein adsorption on graphene for cryo-EM using low-energy hydrogen plasmas. Nat Methods 11:649–652. https://doi.org/10. 1038/nmeth.2931

32. Göringer HU, Stark H, Böhm C, Sander B, Golas MM (2011) Three-dimensional reconstruction of Trypanosoma brucei editosomes

using single-particle electron microscopy. Methods Mol Biol 718:3–22

33. Dykstra MJ, Reuss LE (2003) Biological electron microscopy. Theory, techniques, and troubleshooting, 2nd edn. Springer US, Boston, MA

34. Grassucci RA, Taylor DJ, Frank J (2007) Preparation of macromolecular complexes for cryo-electron microscopy. Nat Protoc 2:3239–3246. https://doi.org/10.1038/nprot.2007.452

35. Grassucci RA, Taylor D, Frank J (2008) Visualization of macromolecular complexes using cryo-electron microscopy with FEI Tecnai transmission electron microscopes. Nat Protoc 3:330–339. https://doi.org/10.1038/nprot.2007.474

36. Cheng A, Eng ET, Alink L, Rice WJ, Jordan KD, Kim LY, Potter CS, Carragher B (2018) High resolution single particle cryo-electron microscopy using beam-image shift. J Struct Biol 204:270–275. https://doi.org/10.1016/j.jsb.2018.07.015

37. Cheng A, Tan YZ, Dandey VP, Potter CS, Carragher B (2016) Strategies for automated CryoEM data collection using direct detectors. Methods Enzymol 579:87–102. https://doi.org/10.1016/bs.mie.2016.04.008

38. Schorb M, Haberbosch I, Hagen WJH, Schwab Y, Mastronarde DN (2019) Software tools for automated transmission electron microscopy. Nat Methods 16:471–477. https://doi.org/10.1038/s41592-019-0396-9

39. Zivanov J, Nakane T, Forsberg BO, Kimanius D, Hagen WJ, Lindahl E, Scheres SH (2018) New tools for automated high-resolution cryo-EM structure determination in RELION-3. elife 7:e42166. https://doi.org/10.7554/eLife.42166

40. Tegunov D, Cramer P (2018) Real-time cryo-EM data pre-processing with warp. Nat Methods 16(11):1146-1152. https://doi.org/10.1038/s41592-019-0580-y

41. Punjani A, Rubinstein JL, Fleet DJ, Brubaker MA (2017) cryoSPARC: algorithms for rapid unsupervised cryo-EM structure determination. Nat Methods 14:290–296. https://doi.org/10.1038/nmeth.4169

42. Wagner T, Merino F, Stabrin M, Moriya T, Antoni C, Apelbaum A, Hagel P, Sitsel O, Raisch T, Prumbaum D, Quentin D, Roderer D, Tacke S, Siebolds B, Schubert E, Shaikh TR, Lill P, Gatsogiannis C, Raunser S (2019) SPHIRE-crYOLO: a fast and accurate fully automated particle picker for cryo-EM. Commun Biol 2:218

43. Mastronarde DN (2005) Automated electron microscope tomography using robust prediction of specimen movements. J Struct Biol 152:36–51. https://doi.org/10.1016/j.jsb.2005.07.007

44. Palovcak E, Wang F, Zheng SQ, Yu Z, Li S, Betegon M, Bulkley D, Agard DA, Cheng Y (2018) A simple and robust procedure for preparing graphene-oxide cryo-EM grids. J Struct Biol 204:80–84. https://doi.org/10.1016/j.jsb.2018.07.007

45. Fernández-Tornero C, Moreno-Morcillo M, Rashid UJ, Taylor NMI, Ruiz FM, Gruene T, Legrand P, Steuerwald U, Müller CW (2013) Crystal structure of the 14-subunit RNA polymerase I. Nature 502:644. https://doi.org/10.1038/nature12636

46. Engel C, Sainsbury S, Cheung AC, Kostrewa D, Cramer P (2013) RNA polymerase I structure and transcription regulation. Nature 502:650. https://doi.org/10.1038/nature12712

47. Dubochet J, Adrian M, Chang JJ, Homo JC, Lepault J, McDowall AW, Schultz P (1988) Cryo-electron microscopy of vitrified specimens. Q Rev Biophys 21:129–228

48. Russo CJ, Scotcher S, Kyte M (2016) A precision cryostat design for manual and semi-automated cryo-plunge instruments. Rev Sci Instrum 87:114302. https://doi.org/10.1063/1.4967864

# Part IV

## Ribosome Assembly, Transport and RNP Complexes

# Chapter 7

# Eukaryotic Ribosome assembly and Nucleocytoplasmic Transport

## Michaela Oborská-Oplová, Ute Fischer, Martin Altvater, and Vikram Govind Panse

*This chapter is dedicated to the memory of our former graduate student and friend Dr. Cohue Peña.*

## Abstract

The process of eukaryotic ribosome assembly stretches across the nucleolus, the nucleoplasm and the cytoplasm, and therefore relies on efficient nucleocytoplasmic transport. In yeast, the import machinery delivers ~140,000 ribosomal proteins every minute to the nucleus for ribosome assembly. At the same time, the export machinery facilitates translocation of ~2000 pre-ribosomal particles every minute through ~200 nuclear pore complexes (NPC) into the cytoplasm. Eukaryotic ribosome assembly also requires >200 conserved assembly factors, which transiently associate with pre-ribosomal particles. Their site(s) of action on maturing pre-ribosomes are beginning to be elucidated. In this chapter, we outline protocols that enable rapid biochemical isolation of pre-ribosomal particles for single particle cryo-electron microscopy (cryo-EM) and in vitro reconstitution of nuclear transport processes. We discuss cell-biological and genetic approaches to investigate how the ribosome assembly and the nucleocytoplasmic transport machineries collaborate to produce functional ribosomes.

**Key words** Budding Yeast, Ribosome Assembly, Nuclear Import, Nuclear Export, preribosome structure

---

## 1   Introduction

Eukaryotic ribosome assembly takes place across multiple cellular compartments: the nucleolus, the nucleoplasm and the cytoplasm (Fig. 1). This dynamic and energy consuming process requires the coordination of three RNA polymerases (I, II, and III), the RNA splicing, and nucleocytoplasmic transport machineries [1]. Despite this complexity, ribosome biogenesis is an incredibly efficient process, with yeast producing up to 60 ribosomes every second [2].

The small subunit (SSU) processome is the first ribosome precursor assembled cotranscriptionally in the nucleolus through stepwise association with UTP-A, UTP-B, and UTP-C complexes

Karl-Dieter Entian (ed.), *Ribosome Biogenesis: Methods and Protocols*, Methods in Molecular Biology, vol. 2533, https://doi.org/10.1007/978-1-0716-2501-9_7, © The Author(s) 2022

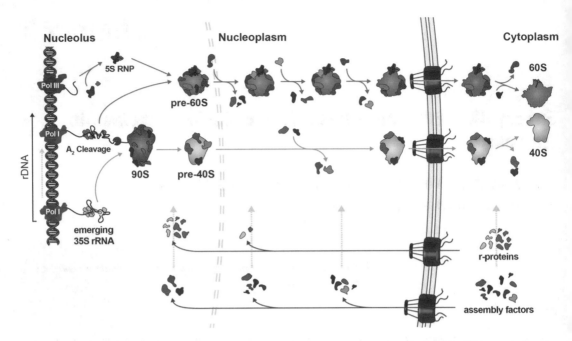

**Fig. 1** Current model for eukaryotic ribosome assembly. Transcription of primary 35S rRNA transcript, the common precursor of 18S, 5.8S, and 25S rRNAs, by Pol I from rDNA repeats together with cotranscriptional joining of U3 snoRNP, r-proteins and 40S assembly factors form the 90S ribosomal precursor. 5S rRNA is transcribed separately by Pol III for assembly of 5S RNP before joining the 60S pre-ribosome. Cotranscriptional cleavage of 35S rRNA at A2 site separates the 60S and 40S r-subunit maturation pathways. Pre-ribosomal particles undergo a cascade of maturation steps in the nucleoplasm by transient association with assembly factors until reaching nuclear export competency. Once exported to the cytoplasm, last maturation events and quality control steps can occur resulting into functional r-subunits production. (Adapted from Peña et al. 2017)

and U3 snoRNP [1, 3]. Cryo-electron microscopy (cryo-EM) studies are revealing how UTP-A, UTP-B complexes, U3 snoRNP and additional biogenesis factors encapsulate and guide pre-rRNA folding in a hierarchical 5′-to-3′-oriented manner [4–7]. During nucleolar maturation, the 5′ domain of the 18S rRNA achieves a mature conformation, and the central domain is correctly positioned relative to the 5′ domain. In contrast, the 3′ major domain is buried within the SSU processome core, and its conformation is distinct as in the mature 40S subunit. Release of the 40S pre-ribosome requires endonucleolytic cleavages within the pre-rRNA [8–11], the release of U3 snoRNA and associated proteins catalyzed by the RNA helicase Dhr1 and its cofactor Utp14 [12, 13]. The RNA exosome mediates degradation of 5′-ETS (external transcribed spacer) rRNA within the 5′-ETS rRNA–UTP complex to disassemble and recycle the UTPs for a new round of 40S assembly [14].

Following 40S preribosome release the growing 27S pre-rRNA associates with 60S-specific r-proteins and maturation factors to initiate 60S pre-ribosome assembly. Cryo-EM structures of early states of the 60S pre-ribosome suggest a sequence of events during nucleolar 60S assembly. Early states the nucleolar 60S pre-ribosome show a characteristic arch-like morphology, whereas the later states adopt a compact shape closer to a mature 60S subunit. The 5' domains (I and II) within 27S pre-rRNA adopt a near mature conformation, and connect with the 3' terminal domain VI, thus forming the solvent-exposed backside of the 60S subunit. In all states, the pre-rRNA spacer ITS2, located in the 27S pre-rRNA between 5.8S and 25S rRNA, and the associated ITS2 factors form the "foot" structure. The central domains III, IV and V, which form the subunit interface, are not visible in the early states. Although cotranscriptional assembly of the 60S pre-ribosome occurs in a sequential manner, it undergoes nonlinear compaction of domains I, II, and VI, which then allows domains III, IV, and V to fall onto the arch-like structure, thus preparing the pre-ribosomal cargo for nuclear export [15–17].

In yeast, before every cell division, ~200,000 pre-ribosomes are transported to the cytoplasm through ~200 NPCs (nuclear pore complexes) by the exportin Crm1 that recognizes nuclear export sequences (NESs) on cargos and interacts with the FG-rich (phenylalanine/glycine-rich) meshwork of the NPC transport channel [18–22]. Nmd3 is the only identified essential adaptor for Crm1-mediated 60S pre-ribosome export [23, 24]. In contrast, no essential NES-containing export adaptor has been identified for 40S pre-ribosome export. 40S pre-ribosome bound shuttling assembly factors Ltv1 and Rio2 can recruit Crm1 in the presence of RanGTP through a leucine-rich NES. Pre-ribosomes also employ multiple export factors (Mex67-Mtr2, Arx1, Ecm1, Bud20) that directly interact with the FG-meshwork of the transport channel [1, 21, 22]. In addition, a non-FG pathway involving the mRNA export factor Gle2 also facilitates 60S pre-ribosome export [25].

Exported pre-ribosomes undergo final maturation and proofreading before initiating translation [26]. Cytoplasmic proofreading of 60S pre-ribosomes involves release of assembly factors that block binding of r-proteins, interactions with translation factors, or pairing with the 40S. Tif6 prevents binding of immature 60S pre-ribosomes to mature 40S subunits, ensuring that only properly assembled subunits engage in translation. Quality control of the 40S pre-ribosome relies on assembly factors that prevent the premature binding of initiation factors, mRNA, tRNA, and the 60S subunit. Ltv1 and Enp1 directly bind uS3 on its solvent side, thereby blocking the mRNA channel opening. Rio2, Tsr1, and Dim1 bind the subunit interface, thus preventing joining of the mature 60S subunit and translation initiation factor eIF1A. Nob1 and Pno1 block the binding of eIF3, thereby interfering with translation initiation [27]. After release of Rio2, Tsr1, and Dim1 initiated by the reorganization of the beak structure, the 40S pre-ribosome becomes competent to interact with a mature 60S subunit. This translation-like interaction is thought to test the ability of a 40S pre-ribosome to engage with a mature 60S subunit, and only then triggers Nob1 to cleave 20S pre-RNA to mature 18S rRNA in vitro [28, 29]. Cryo-EM studies are revealing how these late factors interact with the 40S pre-ribosome and have provided a structural framework for the ordering of cytoplasmic maturation events [30–32].

In addition to >200 assembly factors, ribosome assembly relies on efficient nucleocytoplasmic transport [1]. All r-proteins and assembly factors need to be imported into the nucleus, and correctly assembled pre-ribosomal particles need to be transported through nuclear pore complexes into the cytoplasm. How the ribosome assembly machinery collaborates with the cellular trafficking pathways is currently under intense investigation. Here, we outline biochemical approaches that permit rapid screening and analyses of pre-ribosomal particles for single particle cryo-EM studies, and reconstitution of nucleocytoplasmic transport processes. We discuss genetic and cell-biological approaches that will enable the unveiling of the functional interface between the ribosome assembly and nucleocytoplasmic machineries.

# 2    Materials, Reagents, and Yeast Media

## 2.1    Material (Listed in Alphabetical Order)

1. 15 mL Centrifuge tube (Greiner Bio-One, 188271)
2. 20 mL Luer Solo, Inject (Braun, 4606205V)
3. 50 mL Centrifuge tube (Greiner Bio-One, 227261)
4. 50 mL Magnetic Separation Rack (New BioLabs, S1507S)
5. Centrifuge 5804 R (Eppendorf, 5805 000.327).
6. Centrifuge Sorvall RC3BP with H-6000A Rotor (Thermo-Scientific, 75007530, 11250).
7. Cover glasses (VWR, 631-0137).
8. DynaMag™—Spin Magnet (Invitrogen, 12320D).
9. Fluorescence microscope Leica DM6000 B (Leica).
10. Incubator IFE 600 (Memmert).
11. Incubator shaker ISF1-X (Kuhner).
12. Inoculation loop (Greiner, 731101).
13. Membrane filters 0.45 mm (Millipore, HAWP04700).
14. Microcentrifuge 5415R (Eppendorf, 022621408).
15. Microscope slides (VWR, 631-1550).
16. Planetary mill Pulverisette 6 (Fritsch, 06.2000.00).
17. Spectrophotometer Ultrospec 2100 pro (GE Healthcare, 80-2112-21).

18. Stainless Steel Grinding Balls (Fritsch, 55.0200.10).

19. Stainless Steel Grinding Bowls, 80 mL (Fritsch, 50.4100.00).

20. Sterifil Aseptic System (Millipore, XX1104700).

21. Syringe filter, pore size: 2.7 μm (GE Healthcare, 6888-2527).

22. Syringe filter pore size: 1.6 μm (GE Healthcare, 6882-2516).

23. Thermomixer comfort (Eppendorf).

**2.2  Reagents (Listed in Alphabetical Order)**

1. Acetone (Merck, 1.00014.1000).

2. AcTEV protease (Invitrogen, 12575015).

3. Beta-mercaptoethanol (CalBioChem, 444203).

4. CaCl2(Sigma-Aldrich, 22,350-6).

5. cOmplete protease inhibitor cocktail tablets, EDTA free (Roche, 11873580001),

6. Coomassie Brilliant Blue R-250 (ThermoScientific, 20,278).

7. Difco Agar (BD, 214530).

8. Dithiothreitol (DTT) (AppliChem, A1101).

9. Dynabeads™ M-270 Epoxy (Invitrogen, 14301).

10. Glucose (Sigma-Aldrich, G8270).

11. Glutathione Sepharose 4 Fast Flow (GE Healthcare, 17-5132-01).

12. Glycerol (AppliChem, A1123).

13. HEPES (Sigma-Aldrich, H4034).

14. IgG from rabbit serum (Sigma-Aldrich, I5006).

15. KOAc (Sigma-Aldrich, P1147).

16. LDS sample buffer (Invitrogen, NP0008).

17. $MgCl_2$ (Fluka, 63072).

18. $Mg(OAc)_2$ (Sigma-Aldrich, M5661).

19. NaCl (Merck, 1064045000).

20. $NH_4Cl$ (Sigma-Aldrich, A9434).

21. NuPAGE 4–12% Bis–Tris (Novex, NP0321BOX).

22. Phenylmethanesulfonyl fluoride (PMSF) (AppliChem, A0999).

23. Polyvinylpyrrolidone (K90) (AppliChem, A6393).

24. Sodium phosphate (Sigma-Aldrich, 342483).

25. TCA (Sigma-Aldrich, T6399).

26. Tris–HCl (Sigma-Aldrich, T3253).

27. Triton X-100 (Merck, 1086431000).

28. Tween 20 (Sigma-Aldrich, P9416).

**2.3 Yeast Media**

1. Synthetic complete (SC) media: 0.69% yeast nitrogen base without amino acids (ForMedium, CYN0410) 2% glucose (Sigma-Aldrich, G8270) 0.6–0.8% appropriate drop-out supplements complete mixtures (ForMedium).

2. SC plates (SC, 2% agar).

3. Yeast-extract peptone dextrose (YPD) media: 1% yeast extract, (ForMedium, YEM03), 2% peptone (ForMedium, PEP03), 2% glucose (Sigma-Aldrich, G8270).

4. YPD plates (YPD, 2% agar).

## 3    Pre-ribosome Isolation for Single Particle Cryo-Electron Microscopy

During the last decade, affinity-purification protocols combined with sensitive mass spectrometry have dramatically altered our understanding of eukaryotic ribosome assembly [33]. By employing the powerful "tandem affinity-purification" (TAP), several groups have unravelled the compositions of the 90S, 60S, and 40S pre-ribosomes and thus expanded the inventory of the assembly machinery and ordered the 40S and 60S maturation pathways [34–40]. Recently, improvement in these biochemical approaches together with advances of cryo-EM have driven structural studies of pre-ribosomal particles, thus providing high-resolution snapshots of the process of eukaryotic ribosome assembly [4–6, 15–17, 30–32, 41, 42] (Fig. 2a, b).

**3.1 Preparing Yeast Cells for Cryogenic Lysis (Modified from Rout Lab Protocol: Harvesting Cells and Making Yeast Noodles [43])**

Resuspension Buffer: 1.2% PVP-40 (polyvinylpyrrolidone), 20 mM HEPES pH 7.4, Supplemented with 1:100 complete protease inhibitor cocktail tablet (Roche), 2 mM PMSF, 1 mM DTT (*see* **Note 1**).

*3.1.1 Buffers and Solutions*

*3.1.2 Yeast Cell Preparation*

1. Grow cell culture to $OD_{600} = 2.5$–3.5 in complete media/ 1.5–2.0 in synthetic media.

2. Spin cultures down ($4500 \times g$, 15 min, 4 °C).

3. Resuspend pellet in 50 mL $ddH_2O$ on ice. Put resuspended solution into 50 mL Falcon tube(s) and spin down ($4500 \times g$, 5 min, 4 °C). Repeat this step.

4. Resuspend pellet on ice in a volume of resuspension buffer equal to the volume of the pellet. Spin down ($4500 \times g$, 15 min, 4 °C). Aspirate all liquid from the pellet.

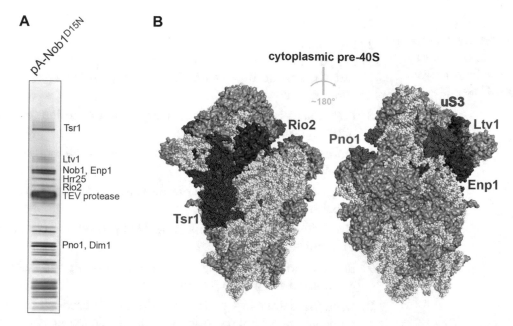

**Fig. 2** Purification and structure of a late 40S pre-ribosome. (**a**) Protein composition of 80S ribosomes Nob1-D15N particles, purified via ProteinA (pA)-tag. Proteins were separated by SDS-PAGE and visualized by silver staining. Labelled protein bands were characterized by mass spectrometry. (**b**) Front and back view of cryo-EM structure of a cytoplasmic 40S preribosome (PDB: 6FAI). The 20S rRNA is shown in light gray, r-proteins in dark gray—except of uS3 in yellow. Assembly factors are shown in color: Tsr1 in orange, Rio2 in blue, Pno1 in green, Ltv1 in purple, and Enp1 in red. (Adapted from Scaiola et al. 2018)

5. Spin just the pellet down again (4500 × *g*, 2 min, 4 °C) to remove the residual buffer (repeat if needed).

6. Pellet should be fairly dry and resemble a thick paste.

7. Fill up a Styrofoam box with a liquid nitrogen and prepare a metal holder next to it.

8. Use a metal clamp to precool and fill up completely a 50 mL Falcon tube with liquid nitrogen using and fix the tube to a metal holder.

9. With a spatula, scoop out cell paste and place into a 20 mL syringe. Press out the cell paste into the liquid nitrogen in the Falcon tube. Avoid touching the liquid nitrogen directly with the tip of the syringe to prevent syringe clogging.

10. When all cell paste is gone, remove liquid nitrogen from the tube (poke holes into cap of Falcon tube, screw on the cap and turn tube upside down to pour out the liquid nitrogen).

11. Do not tighten the tube completely, in order to allow liquid nitrogen vapor to escape. Store tubes at −80 °C.

*3.1.3  Cryogenic Lysis of Yeast Cells (See Also **Note 2**) (Modified from Rout Lab Protocol: Cryogenic Lyses of yeast Cells [43])*

1. Fill a rectangular ice bucket with liquid nitrogen.

2. Pre-chill everything. Immerse the 80 mL stainless steel grinding jars, the stainless steel lid, the grinding balls, steel spoon and the storage tube, with the frozen yeast noodles, in the liquid nitrogen.

3. Pre-cooling is finished when nitrogen bath is no longer bubbling vigorously.

4. Once everything is chilled pour the noodles into the grinding jar.

5. Weigh the grinding jar with noodles and then adjust the counterbalance weight.

6. Use 7–8 of the 20 mm stainless steel balls based on the amount of noodles.

7. Be sure no liquid nitrogen is in the grinding jar prior to grinding to avoid an explosion.

8. Grinding is done in 4 cycles, each cycle composed of 500 rpm, 3 min and in reverse rotation 500 rpm, 2 min (*see also* **Note 3**).

9. Between each cycle the jars are removed and cooled in liquid nitrogen. Do not remove the lid (removal of lid may result in cell loss). To ensure lid is chilled use an empty Falcon tube to pour liquid nitrogen over the top of the grinding jar while the bowl of the grinding jar cools in the liquid nitrogen bath. Do not submerge the jar completely as this will allow liquid nitrogen into the grinding bowl and may also result in cell loss.

10. When 4 cycles are complete, carefully remove powder from the balls with a pre-cooled spatula and transfer the powder into a new prechilled 50 mL Falcon tube (if there is powder stuck to the side of the jar repeat 1 grinding cycle) (*see* **Note 4**).

11. Jars and balls are cleaned with warm water.

12. Frozen ground cells are stored at −80 °C.

*3.1.4  Isolating Pre-ribosomes Using Magnetic Beads (Modified from Oeffinger et al. 2007 [43])*

M-IgG Buffer: 20 mM HEPES pH 7.4, KOAc, 40 mM NaCl, 0.5% Triton-X, 0,1% Tween 20.

Supplemented with (*see* **Note 1**) 2 mM PMSF, 1 mM DTT, 2–10 mM $MgCl_2$ (optional).

Buffers and Solutions

Method (*See Also* **Notes 5–8**)

1. Transfer 2–5 g of ground yeast cells, to a pre-cooled 50 mL falcon, and put it into liquid nitrogen.

2. Pour 40 mL M-IgG Buffer + Detergents into cooled sterile glass beaker with sterile magnet fish and start mixing.

3. Cool down and sterilize metal sieve in liquid nitrogen.

4. Add yeast powder slowly through the sieve into mixing buffer (avoid freezing of clumps).

5. Allow powder to resuspend completely in buffer (5–10 min).

6. Transfer yeast lysate to 50 mL Falcon tube. Spin down (4500 × $g$, 5 min, 4 °C) to get rid of big chunks.

7. Meanwhile take 100 µL bead slurry and wash 3× with 1 mL M-IgG Buffer + Detergents using Magnet rack to wash away buffer and resuspend in 1 mL M-IgG Buffer + Detergents.

8. Filter lysate with 60 mL syringe through 2.7 µM Whatman filter slowly into new 50 mL Falcon (do not push too hard, rather exchange the filter for new one).

9. Repeat with 60 mL syringe through 1.6 µM Whatman filter into new 50 mL Falcon (stop as soon as white foam comes out).

10. Add beads to clarified yeast lysate, seal with parafilm and incubate 30 min at 4 °C on rotating wheel.

11. Collect beads with magnetic rack, wait for complete bead binding (solution clears up).

12. Collect flow-through in a new Falcon tube and repeat bead collection to avoid loss of the beads.

13. Resuspend all collected beads in 1 mL M-IgG Buffer + Detergents and transfer it into 1.5 mL tube.

14. Wash the beads 3× with 1 mL M-IgG Buffer + Detergents using magnetic rack.

15. Wash the beads further 3–5× with 1 mL M-IgG Buffer without Detergents (to get rid of foaming).

16. Resuspend beads in 50–75 µL M-IgG buffer without Detergents.

17. Add 0.5 µL (10 U) TEV protease (Sigma, 20 U/L), seal with parafilm and incubate overnight at 4 °C on rotating wheel.

18. Collect flow-through (purified sample) in new tube using magnetic rack.

19. Use 5 µL sample per EM Copper Grid.

20. To analyze samples, proceed with TCA precipitation, RNA extraction, Silver gel, or RNA gel.

21. Boil beads in 25–50 µL 2× LDS and collect LDS in new tube (using magnetic rack) for TEV cleavage control.

### 3.2 Nuclear Import Assays for Ribosomal Proteins

It is assumed that like a typical import cargo, RanGTP dissociates the r-protein from the importin after arriving in the nuclear compartment. However, r-proteins contain disordered regions, which make them prone to non-specific interactions with other nucleic acids, aggregation and degradation in their non-assembled state. During a single 90 min generation time ~14 million r-proteins synthesized in the cytoplasm, need to be targeted to the yeast nucleus and handed over to the ribosome assembly machinery [1, 44]. Thus, safe and efficient transport of r-proteins to their rRNA binding site is a logistical challenge.

A number of groups have uncovered dedicated chaperones that interact with newly synthesized r-proteins in the cytoplasm [44–55]. The dedicated chaperone–r-protein complexes recruit the import machinery and are transported to the nucleus where they are released by the action of RanGTP.

A different mechanism is employed by the r-protein eS26 to reach the 90S pre-ribosome. Like a typical import cargo protein, eS26 uses importins for targeting to the nucleus. However, after reaching the nuclear compartment, eS26 is removed from the importin by an unloading factor, the escortin Tsr2, without the aid of RanGTP. Tsr2 shields eS26 from proteolysis and enables its safe transfer to the 90S pre-ribosome [56]. Below, we outline a step-by step protocol to investigate the canonical RanGTP dependent disassembly of a Pse1–Slx9 complex (Fig. 3a), and non-canonical Tsr2 dependent disassembly of a Kap123–eS26 complex (Fig. 3b). Slx9 is a predominantly nuclear localized protein, yet it shuttles between the nucleus and the cytoplasm [57, 58]. The import receptor transports Slx9 to the nuclear compartment, where Slx9 facilitates assembly of a Crm1-export complex and efficient export of 40S pre-ribosomes from the nucleus [57–60].

*3.2.1  A. RanGTP Mediated Disassembly of a Pse1–Slx9 Complex*

PBS-KMT buffer (pH 7.3): 150 mM NaCl, 25 mM Sodium phosphate, 3 mM KCl, 1 mM $MgCl_2$, 0,1% Tween 20.

Buffers and Solutions

Method

1. Pipet 50 µL of GSH-Sepharose slurry (per reaction) into a 1.5 mL reaction tube and wash 3 times with 1 mL PBS-KMT buffer, spin down in between for 30 s at 850 x g . Wash GSH-Sepharose beads for all reactions together.

2. Meanwhile thaw recombinant GST-Pse1 and GST-alone sample on ice.

3. Centrifuge the GST-Pse1 and GST-alone or lysates for 10 min at 4 °C at 16,000 x g to pellet aggregates and store the tubes on ice until use.

4. Add 12 µg GST-Pse1 or GST-alone (per reaction) to washed GSH-Sepharose beads suspended in 500 µL of PBS-KMT buffer.

5. Incubate on a rotating platform for 1 h at 4 °C to immobilize GST-Pse1 or GST-alone on GSH-Sepharose beads.

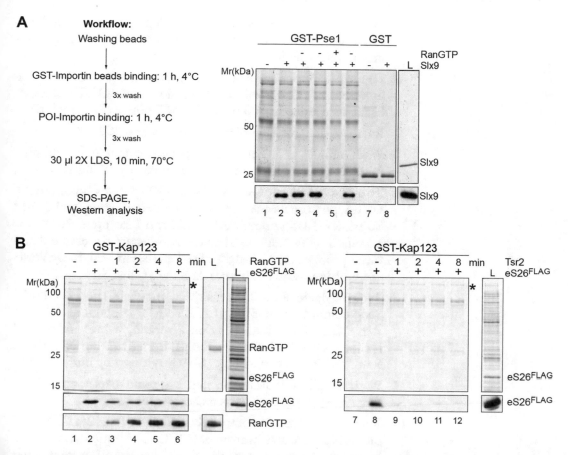

**Fig. 3** In vitro binding assays for nuclear import. (**a**) RanGTP-dependent release of Slx9 from Pse1 importin. Left panel: Workflow overview of the importin binding assay. POI = protein of interest. Right panel: GST–Pse1 complex formation with Slx9 dissociated in the RanGFP-dependent manner. GST–Pse1 (lanes 1–6) or GST alone (lanes 7–8) was immobilized on Glutathione Sepharose, washed with PBS-KMT and incubated with 4 μM Slx9 for 1 h at 4 °C (lanes 2–4 and 6). Pse1-Slx9 complex was subsequently incubated with 1.5 μM RanGTP under same conditions (lane 5). After washing with PBS-KMT, bound proteins were eluted in SDS sample buffer, separated by SDS-PAGE and visualized by Coomassie Blue staining and Western analyses using α-Slx9 antibodies. L = input. (**b**) RanGTP-independent release of eS26 from Kap123 importin. Immobilized GST-Kap123 on Glutathione Sepharose was washed and incubated with 4 μM eS26$^{FLAG}$ for 1 h at 4 °C. GST-Kap123:eS26$^{FLAG}$ complex was washed and incubated with either buffer alone (lane 2 and 8), 0.375 μM His$_6$-Ran$^{QL}$GTP (left panel lanes 3–6) or 0.375 μM His$_6$-Tsr2 (right panel lanes 9–12). Samples were withdrawn at the indicated time points and washed with PBS-KMT. Bound proteins were eluted in SDS sample buffer, separated by SDS-PAGE and visualized by Coomassie Blue staining and Western analyses using α-eS26 and α-RanGTP antibodies. L = input. GST-Kap123 is indicated by asterisk. (Adapted from Schütz et al. 2014)

6. Wash samples as indicated in **step 1** to remove unbound protein. Keep samples on ice between each washing step.

7. To assess the amount of GST-Pse1 or GST-alone bound to the GST-Sepharose beads remove supernatant completely. Add 30 μL 2× LDS sample buffer, mix and heat up at 70 °C for

10 min to elute the bound proteins. Separate the eluted denatured proteins on an 12–15% SDS-PAGE and analyze by Coomassie Blue staining.

8. To form an importin–protein complex, add 3–6 μM Slx9 to the immobilized GST-Pse1 or GST-alone on GSH-Sepharose beads suspended in 500 μL PBS-KMT buffer (from **step 6**).

9. Incubate on a rotating platform for 1 h at 4 °C.

10. Wash samples as indicated in **step 1** to remove unbound protein. Samples are kept on ice between each washing step.

11. To assess the amount of GST-Pse1–Slx9 complex bound to the GST-Sepharose beads remove supernatant completely. Add 30 μL 2× LDS sample buffer, mix and heat up at 70 °C for 10 min to elute the bound proteins. Separate the eluted denatured proteins on a 12–15% SDS-PAGE and analyze by Western blotting using antibodies directed against Slx9.

12. To investigate RanGTP sensitivity, incubate the GST-Pse1–Slx9 complex with 500 μL PBS-KMT containing 1.5 μM Ran$^{QL}$GTP for 1 h at 4 °C on a rotating wheel. In parallel incubate GST-Pse1–Slx9 in 500 μL PBS-KMT buffer without Ran$^{QL}$GTP to assess whether Slx9 is released by buffer alone.

13. Wash samples as indicated in **step 1** to remove released protein. Keep samples on ice between each washing step.

14. Remove supernatant completely, and add 30 μL 2× LDS sample buffer, mix and heat up at 70 °C for 10 min to elute the bound proteins. Separate the eluted denatured proteins on a 12–15% SDS-PAGE and analyze by Coomassie Blue staining and Western blotting using antibodies directed against Slx9.

### 3.2.2 Tsr2 Mediated Disassembly of a Kap123–eS26$^{FLAG}$ Complex (See Also Notes 9–14)

1. Pipet 50 μL of GSH-Sepharose slurry (per reaction) into a 1.5 mL reaction tube and wash 3 times with 1 mL PBS-KMT buffer, spin down in between for 30 s at 850 × *g*. Wash GSH-Sepharose beads for all reactions together.

2. Meanwhile thaw recombinant GST-Kap123 and GST-alone sample on ice.

3. Centrifuge the GST-Kap123 and GST-alone or lysates for 10 min at 4 °C at 16,000 × *g* to pellet aggregates and store the tubes on ice until use.

4. Add 12 μg GST-Kap123 or GST-alone to washed GSH-Sepharose beads suspended in 500 μL of PBS-KMT buffer.

5. Incubate on a rotating platform for 1 h at 4 °C to immobilize GST-Kap123 or GST-alone on GSH-Sepharose beads.

6. Wash samples as indicated in **step 1** to remove unbound protein. Keep samples on ice between each washing step.

7. The amount of GST-Kap123 or GST-alone bound to the GST-Sepharose beads can be assessed at this stage. For this, remove supernatant completely. Add 30 μL 2× LDS sample buffer, mix and heat up at 70 °C for 10 min to elute the bound proteins. Separate the eluted denatured proteins on a 12–15% SDS-PAGE and analyze by Coomassie Blue staining.

8. To form importin–protein incubate the immobilized GST-Pse1 or GST-alone on GSH-Sepharose beads with 3–6 μM eS26$^{FLAG}$ in 500 μL PBS-KMT buffer from **step 6**.

9. Incubate on a rotating platform for 1 h at 4 °C.

10. Wash samples as indicated in **step 1** to remove unbound protein. Samples are kept on ice between each washing step.

11. To assess the amount of GST-Kap123–eS26$^{FLAG}$ complex bound to the GST-Sepharose beads, remove supernatant completely. Add 30 μL 2× LDS sample buffer, mix and heat up at 70 °C for 10 min to elute the bound proteins. Separate the eluted denatured proteins on a 12–15% SDS-PAGE and analyze by Western blotting using antibodies directed against FLAG tag.

12. To investigate Tsr2 dependent disassembly of the complex from **step 10**, incubate the GST-Kap123–eS26$^{FLAG}$ complex with 500 μL PBS-KMT containing 1.5 μM Tsr2. In parallel, incubate GST-Kap123–eS26$^{FLAG}$ with 500 μL of PBS-KMT buffer as a control to assess whether eS26$^{FLAG}$, is released by buffer itself.

13. Wash samples as indicated in **step 1** to remove released protein. Keep samples on ice between each washing step.

14. Remove supernatant completely, and add 30 μL 2× LDS sample buffer, mix and heat up at 70 °C for 10 min to elute and denature the bound proteins. Separate the eluted denatured proteins on a 12–15% SDS-PAGE and analyze by Coomassie Blue staining and Western blotting using antibodies directed against FLAG tag.

*3.2.3 Cell Biological Assays for r-protein Nuclear Import*

It is complicated to monitor the nuclear targeting of r-proteins in vivo since at steady state they reside in the cytoplasm. Therefore, one strategy is to uncouple r-protein nuclear import from their export by selectively impairing recruitment to the pre-ribosome. Fusing GFP to either the N- or C- terminus can prevent r-protein incorporation into the pre-ribosome. These non-functional proxy constructs can be employed to determine nuclear localization signals within r-proteins [56]. Further, by monitoring their mislocalization to the cytoplasm in different importin-deficient (Table 1) and/or mutant strains, these non-functional r-protein fusions (listed in Table 3) can pinpoint their nuclear pathway(s).

**Table 1**
**Yeast strains used for ribosomal nuclear import studies**

| Name | Genotype | Source |
|------|----------|--------|
| *srp1-31/kap60-31 ts* | *MATa ade2-1ura3-1his3-11trpl-1leu2-3,112canJ-100A srp1:: LEU2 +316-srp1-31* | Yano et al. 1994 [61] |
| *srp1-54/kap60-54 ts* | *MATa ade2-1ura3-1his3-11trpl-1leu2-3,112canJ-100A srp1:: LEU2 +316-srp1-54* | Yano et al. 1994 [61] |
| *rsl1-1/kap95-1* | *MATα ura3-52 leu2delta1 ade2 ade3 rsl1-1 rna1-1 ts* | Koepp et al. 1996 [62] |
| *kap104Δ* | *MATα trp1 ura3 leu2 lys2 KAP104::HIS* | Aitchison et al. 1996 [63] |
| *sxm1Δ/kap108Δ* | *MATa ura3-52 his3Δ200 trp1-1 leu2-3,112 lys2-801 sxm1:: his3::TRP1* | Sydorskyy et al. 2003 [64] |
| *mtr10/kap111 shuffle* | *MATα, ade2, his3, leu2, trp1, ura3, mtr10:HIS3 +pRS316-URA3-MTR10* | Senger et al. 1998 [65] |
| *kap114Δ* | *MATα, ura3-52, leu2Δ1, his3Δ200, trp1Δ63, kap114::TRP1* | Greiner et al. 2004 [66] |
| *nmd5Δ/ kap119Δ* | *MATα ura3-52 his3Δ200 trp1-1 leu2-3,112 lys2-801 nmd5:: HIS3* | Sydorskyy et al. 2003 [64] |
| *kap120Δ* | *MATα ura3 leu2 his3 trp1 KAP120::TRP1* | Schlenstedt laboratory |
| *pse1-1/kap121-1* | *MATa leu2 trp1 URA3::pse1-1 PSE1::HIS3* | Seedorf et al. 1997 [67] |
| *pdr6Δ/kap122Δ* | *MATa ura3 his3 leu2 pdr6::KANMX* | Open Biosystems |
| *kap123Δ* | *MATα ura3 leu2 his3 KAP123::TRP1* | Schlenstedt et al. 1997 [68] |
| *msn5/kap142* | *MATa; ura3Δ0 leu2Δ0 his3Δ1 met15Δ0 delta-msn5::KANMX6* | Euroscarf |

**3.3  Nuclear Export Assays for Pre-ribosomes**

*3.3.1  Monitoring Nuclear Export of Pre-ribosomes (See Also Notes 15 and 16)*

Transport of 60S and 40S pre-ribosomes from the nucleus into the cytoplasm can be investigated by monitoring the localization of r-protein fusions with GFP (uL23-GFP, uL5-GFP, uL18-GFP for the 60S subunit and uS5-GFP for the 40S subunit) in distinct mutant strains [72–75]. These r-protein fusions are stably incorporated into pre-ribosomes, and their steady-state localization in wild type (WT) cells is cytoplasmic. Nuclear accumulation of these reporters indicates either an early pre-ribosome assembly and/or export defect. Next to the r-protein GFP reporters, nuclear accumulation of GFP fused export adaptor factors serve as reporters for impairment in late assembly steps and/or of export of 60S (Nmd3-GFP) and 40S (Rrp12-GFP and Rio2-GFP) pre-ribosomes, respectively (Fig. 4).

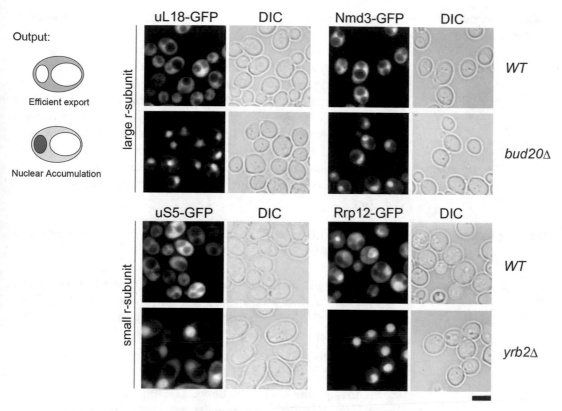

**Fig. 4** Monitoring ribosome export defect by fluorescence microscopy. GFP-reporters for large r-subunit (uL18-GFP or Nmd3-GFP) and small r-subunit (uS5-GFP or Rrp12-GFP) were transformed into WT or indicated mutant strains and they localization was analyzed by fluorescence microscopy. Scale bar = 5 μm. Output of the experiment is indicated on the left scheme: accumulation of the reporter in the nucleus in case of export defect as seen for *bud20Δ* and *yrb2Δ*

Method

1. Transform yeast strains with the reporter plasmids (uL18-GFP, uS5-GFP) and plate on appropriate media.

2. The transformants expressing reporters are grown in appropriate liquid media (for mutants at permissive temperature) until saturation (overnight).

3. The next day, dilute cells into 10 mL fresh media and grown until mid-log phase for at least 2–3 divisions. (In the case of cold or temperature sensitive mutants, shift the cultures to the appropriate restrictive temperature after 2–3 divisions of growth at permissive temperature).

4. Pellet cells by centrifugation in a 15 mL Falcon tube ( $450 \times g$, 3 min) and wash once with 10 mL dH$_2$O.

5. Pour off the supernatant and resuspend the cell pellet in remaining liquid.

6. Place 2 μL of cell suspension on a slide, press a coverslip over before inspection under a fluorescence microscope.

*3.3.2 Reconstitution of Crm1-Nuclear Export Complexes In Vitro*

In actively growing yeast cells, every minute ~25 pre-ribosomal particles are exported into the cytoplasm [2]. The exportin Crm1 (yeast Xpo1) plays an essential role in transporting pre-ribosomes into the cytoplasm. To initiate export, Crm1, in the presence of RanGTP recognizes a nuclear export signal (NES) on adaptor proteins bound to pre-ribosomes, and cooperatively forms a Crm1-export complex [1, 23, 24, 76, 77]. In vitro binding assay with recombinant Crm1 and Ran$^{QL}$ are used to analyze potential NES containing export adaptors of preribosomal subunits [58]. Here, using Ltv1:Crm1:Ran$^{QL}$GTP as an example to outline a protocol for assembly of a trimeric Crm1-export complex in vitro (Fig. 5a).

*Buffers and Solutions*

PBS-KMT buffer (pH 7.3): 150 mM NaCl, 25 mM sodium phosphate, 3 mMKCl, 1 mM MgCl$_2$ Tween-20.

*Method (See Also* **Notes 17–21***)*

1. Pipet 50 μL of GSH-Sepharose slurry (per reaction) into a 1.5 mL reaction tube and wash 3 times with 1 mL PBS-KMT buffer; spin down in between for 30 s at 850 × $g$. Wash GSH-Sepharose beads for all reactions together.

2. In meanwhile thaw GST-fusion proteins (GST-Ltv1, GST-Ltv1$^{\Delta NES}$) and GST sample on ice.

3. Centrifuge the GST-Ltv1 and GST-alone or lysates for 10 min at 4 °C at 16,000 × $g$ to pellet aggregated proteins and store the tubes on ice until use.

4. Add 12 μg GST-Ltv1 protein or GST-alone to washed GSH-Sepharose beads suspended in 500 μL PBS-KMT buffer.

5. Incubate on a rotating platform for 1 h at 4 °C to immobilize GST-Ltv1 and GST-alone on GSH-Sepharose beads.

6. Wash samples as indicated in **step 1** to remove unbound protein. Keep samples on ice between each washing step.

7. The amount of GST-Ltv1 or GST-alone bound to the GST-Sepharose beads can be assessed at this stage. For this, remove supernatant completely, add 30 μL 2× LDS sample buffer, mix and heat up at 70 °C for 10 min to elute the bound proteins. Separate the eluted denatured proteins on a 12–15% SDS-PAGE and analyze by Coomassie Blue staining.

8. Thaw on ice and centrifuge substrate proteins (Ran$^{QL}$GTP and Crm1) at 10 min at 4 °C at 16,000 × $g$ to pellet aggregated proteins.

9. Add simultaneously 2 μM Ran$^{QL}$GTP and 50 nM Crm1 to GSH-Sepharose beads immobilized GST-Ltv1 or GST-alone and suspended in 500 μL PBS-KMT buffer. In parallel, as controls, incubate immobilized GST-Ltv1 with Crm1 and Ran$^{QL}$GTP separately.

10. Incubate on a rotating platform for 1 h at 4 °C.

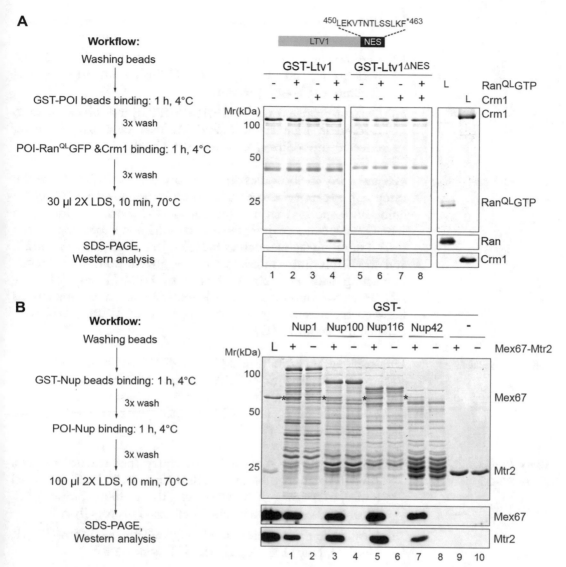

**Fig. 5** In vitro binding assays for nuclear export. (A) Ltv1 NES-dependent export complex formation. Left panel: Workflow overview of the binding assay. POI = protein of interest. Right panel: GST-Ltv1 or GST-Ltv1 lacking NES sequence (450-463aa) was immobilized on the Glutathione Sepharose, washed with PBS-KMT and incubated with buffer alone (lanes 1 and 5), buffer with 2μM His6-Ran$^{QL}$GTP (lanes 2 and 6), 50nM Crm1-His6 (lanes 3 and 7) or 50nM Crm1-His6 and 2μM His6-Ran$^{QL}$GTP simultaneously (lane 4 and 8) for 1h at 4°C. Bound proteins were washed with PBS-KMT, eluted in 2XLDS sample buffer, separated by SDS-PAGE and visualized by Coomassie Blue staining and Western analyses using α-RanGTP and α-Crm1 antibodies. L = input. Adapted from Fischer et al., 2015. (B) Heterodimeric transport receptor Mex67-Mtr2 interacts with FG repeat sequences of different nucleoporins. Left panel: Workflow overview of the binding assay. POI = protein of interest. Right panel: Indicated GST-Nucleoporin fusion proteins were immobilized on Glutathione Sepharose and washed with PBS-KMT before 1 h incubation with 3.6 μg His6-Mex67-Mtr2 at 4°C. Bound proteins were washed, eluted with 2X LDS buffer and analyzed by SDS-PAGE followed by Coomassie staining or Western blotting using α-Mex67/Mtr2 antibody. L = Load; Asterisks indicate Mex67 bands. Adapted from Altvater et al., 2012

11. Wash samples as indicated in **step 1** to remove unbound protein. Keep samples on ice between each washing step.

12. Remove supernatant completely. Add 30 μL 2× LDS sample buffer, mix, and heat up at 70 °C for 10 min to elute and denature the bound proteins.

13. Separate proteins on a 12–15% SDS-PAGE and subject them to Coomassie Blue staining and Western blot analysis using directed antibodies against Ran and Crm1.

*3.3.3 FG-Repeat Binding Assay*

40S and 60S pre-ribosomes are transported through NPC into the cytoplasm by export factors that interact transiently with FG-repeat lining nucleoporins that line the transport channel. In addition to RanGTP-dependent exportins such as Crm1 and Exp5 [23, 24, 78] several shuttling factors such as Mex67-Mtr2, Arx1, Ecm1, Bud20, and Rrp12 promote nuclear export of pre-ribosomes by directly interacting with FG-rich meshwork of NPC [1, 57, 71, 79–82]. Here, we outline a protocol that demonstrates interactions between the heterodimeric transport receptor Mex67-Mtr2 with FG-rich nucleoporins (Fig. 5b).

Buffers and Solutions

Universal buffer (Künzler and Hurt, 1998 [83]): 20 mM HEPES–KOH, pH 7.0, 100 mM KOAc, 2 mM Mg(OAc, 0,1% Tween 20, 10% glycerol. Supplemented with (*see* **Note 1**) 1 complete protease inhibitor cocktail tablet (Roche) per 100 mL 5 mM ß-mercaptoethanol.

Method (*See Also* **Notes 22–28**)

1. Wash 80 μL of GSH-Sepharose slurry (per reaction) into a 1.5 mL reaction tube and wash 3 times with 1 mL universal buffer; spin down in between for 30 s at 3000 rpm at 4 °C. Wash GSH-Sepharose beads for all reactions together.

2. Meanwhile thaw lysates containing GST-nucleoporins (Nup1, Nup100, Nup116, Nup42) or GST alone on ice.

3. Centrifuge the lysates for 10 min at 4 °C at 16,000 × $g$ to pellet aggregated proteins and store the tubes on ice until use.

4. Add 1 mL of each lysate to washed GSH-Sepharose beads (combine GSH-Sepharose beads for reactions with same GST-fusion protein) (*see* **Note 22**).

5. Incubate tubes on a rotating platform for 1 h at 4 °C to immobilize GST and GST fusion protein on GSH-Sepharose beads.

6. Wash samples 3× (850 × $g$, 30 s, 4 °C) with 1.5 mL universal buffer and resuspended in 1 mL buffer each.

7. Split beads, by pipetting 500 μL, into two new 1.5 mL eppendorf tubes.

8. Add 1–5 µg of recombinant affinity-purified His$_6$-tagged protein (3.6 µg for Mex67-Mtr2) or respective volume of buffer as negative control to the GST-/GST-nucleoporin-coated beads and fill up to 1 mL with universal buffer.

9. Incubate tubes on a rotating platform for 1 h at 4 °C.

10. Wash beads 3× (850 × $g$, 30s, 4 °C) with 1 mL universal buffer, remove supernatant completely. Elute the bound proteins by adding 80 µL 2× LDS buffer and heating at 70 °C for 10 min.

11. Spin down beads and analyze the supernatant by SDS-PAGE, Coomassie Blue staining and Western analysis using directed antibodies against Mex67-Mtr2 (*see* **Note 28**).

**3.4  Genetic Analyses of Nuclear Export**

Pre-ribosomal particles are among the largest and most abundant cargoes that need to cross the permeability barrier of the NPC. Rapid transit through the NPC is especially important, as any delay within the channel may hinder transport of other cargoes. Therefore, pre-ribosomal particles deploy a set of multiple redundant export receptors for their transport to the cytoplasm [1, 21]. High-copy suppressor screens and synthetic lethal interactions and in budding yeast have uncovered ancillary factors that also mediate efficient pre-ribosome nuclear export. These approaches have proved to be powerful tools to either discover new components of the ribosome export machinery or to directly test functional overlap of a factor of interest with the process of nuclear export.

The essential export adaptor Nmd3 was identified as a high copy suppressor of the *bud20Δ* mutant slow growth and 60S pre-ribosome export defect [72]. Further, the *bud20Δ* strain exhibits synthetic lethal or synthetic enhanced growth defects when combined with mutants of established 60S pre-ribosome export factors (*nmd3Δ NES1*, *xpo1-1*, *arx1Δ*, *gle2-1*, and *ecm1Δ*), included *mex67* and *mtr2* mutant alleles (*mex67kraa and mtr2-33*) that are specifically impaired in 60S subunit [72]. These analyses culminated in the discovery of new FG-repeat binding proteins that functions directly to the process of nuclear export of 60S pre-ribosomes.

Similarly, a high-copy suppressor screen aimed at identifying genes that suppress the impaired growth of the *slx9Δ* mutant, led to the discovery of the mRNA and 60S export receptor Mex67-Mtr2 as an auxiliary export receptor for in 40S pre-ribosome export [57]. Mex67-Mtr2 mutants that fail to bind to the 40S pre-ribosome were synthetically lethal when combined with the *slx9Δ* mutant [57]. Further, the *slx9Δ* mutant displayed a synthetic growth defect when combined with a strain expressing Rrp12-GFP.

**Table 2**
**Yeast strains used for ribosomal nuclear export studies**

| Name | Genotype | Source |
|------|----------|--------|
| arx1Δ | MATa ura3 his3 leu2 arx1::KANMX6 | Open Biosystems |
| bud20Δ | MATa ura3 his3 leu2 met15 TRP1 bud20::KANMX | Altvater et al. 2012 [72] |
| ecm1Δ | MATa ura3 his3 leu2 met15 ecm1::KANMX6 | Open Biosystems |
| gle2-1 | MATα gle2-1 ade2-1 ADE3 ura3-1 his3-11,15 leu2-3,112 trpl-1 LYS2 canl-100 | Murphy et al. 1996 [84] |
| mex67 shuffle | MATα ura3 leu2 trp1 mex67::HIS3MX +pRS316-MEX67 | Occhipinti et al. 2013 [25] |
| mtr2 shuffle | MATa ura3 his3 leu2 trp1 ade2 mtr2::HIS3MX +pRS316-MTR2 | Santos-Rosa et al. 1998 [85] |
| nmd3 shuffle | MATa ura3 his3 leu2 met15 delta-nmd3::KANMX6 +pRS316-NMD3 | Panse laboratory |
| slx9Δ | MATα ura3 his3 leu2 TRP1 slx9::KANMX | Faza et al. 2012 [57] |
| yrb2Δ | MATa his3 leu2 ura3 yrb2::KANMX6 | Open Biosystems |

Rrp12 is a 40S pre-ribosome export factor that directly interacts with FG-rich nucleoporins [79]. Finally, Yrb2 that stimulate the assembly of Crm1-export complexes on certain NES-containing cargos by cooperatively binding Crm1 and RanGTP also showed a strong genetic interaction with Slx9 [57]. This genetic link culminated in the identification of a new type of RanGTP binding protein that binds to a specific NES-containing cargo and RanGTP and promotes Crm1 recruitment.

Tables 2 and 3 provide a comprehensive list of mutants and their sources to investigate 60S and 40S preribosome export using standard yeast genetic approaches.

# 4  Conclusions

Diverse approaches in budding yeast have greatly advanced our understanding of ribosome assembly and transport. Genetic perturbation of energy-consuming enzymes can now be combined with biochemical affinity purifications to obtain high-resolution snapshots of the ribosome assembly pathway. We also anticipate that traditional genetic, biochemical, and cell-biological approaches will provide eagerly awaited integration of the ribosome pathway with other biological pathways including nucleocytoplasmic transport, cellular quality control and signaling.

**Table 3**
**Plasmids for genetic studies of nucleo-cytoplasmic transport**

| Name | Description | Source |
|---|---|---|
| pRS425-*ARX1* | *ARX1 2μ LEU2 AMPR* | Panse laboratory |
| pRS426-*BUD20* | *BUD20 2μ URA3 AMPR* | Panse laboratory |
| pRS426-*ECM1* | *ECM1 2μ URA3 AMPR* | Panse laboratory |
| pRS425-*GLE2* | *GLE2 2μ LEU2 AMPR* | Panse laboratory |
| pRS425-*KAP114* | *KAP114 2μ LEU2 AMPR* | Panse laboratory |
| pRS426-MEX67 | *MEX67 2μ URA3 AMPR* | Hung et al. 2008 [69] |
| pRS425-*MTR2* | *MTR2 2μ LEU2 AMPR* | Panse laboratory |
| pRS426-*NMD3* | *NMD3 2μ URA3 AMPR* | Panse laboratory |
| pRS426-*RRP12* | *RRP12 2μ URA3 AMPR* | Panse laboratory |
| pRS425-*SLX9* | *SLX9 2μ LEU2 AMPR* | Panse laboratory |
| pRS425-*YRB2* | *YRB2 2μ LEU2 AMPR* | Panse laboratory |
| pRS426-*XPO1/CRM1* | *XPO1/CRM1 2μ URA3 AMPR* | Hung et al. 2008 [69] |
| pRS315-*mex67ΔC1* | *mex67(Δ525-599aa) CEN LEU2 AMPR* | Strässer et al. 2000 [70] |
| pRS314-*mex67Δloop* | *mex67(Δ409-435aa) CEN TRP1 AMPR* | Yao et al. 2007 [71] |
| pRS314-*mtr2Δloop* | *mtr2(Δ116-137aa) CEN TRP1 AMPR* | Yao et al. 2007 [71] |
| pRS314-*nmd3ΔNES1* | *nmd3ΔNES1 CEN TRP1 AMPR* | Yao et al. 2007 [71] |
| pRS315-*rio2ΔNES* | *rio2ΔNES CEN LEU2 AMPR* | Fischer et al. 2015 [58] |
| pRS315-*slx9-1* | *slx9-1 CEN LEU2 AMPR* | Fischer et al. 2015 [58] |

# 5    Notes

1. Add just before use.

2. Outlined below is a step-by-step protocol to lyse frozen yeast noodles using a planetary ball mill (Pulverisette 6, Fritsch).

3. You MUST hear the balls rattling around in the jar!
   *If there is no rattling*: add or remove balls to the jar until you hear it rattle. It is not considered a grinding cycle unless there is rattling.

4. Typically, ~90% of yeast cells can be disrupted in such procedure.

5. Use cryoprotective gloves for harvesting cells.

6. Work on ice or cold room as much as possible.

7. Prepare powder stock from big culture, store at −80 °C and weight only necessary amount for an experiment.

8. The M-IgG beads are prepared by conjugation of Dynabeads (Invitrogen) with rabbit IgG (Sigma) according to the standard protocol.

9. Plasmids encoding GST-Kap123 and GST-Pse1 [86], $Ran^{QL}$GTP mutant [87] originate from Schlenstedt laboratory. Slx9 [58] and $eS26^{Flag}$ ($His_6$-$eS26^{FLAG}$; [56]) can be requested from Panse laboratory.

10. GST recombinant proteins were expressed in *E.coli* and lysed in PBS-KMT (150 mM NaCl, 25 mM sodium phosphate, 3 mM KCl, 1 mM MgCl2, 0.1% Tween, pH 7.3) buffer. His-tagged proteins were purified in buffer containing 50 mM HEPES pH 7.5, 50 mM NaCl, 10% glycerol. It is possible to use directly *E.coli* lysates containing recombinant proteins without purification steps [56, 86]. $His_6$-tagged importins and $Ran^{QL}$GTP ($His_6$-Gsp1Q71L-GTP) were expressed and purified as previously described [86–88].

11. To prepare *E. coli* lysate BL21 cells was grown overnight in 100 mL LB media at 37 °C and 220 rpm. Diluted in 1 l of LB media to $OD_{600}$ 0.2 and again incubated at the same condition. Cells were harvest at logarithmic growth phase and resuspended in PBS-KMT. After cell lysis and centrifugation supernatant is used for the experiment.

12. To prevent unspecific interactions with GST-tagged proteins or GST it is possible to add *E. coli* lysate to the incubation reaction (100 μL is usually sufficient).

13. The Ran protein mutant used in this assay, $Ran^{QL}$ (Gsp1Q71L), is a GTPase deficient mutant originating from Schlenstedt laboratory. $His_6$-$Ran^{QL}$ is stored in KPi buffer (24.8 mM $KH_2PO_4$, 25 mM, $K_2HPO_4$, 20 mM KCl, 5 mM $MgCl_2$, 2 mM imidazole, 5 mM β-mercaptoethanol, pH 6.8).

14. Antibodies against FLAG tag are commercially available reagent from Sigma (F1804).

15. This assay can be performed with strains containing the reporters growing on solid selective media. In this case, strains typically in stationary phase, are spread on fresh YPD plates to induce ribosome production. After growing the cells for 4–8 h at the appropriate temperature, cells can be scraped from plate using an inoculation loop, mixed with 2 μL $H_2O$ placed on a glass slide and analyzed under a fluorescence microscope.

16. The uL23-GFP and uS5-GFP reporter plasmids with different selection markers (LEU2, URA3, TRP1, and HIS3) originate from the Hurt laboratory [73, 74], the uL5-GFP reporter (LEU2) originates from the Silver laboratory [75], and the

uL18-GFP reporter plasmids (LEU2, URA3, TRP1 and HIS3) can be requested from the Panse laboratory [72]. All the above reporters are expressed under the endogenous promoters. The ribosomal protein uL18 can be C-terminally tagged with GFP at the genomic locus for monitoring the nuclear export of the large pre-ribosomal subunit.

17. Plasmids for yeast Crm1 (Xpo1-His$_6$) and Ran$^{QL}$ mutant (His$_6$-Gsp1Q71L) originate from Schlenstedt lab [87], GST-Ltv1 and GST-Ltv1$^{\Delta NES}$ can be requested from Panse lab [58].

18. Recombinant proteins were expressed in *E. coli* and either purified in PBS-KMT or used as lysate.

19. GST-tagged proteins and His$_6$-Gsp1Q71L was expressed in *E. coli* as described in [87, 88]. Crm1-His$_6$ was expressed in *E. coli* as described in [58]. GST, GST-Ltv1 and GST-Ltv1$^{\Delta NES}$, and Crm1-His$_6$ proteins are stored in PBS-KMT buffer. His$_6$-Gsp1Q71L is stored in KPi buffer (24.8 mM KH$_2$PO$_4$, 25 mM, K$_2$HPO$_4$, 20 mM KCl, 5 mM MgCl$_2$, 2 mM imidazole, 5 mM β-mercaptoethanol, pH 6.8).

20. To prevent unspecific interactions with GST-tagged proteins or GST it is possible to add *E.coli* lysate to the incubation reaction (100 μL is usually sufficient).

21. Antibodies against Ran and Crm1 can be requested in Panse laboratory.

22. For the load: Respective amount of affinity-purified His$_6$-tagged Mex67-Mtr2 is added to final 100 μL 2× LDS, heated at 70 °C for 10 min.

23. All the steps should be carried out at 4 °C or on ice.

24. Cut pipette tip when pipetting beads.

25. Recombinant His$_6$-tagged protein (Mex67-Mtr2) was expressed in BL21 *E. coli* strain, lysed by sonication in lysis buffer (500 mM NaCl, 20 mM Tris–HCl pH 8.0, 0.1% Triton X-100, 1 mM PMSF) and purified using Ni-Sepharose (GE Healthcare) following a standard protocol.

26. The lysates containing GST-tagged nucleoporins (Nup1, Nup100, Nup116, Nup42) or GST alone were expressed in BL21 *E. coli* strain lysed by sonication in universal buffer.

27. Due to different expression levels, different volumes of GST-NUPs lysates may need to be used to uniformly load GSH-Sepharose beads.

28. The antibody directed against Mex67-Mtr2 can be requested from the Panse laboratory [72].

## Acknowledgments

V.G.P. is supported by grants from the Swiss National Science Foundation, the NCCR RNA & Disease, the Novartis Foundation and the Olga Mayenfisch Stiftung. M.O-O. is a recipient of a doctoral fellowship from the Boehringer Ingelheim Fonds.

## References

1. Pena C, Hurt E, Panse VG (2017) Eukaryotic ribosome assembly, transport and quality control. Nat Struct Mol Biol 24:689–699

2. Warner JR (1999) The economics of ribosome biosynthesis in yeast. Trends Biochem Sci 24:437–440

3. Kressler D, Hurt E, Bassler J (2017) A puzzle of life: crafting ribosomal subunits. Trends Biochem Sci 42:640–654

4. Kornprobst M, Turk M, Kellner N, Cheng J, Flemming D, Kos-Braun I, Kos M, Thoms M, Berninghausen O, Beckmann R, Hurt E (2016) Architecture of the 90S pre-ribosome: a structural view on the birth of the eukaryotic ribosome. Cell 166:380–393

5. Cheng J, Kellner N, Berninghausen O, Hurt E, Beckmann R (2017) 3.2-A-resolution structure of the 90S preribosome before A1 pre-rRNA cleavage. Nat Struct Mol Biol 24:954–964

6. Sun Q, Zhu X, Qi J, An W, Lan P, Tan D, Chen R, Wang B, Zheng S, Zhang C, Chen X, Zhang W, Chen J, Dong MQ, Ye K (2017) Molecular architecture of the 90S small subunit pre-ribosome. elife 6:e22086

7. Chaker-Margot M, Barandun J, Hunziker M, Klinge S (2017) Architecture of the yeast small subunit processome. Science 355:eaal1880

8. Osheim YN, French SL, Keck KM, Champion EA, Spasov K, Dragon F, Baserga SJ, Beyer AL (2004) Pre-18S ribosomal RNA is structurally compacted into the SSU processome prior to being cleaved from nascent transcripts in Saccharomyces cerevisiae. Mol Cell 16:943–954

9. Kos M, Tollervey D (2010) Yeast pre-rRNA processing and modification occur cotranscriptionally. Mol Cell 37:809–820

10. Billy E, Wegierski T, Nasr F, Filipowicz W (2000) Rcl1p, the yeast protein similar to the RNA 3′-phosphate cyclase, associates with U3 snoRNP and is required for 18S rRNA biogenesis. EMBO J 19:2115–2126

11. Horn DM, Mason SL, Karbstein K (2011) Rcl1 protein, a novel nuclease for 18 S ribosomal RNA production. J Biol Chem 286:34082–34087

12. Sardana R, Liu X, Granneman S, Zhu J, Gill M, Papoulas O, Marcotte EM, Tollervey D, Correll CC, Johnson AW (2015) The DEAH-box helicase Dhr1 dissociates U3 from the pre-rRNA to promote formation of the central pseudoknot. PLoS Biol 13:e1002083

13. Zhu J, Liu X, Anjos M, Correll CC, Johnson AW (2016) Utp14 recruits and activates the RNA helicase Dhr1 to undock U3 snoRNA from the Preribosome. Mol Cell Biol 36:965–978

14. Thoms M, Thomson E, Bassler J, Gnadig M, Griesel S, Hurt E (2015) The exosome is recruited to RNA substrates through specific adaptor proteins. Cell 162:1029–1038

15. Kater L, Thoms M, Barrio-Garcia C, Cheng J, Ismail S, Ahmed YL, Bange G, Kressler D, Berninghausen O, Sinning I, Hurt E, Beckmann R (2017) Visualizing the assembly pathway of nucleolar pre-60S ribosomes. Cell 171(1599–1610):e14

16. Sanghai ZA, Miller L, Molloy KR, Barandun J, Hunziker M, Chaker-Margot M, Wang J, Chait BT, Klinge S (2018) Modular assembly of the nucleolar pre-60S ribosomal subunit. Nature 556:126–129

17. Zhou D, Zhu X, Zheng S, Tan D, Dong MQ, Ye K (2019) Cryo-EM structure of an early precursor of large ribosomal subunit reveals a half-assembled intermediate. Protein Cell 10:120–130

18. Winey M, Yarar D, Giddings TH Jr, Mastronarde DN (1997) Nuclear pore complex number and distribution throughout the Saccharomyces cerevisiae cell cycle by three-dimensional reconstruction from electron micrographs of nuclear envelopes. Mol Biol Cell 8:2119–2132

19. Stade K, Ford CS, Guthrie C, Weis K (1997) Exportin 1 (Crm1p) is an essential nuclear export factor. Cell 90:1041–1050

20. Neville M, Rosbash M (1999) The NES-Crm1p export pathway is not a major mRNA export route in Saccharomyces cerevisiae. EMBO J 18:3746–3756

21. Nerurkar P, Altvater M, Gerhardy S, Schutz S, Fischer U, Weirich C, Panse VG (2015) Eukaryotic ribosome assembly and nuclear export. Int Rev Cell Mol Biol 319:107–140

22. Gerhardy S, Menet AM, Pena C, Petkowski JJ, Panse VG (2014) Assembly and nuclear export of pre-ribosomal particles in budding yeast. Chromosoma 123:327–344

23. Ho JH, Kallstrom G, Johnson AW (2000) Nmd3p is a Crm1p-dependent adapter protein for nuclear export of the large ribosomal subunit. J Cell Biol 151:1057–1066

24. Gadal O, Strauss D, Kessl J, Trumpower B, Tollervey D, Hurt E (2001) Nuclear export of 60s ribosomal subunits depends on Xpo1p and requires a nuclear export sequence-containing factor, Nmd3p, that associates with the large subunit protein Rpl10p. Mol Cell Biol 21:3405–3415

25. Occhipinti L, Chang Y, Altvater M, Menet AM, Kemmler S, Panse VG (2013) Non-FG mediated transport of the large pre-ribosomal subunit through the nuclear pore complex by the mRNA export factor Gle2. Nucleic Acids Res 41:8266–8279

26. Panse VG, Johnson AW (2010) Maturation of eukaryotic ribosomes: acquisition of functionality. Trends Biochem Sci 35:260–266

27. Strunk BS, Loucks CR, Su M, Vashisth H, Cheng S, Schilling J, Brooks CL 3rd, Karbstein K, Skiniotis G (2011) Ribosome assembly factors prevent premature translation initiation by 40S assembly intermediates. Science 333:1449–1453

28. Strunk BS, Novak MN, Young CL, Karbstein K (2012) A translation-like cycle is a quality control checkpoint for maturing 40S ribosome subunits. Cell 150:111–121

29. Lebaron S, Schneider C, van Nues RW, Swiatkowska A, Walsh D, Bottcher B, Granneman S, Watkins NJ, Tollervey D (2012) Proofreading of pre-40S ribosome maturation by a translation initiation factor and 60S subunits. Nat Struct Mol Biol 19:744–753

30. Scaiola A, Pena C, Weisser M, Bohringer D, Leibundgut M, Klingauf-Nerurkar P, Gerhardy S, Panse VG, Ban N (2018) Structure of a eukaryotic cytoplasmic pre-40S ribosomal subunit. EMBO J 37:e98499

31. Heuer A, Thomson E, Schmidt C, Berninghausen O, Becker T, Hurt E, Beckmann R (2017) Cryo-EM structure of a late pre-40S ribosomal subunit from Saccharomyces cerevisiae. elife 6:e30189

32. Zhou Y, Musalgaonkar S, Johnson AW, Taylor DW (2019) Tightly-orchestrated rearrangements govern catalytic center assembly of the ribosome. Nat Commun 10:958

33. Rigaut G, Shevchenko A, Rutz B, Wilm M, Mann M, Seraphin B (1999) A generic protein purification method for protein complex characterization and proteome exploration. Nat Biotechnol 17:1030–1032

34. Bassler J, Grandi P, Gadal O, Lessmann T, Petfalski E, Tollervey D, Lechner J, Hurt E (2001) Identification of a 60S preribosomal particle that is closely linked to nuclear export. Mol Cell 8:517–529

35. Harnpicharnchai P, Jakovljevic J, Horsey E, Miles T, Roman J, Rout M, Meagher D, Imai B, Guo Y, Brame CJ, Shabanowitz J, Hunt DF, Woolford JL Jr (2001) Composition and functional characterization of yeast 66S ribosome assembly intermediates. Mol Cell 8:505–515

36. Grandi P, Rybin V, Bassler J, Petfalski E, Strauss D, Marzioch M, Schafer T, Kuster B, Tschochner H, Tollervey D, Gavin AC, Hurt E (2002) 90S pre-ribosomes include the 35S pre-rRNA, the U3 snoRNP, and 40S subunit processing factors but predominantly lack 60S synthesis factors. Mol Cell 10:105–115

37. Dragon F, Gallagher JE, Compagnone-Post PA, Mitchell BM, Porwancher KA, Wehner KA, Wormsley S, Settlage RE, Shabanowitz J, Osheim Y, Beyer AL, Hunt DF, Baserga SJ (2002) A large nucleolar U3 ribonucleoprotein required for 18S ribosomal RNA biogenesis. Nature 417:967–970

38. Fatica A, Cronshaw AD, Dlakic M, Tollervey D (2002) Ssf1p prevents premature processing of an early pre-60S ribosomal particle. Mol Cell 9:341–351

39. Nissan TA, Bassler J, Petfalski E, Tollervey D, Hurt E (2002) 60S pre-ribosome formation viewed from assembly in the nucleolus until export to the cytoplasm. EMBO J 21:5539–5547

40. Schafer T, Strauss D, Petfalski E, Tollervey D, Hurt E (2003) The path from nucleolar 90S to cytoplasmic 40S pre-ribosomes. EMBO J 22:1370–1380

41. Greber BJ, Gerhardy S, Leitner A, Leibundgut M, Salem M, Boehringer D, Leulliot N, Aebersold R, Panse VG, Ban N

(2016) Insertion of the biogenesis factor Rei1 probes the ribosomal tunnel during 60S maturation. Cell 164:91–102

42. Ma C, Wu S, Li N, Chen Y, Yan K, Li Z, Zheng L, Lei J, Woolford JL Jr, Gao N (2017) Structural snapshot of cytoplasmic pre-60S ribosomal particles bound by Nmd3, Lsg1, Tif6 and Reh1. Nat Struct Mol Biol 24: 214–220

43. Oeffinger M, Wei KE, Rogers R, DeGrasse JA, Chait BT, Aitchison JD, Rout MP (2007) Comprehensive analysis of diverse ribonucleoprotein complexes. Nat Methods 4:951–956

44. Pillet B, Mitterer V, Kressler D, Pertschy B (2017) Hold on to your friends: dedicated chaperones of ribosomal proteins: dedicated chaperones mediate the safe transfer of ribosomal proteins to their site of pre-ribosome incorporation. BioEssays 39:1–12

45. Eisinger DP, Dick FA, Denke E, Trumpower BL (1997) SQT1, which encodes an essential WD domain protein of Saccharomyces cerevisiae, suppresses dominant-negative mutations of the ribosomal protein gene QSR1. Mol Cell Biol 17:5146–5155

46. Iouk TL, Aitchison JD, Maguire S, Wozniak RW (2001) Rrb1p, a yeast nuclear WD-repeat protein involved in the regulation of ribosome biosynthesis. Mol Cell Biol 21:1260–1271

47. Schaper S, Fromont-Racine M, Linder P, de la Cruz J, Namane A, Yaniv M (2001) A yeast homolog of chromatin assembly factor 1 is involved in early ribosome assembly. Curr Biol 11:1885–1890

48. West M, Hedges JB, Chen A, Johnson AW (2005) Defining the order in which Nmd3p and Rpl10p load onto nascent 60S ribosomal subunits. Mol Cell Biol 25:3802–3813

49. Koch B, Mitterer V, Niederhauser J, Stanborough T, Murat G, Rechberger G, Bergler H, Kressler D, Pertschy B (2012) Yar1 protects the ribosomal protein Rps3 from aggregation. J Biol Chem 287:21806–21815

50. Kressler D, Bange G, Ogawa Y, Stjepanovic G, Bradatsch B, Pratte D, Amlacher S, Strauss D, Yoneda Y, Katahira J, Sinning I, Hurt E (2012) Synchronizing nuclear import of ribosomal proteins with ribosome assembly. Science 338: 666–671

51. Stelter P, Huber FM, Kunze R, Flemming D, Hoelz A, Hurt E (2015) Coordinated ribosomal L4 protein assembly into the pre-ribosome is regulated by its eukaryote-specific extension. Mol Cell 58:854–862

52. Pillet B, Garcia-Gomez JJ, Pausch P, Falquet L, Bange G, de la Cruz J, Kressler D (2015) The dedicated chaperone Acl4 escorts ribosomal protein Rpl4 to its nuclear pre-60S assembly site. PLoS Genet 11:e1005565

53. Pausch P, Singh U, Ahmed YL, Pillet B, Murat G, Altegoer F, Stier G, Thoms M, Hurt E, Sinning I, Bange G, Kressler D (2015) Co-translational capturing of nascent ribosomal proteins by their dedicated chaperones. Nat Commun 6:7494

54. Rossler I, Embacher J, Pillet B, Murat G, Liesinger L, Hafner J, Unterluggauer JJ, Birner-Gruenberger R, Kressler D, Pertschy B (2019) Tsr4 and Nap1, two novel members of the ribosomal protein chaperOME. Nucleic Acids Res 47(13):6984–7002. https://doi.org/10.1093/nar/gkz317

55. Black JJ, Musalgaonkar S, Johnson AW (2019) Tsr4 is a cytoplasmic chaperone for the ribosomal protein Rps2 in Saccharomyces cerevisiae. Mol Cell Biol 39:e00094-19. https://doi.org/10.1128/MCB.00094-19

56. Schutz S, Fischer U, Altvater M, Nerurkar P, Pena C, Gerber M, Chang Y, Caesar S, Schubert OT, Schlenstedt G, Panse VG (2014) A RanGTP-independent mechanism allows ribosomal protein nuclear import for ribosome assembly. elife 3:e03473

57. Faza MB, Chang Y, Occhipinti L, Kemmler S, Panse VG (2012) Role of Mex67-Mtr2 in the nuclear export of 40S pre-ribosomes. PLoS Genet 8:e1002915

58. Fischer U, Schauble N, Schutz S, Altvater M, Chang Y, Faza MB, Panse VG (2015) A non-canonical mechanism for Crm1-export cargo complex assembly. elife 4:e05745

59. Bax R, Raue HA, Vos JC (2006) Slx9p facilitates efficient ITS1 processing of pre-rRNA in *Saccharomyces cerevisiae*. RNA 12:2005–2013

60. Li Z, Lee I, Moradi E, Hung NJ, Johnson AW, Marcotte EM (2009) Rational extension of the ribosome biogenesis pathway using network-guided genetics. PLoS Biol 7:e1000213

61. Yano R, Oakes ML, Tabb MM, Nomura M (1994) Yeast Srp1p has homology to armadillo/plakoglobin/beta-catenin and participates in apparently multiple nuclear functions including the maintenance of the nucleolar structure. Proc Natl Acad Sci U S A 91:6880–6884

62. Koepp DM, Wong DH, Corbett AH, Silver PA (1996) Dynamic localization of the nuclear import receptor and its interactions with transport factors. J Cell Biol 133:1163–1176

63. Aitchison JD, Blobel G, Rout MP (1996) Kap104p: a karyopherin involved in the nuclear transport of messenger RNA binding proteins. Science 274:624–627

64. Sydorskyy Y, Dilworth DJ, Yi EC, Goodlett DR, Wozniak RW, Aitchison JD (2003) Intersection of the Kap123p-mediated nuclear import and ribosome export pathways. Mol Cell Biol 23:2042–2054

65. Senger B, Simos G, Bischoff FR, Podtelejnikov A, Mann M, Hurt E (1998) Mtr10p functions as a nuclear import receptor for the mRNA-binding protein Npl3p. EMBO J 17:2196–2207

66. Greiner M, Caesar S, Schlenstedt G (2004) The histones H2A/H2B and H3/H4 are imported into the yeast nucleus by different mechanisms. Eur J Cell Biol 83:511–520

67. Seedorf M, Silver PA (1997) Importin/karyopherin protein family members required for mRNA export from the nucleus. Proc Natl Acad Sci U S A 94:8590–8595

68. Schlenstedt G, Smirnova E, Deane R, Solsbacher J, Kutay U, Görlich D, Ponstingl H, Bischoff FR (1997) Yrb4p, a yeast ran-GTP-binding protein involved in import of ribosomal protein L25 into the nucleus. EMBO J 16:6237–6249

69. Hung NJ, Lo KY, Patel SS, Helmke K, Johnson AW (2008) Arx1 is a nuclear export receptor for the 60S ribosomal subunit in yeast. Mol Biol Cell 19:735–744

70. Strasser K, Bassler J, Hurt E (2000) Binding of the Mex67p/Mtr2p heterodimer to FXFG, GLFG, and FG repeat nucleoporins is essential for nuclear mRNA export. J Cell Biol 150:695–706

71. Yao W, Roser D, Kohler A, Bradatsch B, Bassler J, Hurt E (2007) Nuclear export of ribosomal 60S subunits by the general mRNA export receptor Mex67-Mtr2. Mol Cell 26:51–62

72. Altvater M, Chang Y, Melnik A, Occhipinti L, Schütz S, Rothenbusch U, Picotti P, Panse VG (2012) Targeted proteomics reveals compositional dynamics of 60S pre-ribosomes after nuclear export. Mol Syst Biol 8:628

73. Hurt E, Hannus S, Schmelzl B, Lau D, Tollervey D, Simos G (1999) A novel in vivo assay reveals inhibition of ribosomal nuclear export in Ran-cycle and nucleoporin mutants. J Cell Biol 144:389–401

74. Milkereit P, Strauss D, Bassler J, Gadal O, Kühn H, Schütz S, Gas N, Lechner J, Hurt E, Tschochner H (2003) A Noc complex specifically involved in the formation and nuclear export of ribosomal 40 S subunits. J Biol Chem 278:4072–4081

75. Stage-Zimmermann T, Schmidt U, Silver PA (2000) Factors affecting nuclear export of the 60S ribosomal subunit in vivo. Mol Biol Cell 11:3777–3789

76. Seiser RM, Sundberg AE, Wollam BJ, Zobel-Thropp P, Baldwin K, Spector MD, Lycan DE (2006) Ltv1 is required for efficient nuclear export of the ribosomal small subunit in Saccharomyces cerevisiae. Genetics 174:679–691

77. Zemp I, Wild T, O'Donohue MF, Wandrey F, Widmann B, Gleizes PE, Kutay U (2009) Distinct cytoplasmic maturation steps of 40S ribosomal subunit precursors require hRio2. J Cell Biol 185:1167–1180

78. Wild T, Horvath P, Wyler E, Widmann B, Badertscher L, Zemp I, Kozak K, Csucs G, Lund E, Kutay U (2010) A protein inventory of human ribosome biogenesis reveals an essential function of exportin 5 in 60S subunit export. PLoS Biol 8:e1000522

79. Oeffinger M, Dlakic M, Tollervey D (2004) A pre-ribosome-associated HEAT-repeat protein is required for export of both ribosomal subunits. Genes Dev 18:196–209

80. Bradatsch B, Katahira J, Kowalinski E, Bange G, Yao W, Sekimoto T, Baumgartel V, Boese G, Bassler J, Wild K, Peters R, Yoneda Y, Sinning I, Hurt E (2007) Arx1 functions as an unorthodox nuclear export receptor for the 60S preribosomal subunit. Mol Cell 27:767–779

81. Yao Y, Demoinet E, Saveanu C, Lenormand P, Jacquier A, Fromont-Racine M (2010) Ecm1 is a new pre-ribosomal factor involved in pre-60S particle export. RNA 16:1007–1017

82. Bassler J, Klein I, Schmidt C, Kallas M, Thomson E, Wagner MA, Bradatsch B, Rechberger G, Strohmaier H, Hurt E, Bergler H (2012) The conserved Bud20 zinc finger protein is a new component of the ribosomal

60S subunit export machinery. Mol Cell Biol 32:4898–4912

83. Kunzler M, Hurt EC (1998) Cse1p functions as the nuclear export receptor for importin alpha in yeast. FEBS Lett 433:185–190

84. Murphy R, Watkins JL, Wente SR (1996) GLE2, a Saccharomyces cerevisiae homologue of the *Schizosaccharomyces pombe* export factor RAE1, is required for nuclear pore complex structure and function. Mol Biol Cell 7:1921–1937

85. Santos-Rosa H, Moreno H, Simos G, Segref A, Fahrenkrog B, Pante N, Hurt E (1998) Nuclear mRNA export requires complex formation between Mex67p and Mtr2p at the nuclear pores. Mol Cell Biol 18:6826–6838

86. Fries T, Betz C, Sohn K, Caesar S, Schlenstedt G, Bailer SM (2007) A novel conserved nuclear localization signal is recognized by a group of yeast importins. J Biol Chem 282:19292–19301

87. Maurer P, Redd M, Solsbacher J, Bischoff FR, Greiner M, Podtelejnikov AV, Mann M, Stade K, Weis K, Schlenstedt G (2001) The nuclear export receptor Xpo1p forms distinct complexes with NES transport substrates and the yeast Ran binding protein 1 (Yrb1p). Mol Biol Cell 12:539–549

88. Solsbacher J, Maurer P, Bischoff FR, Schlenstedt G (1998) Cse1p is involved in export of yeast importin alpha from the nucleus. Mol Cell Biol 18:6805–6815

# Chapter 8

# Tethered MNase Structure Probing as Versatile Technique for Analyzing RNPs Using Tagging Cassettes for Homologous Recombination in *Saccharomyces cerevisiae*

Fabian Teubl, Katrin Schwank, Uli Ohmayer, Joachim Griesenbeck, Herbert Tschochner, and Philipp Milkereit

## Abstract

Micrococcal nuclease (MNase) originating from *Staphylococcus aureus* is a calcium dependent ribo- and desoxyribonuclease which has endo- and exonucleolytic activity of low sequence preference. MNase is widely used to analyze nucleosome positions in chromatin by probing the enzyme's DNA accessibility in limited digestion reactions. Probing reactions can be performed in a global way by addition of exogenous MNase, or locally by "chromatin endogenous cleavage" (ChEC) reactions using MNase fusion proteins. The latter approach has recently been adopted for the analysis of local RNA environments of MNase fusion proteins which are incorporated in vivo at specific sites of ribonucleoprotein (RNP) complexes. In this case, ex vivo activation of MNase by addition of calcium leads to RNA cleavages in proximity to the tethered anchor protein thus providing information about the folding state of its RNA environment.

Here, we describe a set of plasmids that can be used as template for PCR-based MNase tagging of genes by homologous recombination in *S. cerevisiae*. The templates enable both N- and C-terminal tagging with MNase in combination with linker regions of different lengths and properties. In addition, an affinity tag is included in the recombination cassettes which can be used for purification of the particle of interest before or after induction of MNase cleavages in the surrounding RNA or DNA. A step-by-step protocol is provided for tagging of a gene of interest, followed by affinity purification of the resulting fusion protein together with associated RNA and subsequent induction of local MNase cleavages.

**Key words** RNA, RNP, Ribosome, Structure probing, Enzymatic probing, Micrococcal nuclease, Fusion protein, Chromatin endogenous cleavage, ChEC, *Saccharomyces cerevisiae*

---

Fabian Teubl and Katrin Schwank contributed equally to this work.

Karl-Dieter Entian (ed.), *Ribosome Biogenesis: Methods and Protocols*, Methods in Molecular Biology, vol. 2533,
https://doi.org/10.1007/978-1-0716-2501-9_8, © The Author(s) 2022

# 1  Introduction

Numerous methods have been developed over the years to chemically or enzymatically probe the structure of chromatin and of ribonucleoprotein (RNP) complexes, two major manifestations of nucleic acid–protein complexes in eukaryotic cells [1–4]. Depending on the respective agent or enzyme applied, the accessibility, flexibility, secondary structure, or tertiary fold of the respective nucleic acid components can be analyzed either in vitro or in vivo. Combined with a high throughput sequencing readout these analyses can be performed genome- or transcriptome wide, respectively.

One of the enzymes which are routinely used to characterize nucleosome positions and chromatin states is the micrococcal nuclease (MNase) which is secreted by the bacterium *Staphylococcus aureus*. MNase has endo- and exonucleolytic activity which is strictly dependent on the presence of calcium. It cleaves both DNA and RNA with some preference for single stranded and for A/T- and A/U-rich regions (reviewed in [5–7]. In a typical nucleosome mapping experiment exogenous MNase is added to chromatin to perform a limited digest. Subsequently, positions of DNA cleavages and regions which were less accessible to the enzyme are determined. Information on the exact positioning of nucleosomes on DNA can be deduced if the size of a protected fragment is close to 146 base pairs which are typically protected by a nucleosome core particle [8–10].

Laemmli and colleagues have introduced a variation of this approach which is termed "chromatin endogenous cleavage" (ChEC) [11]. Here, a DNA-binding protein of interest is expressed in *S. cerevisiae* in fusion with MNase which remains inactive in the cell due to low calcium concentrations. Increasing the calcium concentration after cell breakage activates the enzyme which cleaves then close by accessible DNA. The resulting cuts at specific genomic loci can be analyzed by Southern blotting, or by high throughput sequencing for obtaining a genome wide data set [11–14]. ChEC and related MNase tethering approaches [15, 16] provide a valuable alternative to techniques as CHIP-Seq or DAM-ID [17, 18] for mapping of DNA binding sites of specific proteins. In addition, occupancies of fusion proteins at selected genomic loci can be analyzed in a quantitative way [13].

Protein components of RNPs have been as well expressed in fusion with MNase in yeast. They are potentially assembled in vivo at their endogenous location in the respective RNPs. The activation of MNase after cell breakage by the addition of calcium leads then to specific RNA cleavages in proximity to the fusion proteins which can be mapped with nucleotide resolution either by local [19] or by transcriptome wide primer extension analyses [20]. Experiments using a ribosomal model substrate showed that the radius of the enzymatic probe can be customized through introduction of differently sized linkers between the RNP-protein and MNase [19]. Cleavages up to around 6 nm surface distance from the anchor protein could be observed with longer linkers while more proximal cuts were strongly favored when using a short linker. Thus, in analogy to the ChEC methodology, probing of the RNA in proximity of a MNase fusion protein can reveal if, and in which region this protein binds to cellular RNPs. Importantly, additional information about the RNP's folding state in the surrounding of the MNase fusion proteins can be obtained. In this regard, the general accessibility of the substrate for the enzyme's active center and the preference of MNase for single stranded and A/U-rich regions seem to be major determinants of spatially restricted cleavage positions [19, 20]. Consequently, a low number of defined cleavages can be expected in RNP's with a compact fold and thereby low accessibility. A/U-rich loops of spatially flexible hairpins which are often hardly detectable in structural analyses by X-ray crystallography or single molecule cryo-electron microscopy, were observed to be preferred substrates of MNase tethered to RNPs [20].

To further facilitate the application of MNase fusion proteins for both chromatin and RNP research we established a set of vectors that can be used as templates for PCR based chromosomal N- or C-terminal MNase tagging of genes by homologous recombination in *S. cerevisiae*. The tagging cassettes include regions coding for a variety of protein linkers, the MNase itself, a 3x-FLAG affinity tag as well as a heterologous selection marker (*see* Tables 1, 2 and 3). The cassettes were designed in a modular way allowing for straightforward exchange of each of the individual functional elements. This can be used to replace for example the rather strong *RPS28B* promoter present in the N-terminal tagging cassettes with other promoters better reflecting the endogenous expression level of the protein to be tagged. Too high expression levels might cause an excess of free MNase fusion proteins not assembled in RNPs or chromatin. This in turn could favor the appearance of nontethered cleavages. The plasmids further code for a set of different linker regions separating the anchor protein from the MNase in the fusion protein. The resulting protein linker regions vary in length from 6 to 63 amino acids and contain elements of different predicted conformational flexibility [22]. Finally, the cassettes contain sequences coding for the strong 3x-FLAG affinity tag which can be used for detection of the fusion proteins by Western blotting. In addition, the tag enables efficient affinity purification of the fusion proteins before MNase activation. This can be useful to facilitate the downstream analyses of the resulting cleavages in RNPs.

**Table 1**
**Plasmids containing tagging cassettes**

| Database number | Linker modules | Linker length[a] | Tagging | Marker gene | Affinity tag | Promoter |
|---|---|---|---|---|---|---|
| K2372 | – | 12 aa | C-terminal | KlURA3 | 3xFLAG | – |
| K2373 | No MNase encoded! | – | C-terminal | KlURA3 | 3xFLAG | – |
| K2515 | 2xHA | 30 aa | N-terminal | hph[b] | 3xFLAG | pRPS28B |
| K2628 | – | 8 aa | N-terminal | hph[b] | 3xFLAG | pRPS28B |
| K2488 | Flexible linker + long helical linker | 63 aa | C-terminal | KlURA3 | 3xFLAG | – |
| K2489 | Flexible linker + short helical linker | 48 aa | C-terminal | KlURA3 | 3xFLAG | – |
| K2490 | Flexible linker | 31 aa | C-terminal | KlURA3 | 3xFLAG | – |
| K2491 | – | 6 aa | C-terminal | KlURA3 | 3xFLAG | – |
| K2510 | Long helical linker | 42 aa | C-terminal | KlURA3 | 3xFLAG | – |
| K2511 | Short helical linker | 27 aa | C-terminal | KlURA3 | 3xFLAG | – |

[a]The total length of the region between the protein of interest and the tethered MNase is indicated. This includes amino acids encoded by the priming sequences needed for PCR of the tagging cassettes. K2373 does not contain the MNase-coding sequence. Hence, no linker length is indicated for K2373
[b]Hygromycin resistance gene with TEV promoter and CYC1 terminator

**Table 2**
**Amino acid sequences of linker modules referred to in Table 1**

| Linker | Amino acid sequence of the linker |
|---|---|
| Flexible linker | LGGGGSGGGGSGGGGSAAA |
| Long helix | LAEAAAKEAAAKEAAAKEAAAKEAAAKAAA |
| Short helix | LAEAAAKEAAAKAAA |
| 2xHA | YPYDVPDYAGYPYDVPDYA |

In the following, we provide instruction for PCR based MNase tagging of a gene of interest in *S. cerevisiae* using the described plasmid set. We then outline a step-by-step protocol for the analysis of MNase tagged RNPs, including their purification using the built-in 3x-FLAG tag and the subsequent activation of the tethered MNase to induce local RNA cleavages. For the use of generated fusion protein expressing strains in chromatin analyses we refer to recently published protocols [13, 14, 16, 23].

**Table 3**
**Primer design for PCR based homologous recombination**

| Database number | Upstream priming sequence (5′ to 3′)[a] | Downstream priming sequence (5′ to 3′)[a] | Size of the PCR amplicon without overhangs[b] |
|---|---|---|---|
| K2372 | TCCA TGGAAAAGAGAAG | TACGACTCACTA TAGGG | 2.15 kb |
| K2373 | TCCA TGGAAAAGAGAAG | TACGACTCACTA TAGGG | 1.69 kb |
| K2515 | GACATGGAGGCCCAGA | AGCCATGGATCCCC TAG | 2.67 kb |
| K2628 | GACATGGAGGCCCAGA | AGCCATGGATCCCC TAG | 2.61 kb |
| K2488 | TCCA TGGAAAAGAGAAG | TACGACTCACTA TAGGG | 2.31 kb |
| K2489 | TCCA TGGAAAAGAGAAG | TACGACTCACTA TAGGG | 2.26 kb |
| K2490 | TCCA TGGAAAAGAGAAG | TACGACTCACTA TAGGG | 2.21 kb |
| K2491 | TCCA TGGAAAAGAGAAG | TACGACTCACTA TAGGG | 2.14 kb |
| K2510 | TCCA TGGAAAAGAGAAG | TACGACTCACTA TAGGG | 2.24 kb |
| K2511 | TCCA TGGAAAAGAGAAG | TACGACTCACTA TAGGG | 2.20 kb |

[a]The priming sequences for all vectors except K2515 and K2628 are the same as the ones described in [21]
[b]The sizes of the 5′ regions of the oligonucleotides used for PCR which are homologous to the respective genomic sequence have to be added to these rounded values (*see* Subheading 3.1)

# 2    Materials

### 2.1 Template Plasmids for PCR Based Amplification of Tagging Cassettes

1. Plasmids which can be used as templates for amplification of recombination cassettes by PCR are described in Tables 1, 2, and 3. These plasmids and the corresponding sequence information are available upon request. Tables 4 and 5 provide more detailed information on how these plasmids were constructed.

2. Synthetic oligonucleotides required for PCR-based amplification of recombination cassettes are to be designed as outlined below in the methods section. Several manufacturers offer oligonucleotide synthesis services in the required size range (45–80 nucleotides) with sufficient quality in terms of purity and error rate. As example, EXTREmers offered by Eurofins/Genomics were successfully used for the tagging procedure described below.

**Table 4**
**Plasmid construction**

| Name/number | Cloning strategy | Origin |
|---|---|---|
| pGEM-T easy | | Promega |
| pBS1539 | | [21] |
| K643 | | [24] |
| K1743 | | [19] |
| K2116 | Synthetic gene fragment containing a sequence coding for a flexible linker, a long helix, and part of the MNase (5' to 3'): gtcgaccctaggttgggtggtggtggttcaggcggtggtggtagtggcggtggttct gctgtgtcctaggtccgagttggctgaagctgtctcaagaagcagcagccaag aagccgccgcaaagaagctgtcgccaaagaagctgtctcaaagctgtctcctcgag aacgcaacttcaactaataaaattacataaagaacctgcgactttaattaaagcgattgatggt gatacggttaaattaatgtacaaagtcaaccaatgacattcagactatttattggtcgac | Synthetic DNA, Entelechon |
| K2117 | Synthetic gene fragment containing a sequence coding for a flexible linker, a short helix, and part of the MNase (5' to 3'): gtcgaccctaggttgggtggtggtggttcaggcggtggtggtagtggcggtggttct ggctcgagttggctgaagctgtctaaagaagctgcagcaaaggctgtgctctcgagaacgcaactc aactaaaaaattacataaagaacctgcgactttaattaaagcgattgatggtgatacggttaaattaatgtacaaa ggtcaaccaatgacattcagactatttggtcgac | Synthetic DNA, Entelechon |
| K2127 | The plasmid K2116 was digested with the restriction enzyme SalI. The resulting fragment was cloned into vector K643 | |
| K2128 | The plasmid K2117 was digested with the restriction enzyme SalI. The resulting fragment was cloned into vector K643 | This study |
| K2131 | The plasmid K2127 was digested with the restriction enzyme XhoI. Then, the plasmid backbone was religated | This study |
| K2354 | Synthetic DNA in vector pEX-A2 (Eurofins), containing an MNase and 3xFLAG coding sequence (5' to 3'): tccatggaaagagagaagctcggcgcctgagctcacgcaacttcaactaaaaaattacataaagaacctg cgactttaattaaagcgattgatggtgatacggttaaattaatgtacaaaggtcaaccaatgacattcag | Synthetic DNA, Eurofins genomics |

(continued)

| | | |
|---|---|---|
| | actattattggtcgacacacctgaaacaagcatcctaaaaaggtgtagagaaatatgtgtcctgaagcaa<br>gtgcatttaccaaaaaatgtagaaaatgcaaagaaaatgaagtcgaattcgacaaggtcaaagaa<br>ctgataaatatggacgtgggctggcgtatatttatgctgatggaaaatggtaaacgaggcctagttcgtca<br>aggcttggctaagttgcttatgtttacaaacttaacatacacatgaacacacatttaagaaaagtgaagc<br>acaagcgaaaaagagaaattaaatatttggagcgaagacaacgctgattcaggtagatctgagctcg<br>actacaagaccatgacgggtgattataagatcatgacatcgaggatgacgatgacaagtgaaagctt | |
| K2372 | The plasmid K2354 was digested with the restriction enzymes NcoI/HindIII.<br>The resulting fragment was cloned into vector pB1539 | This study |
| K2373 | The plasmid K2372 was linearized with the restriction enzyme SacI. Then,<br>the plasmid backbone was religated. This construct lacks the MNase coding sequence | This study |
| K2455 | Synthetic DNA in vector pEX-K2 (Eurofins), containing a Hygromycin<br>resistance cassette under control of the heterologous TEF promoter and<br>CYC1 terminator (5′ to 3′):<br><br>gcatgcaccggtttttctggtggtgctttcaatgcggaatccgtcacatccgaaaatttcagagggcttcacttagcgt<br>cgcagatcccagtagtcgccagatgctttgaaaaaagagctcg+ggccgcagcttgcctcgtccccgccg<br>ggtcaccggccagcgacatggagcccagaataccctccttgacagtcttgacgtgcgagctcagggc<br>atgattgactgtcgcccgtacatttagcccatacatcccatgtataatcatttgatcggggaacgtccctcacagacg<br>cacgggcggaagcaaaattacggtctcctcgctacagacctgcgagcaggggaacgtcccctcacagacg<br>cgttgaattgtccccacgccgcgccccctgtagagaaataaaggttaggatttgccactgagttcttcatata<br>cttccttttaaaattcgtctaggatacagttctcacatcacatccgaacataaacaaccatggtaaaaagcctga<br>actcaccgcgacgtctgtcgagagtttctgatcgaaaagttcacgacgctccgacctgatgcagctctcg<br>gaggcggaagaatcctgtgtttcagtttgatgtaggaggcgtggatatgttctgcggtaatagctgcg<br>ccgatggttttcacaagatcgttgttttatcggcacttgcatcggccgcgctccgattccgga<br>agtgcttgacgttgcattggggattcagcgagacgaactgaccccgcagcggggtgcacaggg<br>tgtcacgttgcaagacctgcgaaaccgaactgccccgcgttcacagccggtcgcggagg<br>ccatggatcgactgctcgcgggcatcttgcgggcgatcccacggcgctcggacc<br>gcaaggaatcgtcaatacactacatggcgtgatttcatatgcggattcgtatcccatgtgt<br>atcactggcaaactgtgatggacgacaccgtcagtgcgtcgtcgcgaggctcgatgag<br>ctgatcttgggcgaggactgccccgaagtcggcacctgtgcacgcggatttcggctcca<br>acaatgtctgacgacaagctgccacatcttcttcttggaggcgtgttggcttgtatggagcagc<br>gggattcccaatacgaggtcgccaacatctttcttggaggcgtgagtggctcggtcgta<br>tatgctccgcattggtcttgaccaactcttattcagagcttggttgacgcagctttggacggcgtgggcgtacacaa<br>gcgcaggggtgatggacgcaagcgaatgctccgatccgagccggcggactgtgggcgtacacaa<br>tcgcccgcagaagcgcggccgtctggaccgatggctgctgtgtagaagtactgccgatagtggaa |

**Table 4**
**(continued)**

| Name/number | Cloning strategy | Origin |
|---|---|---|
| | accgacgcccccagcactcgtccgagggcaaaggaataaatctagagtcagtaagttatgtc acgcttacattcacgcccctccccccacatccgcttcaaccgaaaaggaagagttagacaacc tgaagttcaggtccctatttattttttatagttagttattaagaacgttatttatttcaaatttttctttttctg tacagacggcgttacgcatgtaacattatactgaaaacctgctgagaaggtttgggacgctcga aggctttaagggcccctcgagggcgctagtaagccgatccattaccgacatttgggcgtat acgttgacatgttcatgtatgtatctgtatttaaaacacttttgtattattttcctcatatatgttataggtttatacg gatgatttaattaattacttcaccacctttatttcaggctgatatcttagcctttgttactagttagaaaagacat ttttgctgtcagtcactgcaagagattctttgctggcatttcttctagaagcaaaaagagcgatgcgtctttc cgctgaaccgttccagcaaaaagactaccaacgcaatatggattgtcagaatcatataaagaga agcaaataactccttgtcttgtcattataatcttccttgttagtcgaatatcatatagaagtcatcga aatagatattaagaaaacaaactgtacaatcaatcaatcaatacataaatggtaccctaggg gatccctgcagaagcttatgcat | |
| K2456 | The plasmid K2455 was digested with the restriction enzymes NsiI/SphI. The resulting fragment was cloned into the pGEM-T easy vector | This study |
| K2458 | The plasmid K1743 was digested with the restriction enzymes KasI/PstI. The resulting fragment containing the pRPS28B promoter was cloned into vector K2456 | This study |
| K2460 | Genomic DNA deriving from *S. cerevisiae* was amplified using the oligos O4246/O4247. The PCR amplicon was digested with the restriction enzymes SphI/SacI. The resulting fragment was cloned into vector K2458 | This study |
| K2488 | The plasmid K2127 was amplified using the oligos O4299/O4301. The resulting PCR amplicon was digested with the restriction enzymes NcoI/NheI. The resulting fragment was cloned into vector K2372 | This study |
| K2489 | The plasmid K2128 was amplified using the oligos o4299/O4301. The resulting PCR amplicon was digested with the restriction enzymes NcoI/NheI. The resulting fragment was cloned into vector K2372 | This study |
| K2490 | The plasmid K2131 was amplified using the oligos O4299/O4301. The resulting PCR amplicon was digested with the restriction enzymes NcoI/NheI. The | This study |

| | | |
|---|---|---|
| K2491 | The plasmid K2131 was amplified using the oligos O4300/O4301. The resulting PCR amplicon was digested with the restriction enzymes NcoI/NheI. The resulting fragment was cloned in K2372 | This study |
| K2510 | The plasmid K2488 was linearized with the restriction enzyme AvrII. Then, the plasmid backbone was religated | This study |
| K2511 | The plasmid K2489 was linearized with the restriction enzyme AvrII. The plasmid backbone was religated | This study |
| K2514 | Synthetic gene fragment containing a sequence coding for a 3xFLAG tag, the MNase and a 2xHA tag (5' to 3'): <br><br> taatacgactcactataggctcgagggcgccggtaccatgactacaaagaccatgacggtgattataagatca tgacatrgattacaaggatgacgatgacaaggctagcatgaacgcaactcaactaaaaattacataaag aacctgcgactttaattaaagcgattgatggtgtatacggttaaattaa tgtacaaaggtcaaccaatgacattcagactattattggtggacacacctgaaacaaagcatcctaaaaaggtgtgagaaatat ggtcctgaagcaagtgcatttaccaaaaaatgtagaaaatgcaagaaaaattgaagtcgagttcgacaaggtc aaagaactgataaatatggacgtgggctcggtatatttatgtcgatggaaaaatggtaaacgaagccttag ttcgtcaaggcttggctaaagttgcttatgtttacaaactaacaataacacatgaacaacatttaagaaaaagtgaagcacaagcgaaaaaaga gaaattaaatatttggagcgaagacaacgctgattcaggtgtcgaccct aggagctacccatacgatgttcctgactatcgggctatccctatgacgtcccgactatgcactaggggg atccatggtaagagaaatagatccaatttcgcattcaggaaggactgcaaagaaagaacacgaagattc ctrgttagaaggcaatgttttccaaaatgcaccggaagatatggatgaaataccatatatagcgcaaaaggct catcctcgcagctatagtgtcacctaaat | Synthetic DNA, Eurofins genomics |
| K2515 | The plasmid K2514 was digested with the restriction enzymes KpnI/PstI. The resulting plasmid was cloned in K2460 | This study |
| K2628 | The plasmid K2515 was linearized with the restriction enzyme AvrII. Then, the plasmid backbone was religated | This study |

**Table 5**
**Oligonucleotides used for plasmid construction**

| Database number | Sequence (5' to 3') |
|---|---|
| O4299 | GCGCGGATCCATGGAAAAGAGAAGCCCTAGGTTGGGTGGTGG |
| O4300 | ACACGCGCGGATCCATGGAAAAGAGAAGCAACGCAACTTCAACTAAAAAATTACA |
| O4301 | TCGTTTACCATTTTTCCATCAGC |
| O4246 | TTTTTTGCATGCAATCTGGGGACTGTATTAATC |

***2.2 Generation by PCR of Tagging Cassettes for Homologous Recombination***

1. Proofreading DNA Polymerase for PCR reactions with buffers provided by the manufacturer.

2. dNTP solution mix containing each dNTP in 10 mM concentration (NEB), stored at −20 °C.

3. 10 M lithium chloride.

4. >99.8% ethanol (p.a.).

***2.3 Transformation of Competent Yeast Cells and Screening for Positive Clones***

1. Material required for transformation of yeast cells and denaturing extraction of proteins as described in detail in [25].

2. Material for size separation of DNA by native agarose gel electrophoresis according to [26].

3. YPD-Hygromycin plates: 1% (w/v) yeast extract (Difco Laboratories), 2% (w/v) Bacto Peptone (Difco Laboratories), 2% (w/v) glucose, 2% (w/v) agar. The medium is autoclaved for 20 min and supplemented with 200 μg/mL hygromycin B (ThermoFisher Scientific) before casting the plates. A 200 mg/mL stock solution of hygromycin B can be sterilized by filtration through a filter with a pore size of 0.22 μm (Sarstedt) and stored at −20 °C.

4. SC-URA plates: 0.67% (w/v) YNB with nitrogen (Sunrise Science Products), 0.062% (w/v) CSM Ura-Leu-Trp powder (Sunrise Science Products), 2% (w/v) glucose, 2% (w/v) agar. The medium is autoclaved for 20 min and supplemented with 100 mg/L leucine (Sunrise Science Products) and 50 mg/L tryptophan (Sunrise Science Products) before casting the plates. Stock solutions (50x) of these amino acids can be sterilized by filtration through a filter with a pore size of 0.22 μm (Sarstedt) and stored at 4 °C.

5. YPD medium: 1% (w/v) yeast extract (Difco Laboratories), 2% (w/v) Bacto peptone (Difco Laboratories), 2% (w/v) glucose. The medium is autoclaved for 20 min.

6. Material for SDS polyacrylamide electrophoresis and subsequent transfer of proteins to a PVDF membrane by the Western blotting approach according to [26].

7. Immobilon-P PVDF membrane for Western blotting (Carl Roth).

8. Primary anti-Flag-Tag antibody: Rat monoclonal anti-DYKDDDDK antibody, clone L5, 2 mg/mL (Agilent Technologies).

9. Peroxidase coupled secondary antibodies: Peroxidase-AffinityPure goat anti-rat IgG + IgM (H + L) (Dianova).

10. Buffer PBS: 137 mM sodium chloride; 2.7 mM potassium chloride, 10 mM disodium hydrogen phosphate, 2 mM potassium dihydrogen phosphate.

11. Buffer PBS-T: PBS with 0.05% Tween 20.

12. Dry milk powder.

13. BM-Chemiluminescence blotting substrate (Sigma-Aldrich) and an appropriate imaging system for chemiluminescence reactions.

**2.4 Yeast Culture and Preparation of Cellular Extracts**

1. YPD medium: 1% (w/v) yeast extract (Difco Laboratories), 2% (w/v) Bacto peptone (Difco Laboratories), 2% glucose. The medium is autoclaved for 20 min.

2. Protease inhibitor stock solution (100x concentrated): 200 mM benzamidine and 100 mM PMSF in ethanol p.a., stored at −20 °C.

3. Buffer AG100: 20 mM Tris–HCl pH 8.0, 100 mM potassium chloride, 5 mM magnesium acetate, 5 mM EGTA. Cool down the buffer to 4 °C and adjust it to 1x protease inhibitor concentration shortly before usage.

4. 40 U/μL recombinant RNasin ribonuclease inhibitors (Promega), stored at −20 °C.

5. Glass beads with 0.75–1.0 mm diameter (Carl Roth).

6. Vibrax-VXR rotary shaker (IKA).

7. Protein assay dye reagent (Bio-Rad), stored at 4 °C.

8. Buffer AE+: 20 mM EDTA, 50 mM sodium acetate pH 5.3, stored at 4 °C.

**2.5 Purification of Preribosomal Particles from Cellular Extracts and Induction of MNase Cleavage**

1. Buffer AG100++: 20 mM Tris–HCl pH 8.09, 100 mM potassium chloride, 5 mM magnesium acetate, 5 mM EGTA, 0.1% (w/v) Tween, 0.5% (w/v) Triton X-100. Cool down the buffer to 4 °C and adjust it to 1× protease inhibitor concentration (*see* Subheading 2.4) shortly before usage.

2. Buffer AE+: *see* Subheading 2.4.

3. Poly-Prep chromatography columns with 10 mL reservoir (Bio-Rad).

4. Buffer AG100: *see* Subheading 2.4.

5. 0.25 M calcium chloride.

6. 1 mL spin columns with 35 μm filter (MoBiTec).

7. Water bath.

8. Turning wheel.

9. ANTI-FLAG ® M2 Affinity Gel (Sigma-Aldrich).

## 3   Methods

### 3.1   Primer Design and Choice of the Template Plasmid for PCR Reactions

Table 1 provides an overview on different plasmids which were created as templates for PCR based amplification of different tagging cassettes. Some of the plasmids are designed for N-terminal and others for C-terminal MNase tagging of a gene of interest in *S. cerevisiae*. Otherwise, the MNase cassettes encoded by the different plasmids differ by the linkers between MNase and the target protein and by the yeast selection markers. Two oligonucleotides have to be designed after choosing one of the plasmids as template for PCR based amplification of a recombination cassette (see for an overview [25, 27, 28]). These two oligonucleotides, in the following referred to as upstream and downstream oligonucleotide, are designed to contain at their 3′-end vector specific priming sequences indicated in the respective columns in Table 3. The priming sequences hybridize with corresponding regions on the plasmid which flank the tagging cassette and thus serve to amplify these cassettes in the PCR reaction. Sequence stretches of the gene of interest are added at the 5′-end of the primers. They should target cellular homologous recombination reactions of the amplified cassette to the gene of interest. For N-terminal tagging more than 40 nucleotides upstream of the start codon of the gene of interest are added 5′ to the upstream priming sequence to generate the upstream oligonucleotide. The start codon of the gene and more than 40 following nucleotides are added in reverse complement orientation to the 5′-end of the downstream priming sequence. Thus, the priming sequence in this downstream oligonucleotide directly follows 3′ after the reverse complement sequence of the start codon (5′-CAT-3′). For C-terminal tagging a stretch of more than 40 nucleotides ending with the last codon before the stop codon of the gene of interest is added 5′ to the upstream priming sequence in the upstream oligonucleotide. For the downstream oligonucleotide, more than 40 nucleotides of sequence just 3′ of the genes stop codon are added 5′ of the priming sequence in reverse complement orientation. Thereby the priming sequence continues directly 3′ after this reverse complement stretch of the genes 3′ untranslated region.

**3.2  Generation of PCR-Based Tagging Cassettes for Homologous Recombination**

1. Approximately 25 ng of the selected plasmid is used as template in PCR reactions.

2. PCR reaction mixtures are prepared with a pair of upstream and downstream oligonucleotides and a proofreading DNA polymerase according to the manufacturer's instructions (*see* **Note 1**). To obtain sufficient amounts of the desired PCR product two to six reactions can be performed in parallel, each with 50 μL reaction volume (*see* **Note 2**).

3. The quantity and size of the PCR products are determined by native DNA agarose gel electrophoresis using 5 μL of the PCR reaction mixture. The expected sizes for tagging cassettes amplified from the different plasmid templates are indicated in Table 1.3.

4. Identical PCR reactions performed in parallel are pooled (*see* **step 1**) and supplemented with 0.1 × volume of 10 M lithium chloride and 2.5 volumes of ice-cold ethanol.

5. The samples are incubated for at least 30 min at −20 °C and subsequently centrifuged at 14,000 × $g$ at 4 °C for at least 20 min.

6. The supernatant is discarded, and the remaining DNA pellet is resolved in 20 μL of water. Native DNA agarose gel electrophoresis [26] using about 10% of the DNA solution can be performed to confirm successful precipitation and to quantify the amount of obtained DNA.

**3.3  Transformation of Competent Yeast Cells and Screening for Positive Clones**

1. Yeast strains used for transformation with tagging cassettes based on plasmids K2515 and K2628 should not carry a hygromycin resistance marker gene. Yeast strains used for transformation with tagging cassettes based on K2372, K2373, K2488, K2489, K2490, K2491, K2510, and K2511 should have an inactivated URA3 gene. Strains expressing only Flag-tagged bait proteins without MNase can be generated using plasmid K2373. The latter strains can be included in the downstream RNP probing analyses as a negative control testing for MNase independent cleavage events in the RNP of interest.

2. Yeast cells are made chemically competent for transformation as outlined in detail in [25].

3. For homologous recombination, 50 μL of competent yeast cell suspension are transformed with 10 μg of the PCR amplified tagging cassette (*see* Subheading 3.2). Yeast transformation is performed as described in [25].

4. Cells transformed with recombination cassettes based on plasmids K2515 and K2628 are plated on YPD-Hygromycin plates. For all other recombination cassettes, cells are plated on SC-URA plates. Before spreading on YPD-Hygromycin

plates, the transformed cells should regenerate for at least 6 h in 10 mL of liquid YPD medium at 30 °C with shaking. Plates are incubated upside down at 30 °C until appearance of colonies (2–5 days depending on the strain background and plates used).

5. Several [4–10] colonies are individually streaked out in about 1 cm × 1 cm large patches on respective new selective plates and incubated for 16–24 h at 30 °C.

6. The resulting cellular material is used for denaturing protein extraction which is performed according to [25].

7. Proteins extracted from the different clones are then separated by size using SDS polyacrylamide gel electrophoresis followed by Western blotting to a PVDF membrane [26].

8. The membrane is incubated for 1 h at room temperature in 5% (w/v) dry milk powder in PBS.

9. Immunodetection of fusion proteins is performed using rat anti Flag-Tag-antibodies (1:1000 diluted in PBST containing 1% dry milk powder) as primary antibodies and peroxidase coupled goat anti-rat antibodies as secondary antibodies (1:5000 diluted in PBST containing 1% dry milk powder). The membrane is washed three times for 5 min in PBST after each antibody incubation step.

10. Fusion proteins are visualized on the membrane using the BM Chemiluminescence Blotting Substrate according to the manufacturer's instructions.

11. Clones expressing MNase fusion proteins of the expected size can be inoculated in YPD medium starting from the yeast cells streaked out in **step 5** (*see* **Notes 3** and **4**).

*3.4 Yeast Cell Culture and Preparation of Cellular Extracts*

1. Yeast strains expressing MNase fusion proteins are cultured in YPD medium at 30 °C to an $OD_{600}$ of approximately 0.8–1.2. For probing of (pre)ribosomal particles we routinely use culture volumes of 1–4 L for the subsequent analyses. The culture volume should be optimized for other RNPs depending on their respective expression level.

2. Cells are pelleted for 8 min with 9000 × $g$ at room temperature.

3. The supernatant is discarded and the cells are resuspended in 20 mL of ice-cold water per liter of cell culture.

4. The suspension is transferred to a 50 mL reaction tube and centrifuged for 3 min at 4200 × $g$ at 4 °C.

5. The supernatant is discarded. The cell pellet can be frozen at this stage at −20 °C and stored until usage. In this case the cells are thawed on ice before continuing with the next step.

6. At this point all buffers should be ready and cooled down to 4 °C. All subsequent steps are performed at 4 °C, unless stated otherwise.

7. The cells are resuspended in 10 mL of buffer AG100 per liter of cell culture.

8. The cells are centrifuged for 3 min at 4200 × $g$ and 4 °C and the supernatant is discarded.

9. The wet weight of the cellular pellet is determined.

10. For each gram of cells 1.5 mL of buffer AG100 supplemented with RNasin (0.04 U/µL) is added and the cells are resuspended.

11. The cell suspension is distributed in portions of 800 µL to precooled 2 mL reaction tubes loaded with 1.4 g of glass beads.

12. For mechanical disruption of the cells, the tubes are shaken for 7 min at 4 °C on an IKA Vibrax basic shaker at maximum speed. Afterward, the cell suspensions are chilled on ice for 3 min. The procedure is repeated at least three times (*see* **Note 5**).

13. The cell lysate is centrifuged for 5 min at 14,000 × $g$ and 4 °C.

14. The supernatant is pooled in a new 1.5 mL reaction tube and centrifuged for 10 min at 14,000 × $g$ and 4 °C.

15. The supernatant is transferred to a new 1.5 mL reaction tube.

16. The protein concentration of the cleared cell extract is determined with the Bio-Rad protein assay according to the manufacturer's instructions.

17. Here, samples can be taken for downstream RNA analyses. For this, a volume of cellular extract containing 300 µg of protein (= input sample) is added to 500 µL of ice-cold buffer AE+ and stored at −20 °C until usage (*see* **Note 6**).

*3.5 Purification of RNPs from Cellular Extracts and Activation of MNase*

1. The cellular extract prepared in 3.4 is supplemented with 0.1% (w/v) Tween and 0.5% (w/v) Triton X-100 (*see* **Note 7**).

2. Prior to affinity purification, the Anti-Flag M2 affinity matrix is equilibrated with buffer AG100++. For preribosomal particles we usually use 200 µL of matrix suspension containing about 100 µL matrix for cellular extracts prepared from 1 L of yeast cell culture. The suspension is transferred to Poly-Prep chromatography columns, washed once with 10 mL water and four times with 3 mL of buffer AG100++.

3. The equilibrated affinity matrix is transferred to the tube containing the cellular extract (**step 1**) and incubated for 1 h at 4 °C on a turning wheel.

4. The suspension is transferred into a Poly-Prep chromatography column and washed twice with 2 mL of buffer AG100++ and once with 10 mL AG100++.

5. The affinity matrix is suspended in 1 mL AG100 and transferred into a 1.5 mL reaction tube (*see* **Note 8**).

6. The bead suspension is centrifuged for 2 min at $2000 \times g$ and 4 °C. A part of the supernatant is carefully taken off such that the affinity matrix remains in a volume of 200 μL in the reaction tube.

7. In order to activate the MNase, calcium chloride is added to a final concentration of 8 mM.

8. The reaction tube is incubated with gentle shaking. The optimal temperature and incubation time for the RNP analyzed is to be determined in pilot experiments (*see* **Note 9**).

9. 500 μL of ice-cold AE+ is added to stop the reaction. The sample can then be stored at −20 °C until subsequent RNA analyses.

10. RNA extraction and the analyses of MNase-dependent RNA cleavages by either Northern blotting, targeted primer extension reactions or random primer extension analyses followed by high-throughput sequencing can be performed on samples thawed on ice as described in [20].

# 4   Notes

1. For PCR reactions we use routinely Herculase II Fusion DNA Polymerase (Agilent) according to the manufacturer's instructions with the thermocycler programmed to the following settings: Initial melt for 2 min at 95 °C followed by a 35 cycles of 20 s melting at 95 °C, 20 s annealing at 45 °C and elongation for 2 min at 72 °C. Lastly, a final elongation step is performed for 5 min at 72 °C.

2. The template plasmids are designed in a modular way such that respective stretches of homology with the genomic region of interest can be cloned 5′ and 3′ of the plasmids tagging cassettes. Usage of gene fragments of 100–500 nucleotides size, whose synthesis is offered by several companies, and either classical [26] or more recent [29, 30] molecular cloning strategies allow to easily integrate these larger complementary sequence stretches into the plasmids listed in Table 1. In this way, PCR based amplification of the cassette can be avoided. Instead, the newly generated plasmid is amplified in *E. coli*, purified, and the cassette together with the flanking homology stretches can be excised with the appropriate combination of restriction enzymes. Due to larger stretches of homology with the target gene region a clear increase in the number of positive transformants can be expected when using this approach.

3. At least two clones expressing fusion proteins of the expected size should be chosen for further analyses. Identical cleavage pattern among these biological replicates minimizes the risk that the probing results are due to unexpected rare genetic events during homologous recombination.

4. Integration at the expected genomic locus can be further confirmed by PCR analyses on genomic DNA of the selected clone, using one primer pairing in the tagging cassette and another one pairing in reverse orientation at the endogenous genomic locus. In case that in the downstream analyses no cleavage pattern can be observed, the primers should be designed such that the MNase coding sequence is amplified. The identity of the MNase coding sequence can then be confirmed by DNA sequencing.

5. The protein concentration in the crude cell extract can be measured using the Bio-Rad protein assay according to the manufacturer's recommendations, to test the disruption efficiency. Usual protein concentrations at this step should yield >10 mg/mL. If the concentration is lower, the procedure should be repeated until no significant further increase in protein concentration is observed.

6. At this point it is possible to perform RNP probing experiments in cellular extracts without prior affinity purification of the RNP of interest. For this, the cellular extract is supplemented with calcium chloride to a final concentration of 8 mM. After incubation at the desired temperature and time periods (*see* **Note 9**) a volume of cellular extract containing 300 µg protein is transferred to a new tube containing 500 µL of ice-cold buffer AE+. These samples can be stored at −20 °C or directly used for RNA extraction and downstream analyses.

7. For better handling, prepare 10% (w/v) stocks of both Triton X-100 and Tween 20 and use them to adjust the concentrations in the cellular extract.

8. At this point the suspension can be split into two equal volumes which are distributed to two 1.5 mL reaction tubes. They are treated in parallel as described below except that for one of the two reaction tubes **step 7** (addition of calcium chloride) is omitted. This reaction serves then as control to determine calcium and MNase independent cleavages in the RNP analyzed.

9. To determine the optimal temperature and time period for incubation in the presence of calcium several reactions can be performed in parallel for which these parameters are varied. For preribosomal particles with intermediate maturation state we use 15 min incubation at 16 °C. At optimal incubation conditions a substantial amount of target RNA (>20%) should be

cleaved as determined by RNA extraction and northern blotting. Excessive cleavage conditions should be avoided since they may favor disintegration of the analyzed RNP and accumulation of nontethered cleavages.

## Acknowledgments

We thank all members of the chair of Biochemistry III for their support of this work. This work was financially supported by the grant SFB 960 from the "Deutsche Forschungsgemeinschaft" (DFG).

## References

1. Even-Faitelson L, Hassan-Zadeh V, Baghestani Z, Bazett-Jones DP (2016) Coming to terms with chromatin structure. Chromosoma 125:95–110. https://doi.org/10.1007/s00412-015-0534-9

2. Herschlag D (2009) Biophysical, chemical, and functional probes of RNA structure, interactions and folding. Methods Enzymol 468:xv

3. Weeks KM (2010) Advances in RNA structure analysis by chemical probing. Curr Opin Struct Biol 20:295–304. https://doi.org/10.1016/j.sbi.2010.04.001

4. Wu C, Allis CD (2012) Nucleosomes, histones & chromatin. Part B. In: Methods in enzymology, vol 513, 1st edn. Elsevier/Academic Press, Amsterdam/Boston. http://search.ebscohost.com/login.aspx?direct=true & scope=site & db=nlebk & db=nlabk & AN=478429

5. Anfinsen CB, Cuatrecasas P, Taniuchi H (1971) 8 Staphylococcal nuclease, chemical properties and catalysis. In: Hydrolysis, vol 4. Elsevier, pp 177–204

6. Chung H-R, Dunkel I, Heise F, Linke C, Krobitsch S, Ehrenhofer-Murray AE, Sperling SR, Vingron M (2010) The effect of micrococcal nuclease digestion on nucleosome positioning data. PLoS One 5:e15754. https://doi.org/10.1371/journal.pone.0015754

7. Dingwall C, Lomonossoff GP, Laskey RA (1981) High sequence specificity of micrococcal nuclease. Nucleic Acids Res 9:2659–2673. https://doi.org/10.1093/nar/9.12.2659

8. Reeves R (1984) Transcriptionally active chromatin. Biochim Biophys Acta 782:343–393. https://doi.org/10.1016/0167-4781(84)90044-7

9. Tsompana M, Buck MJ (2014) Chromatin accessibility: a window into the genome. Epigenetics Chromatin 7:33. https://doi.org/10.1186/1756-8935-7-33

10. Teif VB (2016) Nucleosome positioning: resources and tools online. Brief Bioinformatics 17:745–757. https://doi.org/10.1093/bib/bbv086

11. Schmid M, Durussel T, Laemmli UK (2004) ChIC and ChEC; genomic mapping of chromatin proteins. Mol Cell 16:147–157. https://doi.org/10.1016/j.molcel.2004.09.007

12. Zentner GE, Kasinathan S, Xin B, Rohs R, Henikoff S (2015) ChEC-seq kinetics discriminates transcription factor binding sites by DNA sequence and shape in vivo. Nat Commun 6:8733. https://doi.org/10.1038/ncomms9733

13. Babl V, Stöckl U, Tschochner H, Milkereit P, Griesenbeck J (2015) Chromatin endogenous cleavage (ChEC) as a method to quantify protein interaction with genomic DNA in Saccharomyces cerevisiae. Methods Mol Biol 1334:219–232. https://doi.org/10.1007/978-1-4939-2877-4_14

14. Grünberg S, Zentner GE (2017) Genome-wide mapping of protein-DNA interactions with ChEC-seq in Saccharomyces cerevisiae. J Vis Exp (124):55836. https://doi.org/10.3791/55836

15. Skene PJ, Henikoff S (2017) An efficient targeted nuclease strategy for high-resolution mapping of DNA binding sites. elife 6:e21856. https://doi.org/10.7554/eLife.21856

16. Hainer SJ, Fazzio TG (2019) High-resolution chromatin profiling using CUT & RUN. Curr Protoc Mol Biol 126:e85. https://doi.org/10.1002/cpmb.85

17. Park PJ (2009) ChIP-seq: advantages and challenges of a maturing technology. Nat Rev

Genet 10:669–680. https://doi.org/10.1038/nrg2641

18. Aughey GN, Cheetham SW, Southall TD (2019) DamID as a versatile tool for understanding gene regulation. Development 146: dev173666. https://doi.org/10.1242/dev.173666

19. Ohmayer U, Perez-Fernandez J, Hierlmeier T, Pöll G, Williams L, Griesenbeck J, Tschochner H, Milkereit P (2012) Local tertiary structure probing of ribonucleoprotein particles by nuclease fusion proteins. PLoS One 7:e42449. https://doi.org/10.1371/journal.pone.0042449

20. Pöll G, Müller C, Bodden M, Teubl F, Eichner N, Lehmann G, Griesenbeck J, Tschochner H, Milkereit P (2017) Structural transitions during large ribosomal subunit maturation analyzed by tethered nuclease structure probing in S. cerevisiae. PLoS One 12: e0179405. https://doi.org/10.1371/journal.pone.0179405

21. Puig O, Caspary F, Rigaut G, Rutz B, Bouveret E, Bragado-Nilsson E, Wilm M, Séraphin B (2001) The tandem affinity purification (TAP) method: a general procedure of protein complex purification. Methods 24: 218–229. https://doi.org/10.1006/meth.2001.1183

22. Arai R, Ueda H, Kitayama A, Kamiya N, Nagamune T (2001) Design of the linkers which effectively separate domains of a bifunctional fusion protein. Protein Eng 14:529–532

23. Griesenbeck J, Wittner M, Charton R, Conconi A (2012) Chromatin endogenous cleavage and psoralen crosslinking assays to analyze rRNA gene chromatin in vivo. Methods Mol Biol 809:291–301. https://doi.org/10.1007/978-1-61779-376-9_20

24. Merz K, Hondele M, Goetze H, Gmelch K, Stoeckl U, Griesenbeck J (2008) Actively transcribed rRNA genes in S. cerevisiae are organized in a specialized chromatin associated with the high-mobility group protein Hmo1 and are largely devoid of histone molecules. Genes Dev 22:1190–1204. https://doi.org/10.1101/gad.466908

25. Knop M, Siegers K, Pereira G, Zachariae W, Winsor B, Nasmyth K, Schiebel E (1999) Epitope tagging of yeast genes using a PCR-based strategy: more tags and improved practical routines. Yeast 15:963–972. https://doi.org/10.1002/(SICI)1097-0061(199907)15:10B<963:AID-YEA399>3.0.CO;2-W

26. Green MR, Sambrook J (2012) Molecular cloning. A laboratory manual, 4th edn. Cold Spring Harbor Laboratory Press, Cold Spring Harbor, NY

27. Janke C, Magiera MM, Rathfelder N, Taxis C, Reber S, Maekawa H, Moreno-Borchart A, Doenges G, Schwob E, Schiebel E, Knop M (2004) A versatile toolbox for PCR-based tagging of yeast genes: new fluorescent proteins, more markers and promoter substitution cassettes. Yeast 21:947–962. https://doi.org/10.1002/yea.1142

28. Schneider BL, Seufert W, Steiner B, Yang QH, Futcher AB (1995) Use of polymerase chain reaction epitope tagging for protein tagging in Saccharomyces cerevisiae. Yeast 11: 1265–1274. https://doi.org/10.1002/yea.320111306

29. Gibson DG, Young L, Chuang R-Y, Venter JC, Hutchison CA, Smith HO (2009) Enzymatic assembly of DNA molecules up to several hundred kilobases. Nat Methods 6:343–345. https://doi.org/10.1038/nmeth.1318

30. Hill RE, Eaton-Rye JJ (2014) Plasmid construction by SLIC or sequence and ligation-independent cloning. Methods Mol Biol 1116:25–36. https://doi.org/10.1007/978-1-62703-764-8_2

# Part V

**RNA Modification**

# Chapter 9

## Chemical Modifications of Ribosomal RNA

### Sunny Sharma and Karl-Dieter Entian

### Abstract

Cellular RNAs in all three kingdoms of life are modified with diverse chemical modifications. These chemical modifications expand the topological repertoire of RNAs, and fine-tune their functions. Ribosomal RNA in yeast contains more than 100 chemically modified residues in the functionally crucial and evolutionary conserved regions. The chemical modifications in the rRNA are of three types—methylation of the ribose sugars at the C2-positionAbstract (Nm), isomerization of uridines to pseudouridines ($\Psi$), and base modifications such as (methylation (mN), acetylation (acN), and aminocarboxypropylation (acpN)). The modifications profile of the yeast rRNA has been recently completed, providing an excellent platform to analyze the function of these modifications in RNA metabolism and in cellular physiology. Remarkably, majority of the rRNA modifications and the enzymatic machineries discovered in yeast are highly conserved in eukaryotes including humans. Mutations in factors involved in rRNA modification are linked to several rare severe human diseases (e.g., X-linked Dyskeratosis congenita, the Bowen–Conradi syndrome and the William–Beuren disease). In this chapter, we summarize all rRNA modifications and the corresponding enzymatic machineries of the budding yeast.

**Key words** rRNA modification, Ribose methylation, Pseudouridylation, Base methylation, Aminocarboxypropylation, Acetylation of cytidines, Methyltransferase

## 1 Introduction

RNA modifications are present in all three kingdoms of life and detected in all classes of cellular RNAs. RNA modifications are diverse, with more than 100 types of chemical modifications identified to date [1]. Ribosomes are molecular assemblies of RNA and proteins and are responsible for the synthesis of all proteins in the cells [2]. Structural and functional analyses of ribosomes have revealed that it is the ribosomal RNA (rRNA) that makes the structural framework of ribosomes and catalyzes the joining of amino acids (peptidyl transfer) during translation, hence making the ribosome a ribozyme [3]. Though the chemical composition of RNA seems to be rather insufficient to provide the structural complexity to RNA, the composition analysis of rRNA has shown that rRNA contains different chemical modifications that are added

Karl-Dieter Entian (ed.), *Ribosome Biogenesis: Methods and Protocols*, Methods in Molecular Biology, vol. 2533, https://doi.org/10.1007/978-1-0716-2501-9_9, © The Author(s) 2022

both co- and posttranscriptionally [4, 5]. Ribosomal RNA (rRNA) contains three types of chemical modifications, methylation of the ribose sugars at the C2-position (Nm), isomerization of uridines to pseudouridines ($\Psi$), and base modifications (methylation (mN) such as acetylation (acN) and aminocarboxypropylation (acpN)) [6]. Mutations in factors involved in rRNA modifications are associated with several rare severe human diseases (e.g., X-linked dyskeratosis congenita, the Bowen–Conradi syndrome, Hutchison Gilford syndrome, and the William–Beuren disease) [7–13]. Emerging evidences indicate that some bases are not always completely modified providing heterogeneity with respect to RNA modification [14–16]. Heterogeneity in rRNA modification has been correlated with disease etiology (cancer) and shown to play a role in cell differentiation (hematopoiesis) [17]. Remarkably, alterations in rRNA modification patterns profoundly affect the preference of ribosomes for cap- versus IRES-dependent translation having major consequences on cell physiology [18, 19]. Here, we summarize all known rRNA modifications of the budding yeast with an emphasis on base modifications (*see* Tables 1, 2, 3 and 4).

In *Saccharomyces cerevisiae*, 18S rRNA of the small subunit contains 14 $\Psi$s, 18 Nms (2′O-methylated Ns), 4 mNs (methylated Ns), and 2 acNs (acylated Ns) (Tables 1 and 2), whereas 25S rRNA of the large subunit contains 30 $\Psi$s, 35 Nms, and 6 base methylations (Tables 3 and 4). Mapping of these modifications has revealed that these modifications cluster in the functionally conserved regions of the ribosomes like the intersubunit and the peptidyl transferase center [6, 20, 21]. Due to technical limitations, the chemical modification profile of rRNA, especially for the base modifications, remained poorly characterized for a long time. Using state-of-the-art RP-HPLC and mass spectrometry together with "reverse genetics," we and others have recently completed the characterization and mapping of the complete set of yeast rRNA modifications, and have identified the corresponding enzymatic machinery involved in adding these modifications to the RNA [16, 22, 23].

## 2    Ribose Methylation

Methylation of 2′-OH of ribose sugar to a 2′-O-methyl-ribose is a characteristic modification in mRNA and many noncoding RNA (ncRNA) including tRNA, rRNA and siRNAs (Fig. 1). Ribose methylation favors a 3′-*endo* conformation of the ribose and since 3′-*endo* conformations are known to stabilize A-form helices, methylation of ribose increases the rigidity of the RNA by promoting base stacking. Furthermore, ribose methylation provides RNA stability against base and nuclease hydrolysis by insulating the otherwise active 2′-OH group. Our recent analyses together with other

**Table 1**
**18S rRNA modifications catalyzed by snoRNPs**

| Modified residue | snoRNA | Modified residue | snoRNA |
|---|---|---|---|
| 2′O-A28 | snR74 | Ψ 106 | snR44 |
| 2′O-A100 | snR51 | Ψ 120 | snR49 |
| 2′O-C414 | U14 (snR128) | Ψ 211 | snR49 |
| 2′O-A420 | snR52 | Ψ 302 | snR49 |
| 2′O-A436 | snR87 | Ψ 466 | snR189 |
| 2′O-A541 | snR41 | Ψ 632 | snR161 |
| 2′O-A562 | snrR40 | Ψ 759 | snR80 |
| 2′O-U578 | snR77 | Ψ 766 | snR161 |
| 2′O-A619 | snR47 | Ψ 999 | snR31 |
| 2′O-A796 | snR53 | Ψ 1181 | snR85 |
| 2′O-A974 | snR54 | Ψ 1187 | snR36 |
| 2′O-C1007 | snR79 | Ψ 1191 | snR35 |
| 2′O-G1126 | snR41 | Ψ 1290 | snR83 |
| 2′O-U1269 | snR55 | Ψ 1415 | snR83 |
| 2′O-G1271 | snR40 | | |
| 2′O-G1428 | snR56 | | |
| 2′O-G1572 | snR57 | | |
| 2′O-C1639 | snR70 | | |

**Table 2**
**18S rRNA modifications catalyzed by specific enzymes**

| Modified residue | Enzymes | snoRNAs |
|---|---|---|
| $m^7G1575$ | Bud23 | |
| $m^1acp^3\Psi1191$ | Nep1, Tsr3 | snR35 |
| $m^6_2A1781$ | Dim1 | |
| $m^6_2A1782$ | Dim1 | |
| $ac^4C1280$ | Kre33 | snR4 |
| $ac^4C1773$ | Kre33 | snR45 |

**Table 3**
**25S and 5.8S rRNA modifications catalyzed by snoRNPs**

| Modified residue | snoRNA | Modified residue | snoRNA |
|---|---|---|---|
| 2′O-A649 | U18 (snR18) | 2′O G2922 | SPB1 |
| 2′O-C650 | U18 (snR18) | 2′O A2946 | snR71 |
| 2′O-C663 | snR58 | 2′O C2948 | snR69 |
| 2′O-G805 | snR39 | 2′O C2959 | snR73 |
| 2′O-A807 | snR59 | Ψ776 | snR80 |
| 2′O-A817 | snR60 | Ψ960 | snR8 |
| 2′O-G867 | snR50 | Ψ966 | snR43 |
| 2′O-A876 | snR72 | Ψ986 | snR8 |
| 2′O-U898 | snR40 | Ψ990 | snR49 |
| 2′O-G908 | snR60 | Ψ1004 | snR5 |
| 2′O-A1133 | snR61 | Ψ1042 | snR33 |
| 2′O-G1142 | ? | Ψ1052 | snR81 |
| 2′O-C1437 | U24 (snR24) | Ψ1056 | snR44 |
| 2′O-A1449 | U24 (snR24) | Ψ1110 | snR82 |
| 2′O-G1450 | U24 (snR24) | Ψ1124 | snR5 |
| 2′O-U1888 | snR62 | Ψ2129 | snR3 |
| 2′O-C2197 | snR76 | Ψ2133 | snR3 |
| 2′O-A2220 | snR47 | Ψ2191 | snR32 |
| 2′O-A2256 | snR63 | Ψ2258 | snR191 |
| 2′O-A2280 | snR13 | Ψ2260 | snR191 |
| 2′O-A2281 | snR13 | Ψ2264 | snR3 |
| 2′O-G2288 | snR75 | Ψ2266 | snR84 |
| 2′O-C2337 | snR64 | Ψ2314 | snR86 |
| 2′O-U2347 | snR65 | Ψ2340 | snR9 |
| 2′O-G2395 | snR190 (predicted) | Ψ2349 | snR82 |
| 2′O-U2417 | snR66 | Ψ2351 | snR82 |
| 2′O-U2421 | snR78 | Ψ2416 | snR11 |
| 2′O-G2619 | snR67 | Ψ2735 | snR189 |
| 2′O-A2640 | snR68 | Ψ2826 | snR34 |
| 2′O-U2724 | snR67 | Ψ2865 | snR46 |
| 2′O-U2729 | snR51 | Ψ2880 | snR34 |
| 2′O-G2791 | snR48 | Ψ2923 | snR10 |
| 2′O-G2793 | snR48 | Ψ2944 | snR37 |
| 2′O-G2815 | snR38 | Ψ2975 | snR42 |
| 2′O-U2921 | snR52 | | |
| *5.8 S RNA* Ψ 73 | snR43 | | |

**Table 4**
**25S and 5S rRNA modifications catalyzed by enzymes**

| Modified residue | Enzyme |
|---|---|
| *25S rRNA* | |
| m$^1$A645 | Rrp8 (Bmt1) |
| m$^1$A2142 | Bmt2 |
| m$^5$C2278 | Rcm1 (Bmt3) |
| m$^5$C2870 | Nop2 (Bmt4) |
| m$^3$U2634 | Bmt5 |
| m$^3$U2843 | Bmt6 |
| *5S rRNA* | |
| Ψ 50 | Pus7 |

groups have identified several partial rRNA modifications in eukaryotes including humans. These observations suggest the existence of a heterogeneous population of ribosomes supporting the "specialized" translation model, which could possibly play an important role during embryonic development [14–16, 22, 24, 25].

**2.1   C/D Box snoRNPs**

All 2'-OH ribose methylation occur at distinct positions in eukaryotic rRNAs (Tables 1 and 3). The respective positions are targeted *via* specific C/D box snoRNAs having complementary guide sequences to the respective rRNAs together with distinguishing sequence elements called boxes C and D.

The methylation guide sequence is located upstream of the box D/D' element and consists of 10–21 nucleotides. The guide sequences direct ribose methylation to the nucleotide base paired to the fifth nucleotide (nt) upstream of the box D or D' sequence (box D + 5 rule) [26]. The C/D box snoRNPs consist of four common core proteins: Fibrillarin (human)/Nop1 (yeast), Nop58, Nop56, and Snu13 [27]. Interestingly, C/D box snoRNPs involved in functions apart from catalysis like U3, U14, U8, U22, snR4, and snR45 also contain additional proteins [27, 28]. Nop1 is a *S-adenosyl methionine* (SAM) dependent methyltransferase and catalyzes the 2'-O methylation reaction. Snu13 binds to the kink-turn (loop-stem structure that includes the canonical C/D elements in the loop portion) in the C/D box of snoRNAs. Nop56 and Nop58 are characterized by extensive coiled-coil domains, likely responsible for heterodimerization and providing stability to the snoRNA.

## 3  Pseudouridylation

Pseudouridylation (ψ) is a C-glycoside rotation isomer of uridine (Fig. 1). Due to rotation, the nitrogen atom at position 1 (N1) forms no longer a glycosidic bond to the ribose and is protonated at physiological pH. Compared to uracil, in pseudouracil both N1 and N3 participate in hydrogen bonding. The N1 proton makes hydrogen bonding with a phosphate group from the same or neighboring nucleotide and provides stability of the structure.

Furthermore, like ribose methylation, pseudouridine also favors a C3-*endo* sugar pucker (the conformation preferred by an A-form RNA helix) and has been shown to increase the thermal stability of RNA by up to 2 °C [29]. Therefore, the presence of ψ also plays an important role in RNA stability that may not be essential, but seemingly provides a significant advantage [5].

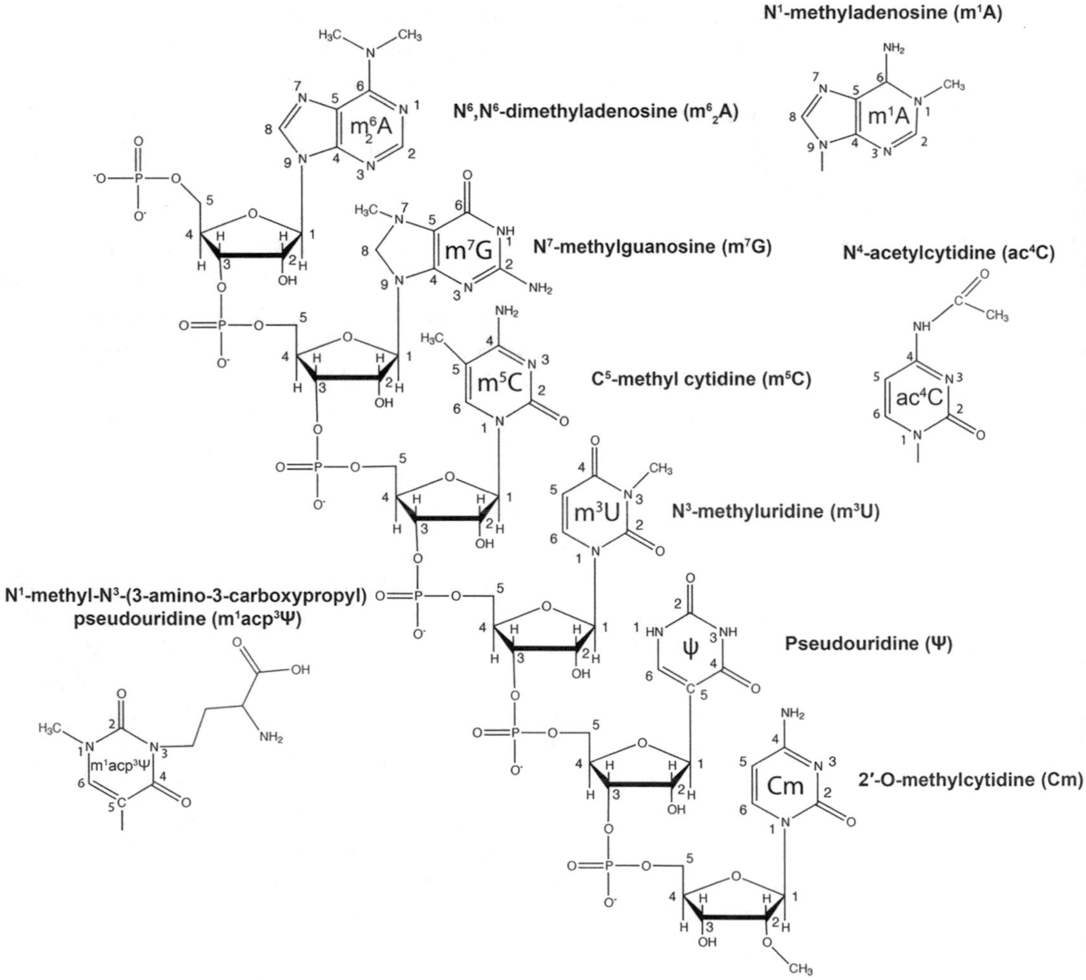

**Fig. 1** Chemical structure of modified bases and 2′O-methylation in yeast rRNAs

**3.1  H/ACA snoRNPs**   The majority of pseudoridines in rRNAs are added *via* specific H/ACA box snoRNPs having complementary guide sequences to the respective rRNAs and contain small sequence elements referred to as boxes H and ACA [30]. Similar to C/D box snoRNAs, substrate targeting involves base pairing through two short guide sequences in a loop portion of the duplex structures (Tables 1 and 2). The guide sequences are 14–15 nucleotides from the H or ACA box. The binding of the substrate places the target uridine in a pseudouridylation pocket between the flanking paired regions [30].

H/ACA snoRNPs contain four core proteins in yeast: Cbf5p (Dyskerin in humans), Gar1, Nhp2, and Nop10. Cbf5 is the catalytic pseudouridine synthase. Although the crystal structure from the eukaryotic H/ACA snoRNP is still missing, the archaeal H/ACA structure has provided noteworthy details about the organization of various core proteins [31]. Cbf5 has been shown to contact the ACA motif and both P1 and P2 stem. Nhp2, the yeast homolog of archaeal L7Ae binds to the K loop structure in the upper half of the RNA. Gar1 does not bind to the RNA directly but rather joins the complex through its interaction with Cbf5. Further structural analyses of Cbf5 have revealed that its interaction with Gar1 is essential for substrate binding and release [27].

# 4  Base Modifications

The rRNAs contain three different types of base modifications—methylation (m), acetylation (ac), and aminocarboxypropylation (acp). Methylation is the most common base modification in rRNA. All four nitrogenous bases of RNA undergo methylation either at nitrogen (N) or carbon (C) atoms. On the other hand, only cytosine bases are acetylated, and aminocarboxypropyl is added either to a uridine or pseudouridine residues in yeast. The base modifications of RNA are primarily catalyzed by snoRNA-independent enzymes with only exception being 18S rRNA acetylation that requires particular C/D box snoRNAs (Tables 2 and 4).

**4.1  Base Methylation**   Methylation of nitrogenous base strongly affect their physical and chemical properties. Methylation promotes base stacking by increasing the hydrophobicity and the polarizability. Furthermore, methylation also influences the structure by increasing steric hindrance, blocking canonical (Watson–Crick) hydrogen bonding and fostering noncanonical Hoogsteen base paring. This presumably helps ncRNA like rRNA to attain and maintain specific conformations, essential for their corresponding function—both with respect to their structure and their enzymatic activity.

### 4.2 Methyl transferases

Methyltransferases are the enzymes that catalyze specific transfer of methyl group form a methyl donor to various substrates. S-*adeno-syl-methionine* (SAM or AdoMet) is the most common methyl donor by virtue of the presence of a charged methylsulfonium center [32]. Methyltransferases that utilize the methyl group of SAM for the methylation reaction are called SAM dependent methyltransferases. Based on their structural analysis, all currently known SAM dependent methyltransferases have been divided into five distinct classes (Class I to Class V) [33].

*Class I methyltransferases* are characterized by a Rossmann-fold like domain and methylate a wide variety of substrates (DNA, RNA and proteins along with other small molecules). Rossmann folds are nucleotide (especially NAD(P)) binding domains that also contain an alternating α/β strands topology in which two Rossmann fold domains are linked into 6 parallel β stands sandwiched by a pair of α-helices [32]. The Rossmann-like fold comprises of alternating β-stranded and α-helical regions, with all strands forming a central relatively planar β-sheet, and helices stuffing two layers, one on each side of the plane.

*Class II methyltransferases* are characterized by a methionine synthase activation domain. The Met synthase activation contains an unusual fold with long, central, antiparallel β-sheet flanked by groups of helices at either end, which makes it structurally distinct from Class I methyltransferases [32].

*Class III methyltransferases* act on ring carbons of the large, planar precorrin substrates during cobalamin biosynthesis (e.g., CbiF) [32].

*Class IV methyltransferases* belong to the SPOUT family and methylate either RNA or proteins [32, 34]. These enzymes contain a six- stranded parallel β sheet flanked by seven α-helices. Interestingly the first three strands of these methyltransferases form half of a Rossmann fold. The active site of SPOUT methyltransferases is located near the subunit interface of a homodimer.

*Class V methyltransferases* contain typical SET domains, discovered originally as conserved domain shared by chromatin remodeling proteins **S**u (var) 3–9, **E** (Z) (short for Enhancer of Zeste) and Trithorax [32]. Most of the currently known SET methyltransferases methylate lysine residues of various nuclear proteins involved in chromatin remodeling and transcriptional regulation. The SAM binding site and the catalytic center of SET domains contains all-β (eight curved β strands forming three small sheets) and knot-like structures like Class IV methyltransferases but based on a different topology [32].

### 4.3 N4- Acetylation of Cytidine (ac⁴C)

Acetylation of cytidine residues is a highly conserved base modification present in 18S rRNA, as well as leucine and serine tRNAs of yeast [35, 36]. Molecular dynamics simulation and in vitro studies using the noninitiator methionine-accepting tRNA of E. *coli* have reported that acetylation of cytidine residues stabilize the C3'-endo puckering conformation of ribose, and stabilizes the G–C base pairing in the RNA, which has been highlighted as an important function of this modification in counteracting mistakes that may occur during translation due to misreading of the isoleucine AUA codon by tRNA$^{Met}$ [37–39]. Interestingly, in the 18S rRNA both ac$^4$C residues [ac$^4$C 1280 (helix 34) and ac$^4$C1773 (helix 45)] are also involved in C-G base pairings that are fundamental for ribosome functionality [6, 40]. The disruption of these base pairing was found to be lethal for yeast cells (unpublished data).

Structural and functional analysis of bacterial RNA acetyltransferase TmcA has revealed that RNA acetyltransferases utilize acetyl-CoA as an acetyl group donor, which is transferred in an ATP-dependent manner to the cytosine residues [41]. RNA acetyltransferases contain an N- terminal RNA helicase domain similar to that of DEAD-box RNA helicases paired with a C- terminal Gcn5-related N-acetyltransferase (GNAT) fold. TmcA is a stand-alone enzyme and does not necessitate auxiliary factors for substrate specificity, which is likely due to similar substrates that it acetylates [42].

In contrast to TmcA, the yeast and higher eukaryotes TmcA homologs Kre33/NAT10 utilize protein factors Tan1 and THUMPD1, respectively, for tRNA acetylation and snoRNAs snR4 and snR45 for 18S rRNA acetylation [28, 43, 44].

### 4.4  3-Amino carboxy propylation acp

The addition of 3-aminocarboxypropyl (acp) to the RNA is another highly conserved modification in eukaryotic cellular RNAs derived from S-adenosyl-L-methionine (SAM) [45]. This modification is mostly added to the uridine and pseudouridine residues and impacts the ability of these bases to establish hydrogen bonding with otherwise complementary adenosine residue [46, 47].

RNA aminocarboxypropyl transferase is a novel class of SAM dependent acp transferase with a significant homology to the SPOUT-class RNA-methyltransferases    [46, 47]. Structure analysis of its archaeal Tsr3 homologs has revealed that these enzymes contains the same fold as in SPOUT- class-RNA methyltransferase [34], but due to a discrete SAM binding arrangement acp transferases transfer the acp instead of the methyl group of SAM to its substrate [47].

## 5  Base Modifications of 18S rRNA

The 18S rRNA of ribosome small subunit (SSU) contains four base methylation: one m$^1$acp3$\Psi$1191, two m$^6_2$A1781, m$^6_2$A1782, and a single m$^7$G1575, and two base acetylation—ac$^4$C 1280 and 1773 (Fig. 1 and Table 3).

### 5.1 Dim1 Catalyzes m62A1781 and m62A1782 dimethylation

The first base methylation analyzed in rRNAs of *S. cerevisiae* were the $m^6_2A1781$ and $m^6_2A1782$ dimethylations [48]. Both dimethylations of adenine residues at carbon atom 6 (C-6) in the 3′ of SSU rRNA are highly conserved and are catalyzed by universally conserved orthologous methyltransferases. In *S. cerevisiae*, Dim1 catalyzes the methylation of both adenine residues [48, 49]. Dim1 is an essential protein and plays a key role in 40S biogenesis. Interestingly, both these dimethylations of 18S are performed in the cytoplasm and it has been shown that 40S subunits lacking dimethylated 18S rRNA are not competent for translation in vitro [48, 49].

Nevertheless, further analysis of this methylation and its corresponding enzymes revealed that the methylation deficient mutant of *dim1* is viable albeit influences the 35S rRNA processing, suggesting that methylations are dispensable for ribosome function in vivo [48, 49].

### 5.2 Bud23 Catalyzes m7G1575 Methylation

Bud23 catalyzes the methylation of nitrogen atom 7 in the guanosine residue at position 1575 ($m^7G1575$) of 18S rRNA [50]. Residue G1575 is highly conserved and interacts with the anticodon loop of the P-site tRNA [40]. Bud23 is a eukaryote specific enzyme and no orthologs have been detected in prokaryotes. It is a nucleolar protein and has been shown to be critical for the efficient export of the small subunit and its cytoplasmic maturation [50]. Intriguingly, as observed for Dim1, the $m^7G1575$ methylation also turned out to be not the essential function of Bud23 as the loss of methylation does not exhibit any 40S processing and export defects. Conspicuously, Bud23 needs the assistance of methyltransferase adaptor protein, Trm112 for the methylation of G1575 [50–52].

### 5.3 Nep1 (Emg1) and Tsr3 Catalyze Ψ1191 Modification (m1 acp3Ψ 1191)

The most interesting modification in the rRNA result in 1-methyl-3-(3-amino-3-carboxypropyl)-pseudouridine ($m^1acp3\Psi1191$) [4]. *S. cerevisiae* 18S rRNA contains a single $m^1acp3\Psi$ hypermodification at residue 1191, located in the decoding center of the 40S subunit, proximal to the P site-tRNA [40]. The $m^1acp3\Psi1191$ modification comprises of three reactions: (1) pseudouridylation, (2) methylation, and finally (3) the addition of 3-amino-3-carboxypropyl [8, 47, 53]. During maturation of 18S rRNA, these modifications are added sequentially. First, snR35 snoRNP catalyzes the pseudouridylation of U1191, thus unlinking the N1 of the U1191 from the glycosidic bond with the ribose sugar [30]. Next, Nep1 (Emg1) methylates this N1 of Ψ1191. Nep1, also described as Emg1 is a highly conserved and an essential pseudouridine-N1-specific methyltransferase [8] with an extended SPOUT-class methyltransferase fold and a pre-organized SAM-binding site [9, 54, 55]. Remarkably, a point mutation in the human Nep1 (Emg1) protein (D86G) has been shown to be responsible for Bowen–Conradi syndrome (BSC mutation) [7]. As already observed in case of Bud23 and Dim1, the methylation appeared not to be the essential function of the Nep1. Instead, the BSC-mutated yeast Nep1 protein showed enhanced dimerization propensity and increased affinity for its RNA-target in vitro. Furthermore, the BCS mutation prevented nucleolar accumulation of Nep1, which could be the reason for reduced growth in yeast and the Bowen-Conradi syndrome [8]. Furthermore, loss of methylation leads to defects in 40S subunits and affects antibiotic sensitivity [8, 56, 57]. Genetic analysis of Nep1 has provided understanding of its possible essential function [56, 58]. Overexpression of Rps19 protein has been demonstrated to suppress the deletion of otherwise essential Nep1 [58]. This has led to the hypothesis that perhaps the essential function of Nep1 is to assist the incorporation of Rps19 protein during 40S biogenesis. Nevertheless, this model awaits the biochemical experiments in its support [59].

Whereas $\Psi$ (snR35) and N1-CH$_3$ (Nep1) are introduced in the nucleus, it was shown that the addition of 3-amino-3-carboxypropyl to the $\Psi$1191 takes place in the cytoplasm [53]. The enzyme responsible for the transfer of 3-amino-3-carboxypropyl (acp) to the N3 atom of $\Psi$1191 was recently identified as Tsr3 [47]. A homologous enzyme was also identified in *E. coli* that catalyzes acp$^3$U modification at position 47 in the variable loop of eight *E. coli* tRNAs [46].

## 5.4 Kre33/NAT10 Catalyzes ac$^4$C1280 and ac$^4$C1773 Acetylation of the 18S rRNA in a snoRNA Dependent Manner

Eukaryotes contain only one cytidine acetyltransferase Kre33 (yeast) and NAT10 (human) that catalyzes both rRNA and tRNA cytidine acetylation [28, 43, 44]. Kre33 contains a N terminal helicase domain fused to the C terminal acetyltransferase domain related to GCN5 [42, 44]. In *S. cerevisiae* Tan1 was initially identified as a protein that is required for acetylation of ac$^4$C formation at position 12 of tRNA-Ser (CGA) [36]. Nevertheless, Tan1 does not contain any catalytic (acetyltransferase) domain for ac$^4$C formation but rather contains the THUMP domain, responsible for tRNA binding.

Interestingly, the acetylation of two cytosine residues in 18S rRNA catalyzed by Kre33 are guided by the two box C/D snoRNAs snR4 and snR45 which are not known to be involved in methylation [28]. This is in contrast to tRNA acetylation where protein Tan1 likely guides Kre33 to the acetylated cytidine [28, 43, 44]. These results highlighted yet another example of an incredible cellular modularity, where a single enzyme is targeted to diverse substrates by means of either protein or RNA adaptors. Both snR4 and snR45 establish extended bipartite complementarity around the cytosines targeted for acetylation [28].

The viability of catalytically deficient Kre33 mutants demonstrated that acetylation of 18S rRNA is dispensable for cell viability. Although both catalytic deficient mutants, kre33-*H545A* and kre33-*R637A* exhibited severe growth defects at 37 °C, similar to what was observed previously for the Tan1 deletion mutant [36, 44]. Since snoRNA deletions did not exhibit this phenotype at 37 °C, we concluded that this is probably due to the loss of tRNA acetylation.

# 6    Base Modifications of 25S rRNA

The 25S rRNA of the ribosome large subunit (LSU) in yeast contains 6 base methylation: two $m^1A$ (1-methyl adenosine), two $m^5C$ (5-methyl cytosine), and two $m^3U$ (3-methyl uridine) (Fig. 1 and Table 4). Two $m^5U$ (5-methyl uridine) methylations were also reported previously but the presence of these in the 25S rRNA have been disproven.

## 6.1    Rrp8 (Bmt1) Catalyzes $m^1$ A 645 Methylation

Rrp8, a protein previously shown to be involved in the processing of 35S rRNA at site A2 [60]. Rrp8 catalyzes $m^1A645$ base methylation of 25S rRNA and is a Class I SAM dependent rRNA methyltransferase [61]. The mapping of $m^1A645$ on the ribosomal RNA revealed that this residue is present in helix 25.1 of domain II of the 25S rRNA. Helix 25.1 is highly conserved in eukaryotes including humans [62]. The in vivo structural probing of 25S rRNA, using both DMS and SHAPE, revealed that the loss of the Rrp8-catalyzed $m^1A$ modification alters the conformation of domain I of yeast 25S rRNA causing translation initiation defects detectable as halfmer formation, likely because of incompetent loading of 60S on the 43S-preinitiation complex [62]. Surprisingly, quantitative proteomic analysis of the yeast $\Delta rrp8$ mutant strain using 2D-DIGE have exhibited that loss of $m^1A645$ impacts production of a specific set of proteins involved in carbohydrate metabolism, translation, and ribosome synthesis [62]. These findings in yeast point to a role of Rrp8 in primary metabolism. In conclusion, the $m^1A$ modification is crucial for maintaining an optimal 60S conformation, which in turn is important for regulating the synthesis of key metabolic enzymes.

## 6.2    Bmt2 Catalyzes A2142 Methylation ($m^1A2142$)

Bmt2 catalyzes the $m^1A2142$ methylation located in helix 65 (H65) of the 25S rRNA [63]. H65 belongs to domain IV of 25S rRNA, which makes most of the intersubunit surface of the large subunit. Interestingly, L2, a highly conserved protein makes physical contact with H65, especially with its SH3-β barrel globular domain. Like Rrp8, Bmt2 also belongs to Class I Rossmann-like fold methyltransferases family [63].

A deletion mutant of *BMT2* was previously identified to extend hibernating life span and to exhibit peroxide sensitivity [64]. A methyltransferase dead mutant (bmt2-*G180R*) and rDNA point mutants (A2142G, A2142C, and A2142T) also exhibited hydrogen peroxide sensitivity. Taken together this indicates that the biosynthetic pathways of this modifications interact with the cellular response toward oxidative stress stimulated by hydrogen peroxide.

**6.3   Rcm1 (Bmt3) and Nop2 (Bmt4) Catalyze $m^5C2278$ and $m^5C2870$ Methylation**

Yeast 25S rRNA contains two $m^5C$ residues at positions 2278 and 2870 [65]. Rcm1 and Nop2 were shown to be responsible for two distinct $m^5C$ methylations of 25S rRNA at position C2278 and C2870, respectively [66]. Both Rcm1 and Nop2 belong to Class I methyltransferases characterized by Rossmann-like folds. Interestingly, biochemical and structural analyses of other RNA cytosine methyltransferases have provided an important insight into their catalytic mechanism [67]. All known RNA cytosine methyltransferases utilize two highly conserved cysteine residues in the motif IV and motif VI for the addition of methyl group at C5 of cytosine [65, 67]. The cysteine in motif VI makes a nucleophilic attack on to the C-6 of cytosine and form a covalent adduct with the RNA, whereas the cysteine of motif IV is important for the release of the substrate [67]. For both Rcm1 and Nop2 exchange of cysteine in motif VI with the alanine led to methyltransferase-dead mutants, whereas replacement of cysteine in motif IV with alanine turned out to be lethal [66].

The lethality of both rcm1 and nop2 motif IV cysteine mutant proteins suggested that due to substitution of cysteines in motif IV, the mutant proteins fail to separate themselves from their corresponding targets and forms a stable protein-rRNA complex. This fixing of the mutant protein then blocks the 25S rRNA processing and probably causes cell death. This model was further supported by suppression of this lethality upon exchange of both motif IV and motif VI cysteine residues together in case of Rcm1 and also Nop2, as this precluded the formation of any covalent complex [66].

Nop2 is an essential protein in *S. cerevisiae* [68]. Previous biochemical analyses using the hypomorphic expression system have shown that Nop2 depletion causes severe defects in the rRNA processing and 60S biogenesis. The viability of the *nop2-C478A* methyltransferase-deadmutant demonstrated, that methylation at C2870 is not the essential function of Nop2. In other words $m^5C2870$ is not essential for viability. Nevertheless, the polysome profiles and Northern-blotting analysis of the methyltransferase-dead mutant of Nop2 demonstrated that loss of $m^5C2870$ strongly impairs the 35S rRNA processing and 60S biogenesis; the phenotypes observed previously upon depletion of Nop2 [66]. Therefore, this suggested that the Nop2 depletion phenotypes observed previously are apparently the result of reduced $m^5C$ modification.

Absence of $m^5C2278$ causes anisomycin hypersensitivity [66]. In contrast to $m^5C2870$, loss of $m^5C$ 2278 did not exhibit any defects in 60S biogenesis and 35S rRNA processing. As far as the biological role of $m^5C2278$ is concerned, loss of $m^5C2278$ in helix 70 (H70) causes anisomycin hypersensitivity, indicating that the loss of this methylation disrupts its optimal conformation. Together with the data from the $m^1A2142$ base modification in helix 65, the anisomycin hypersensitivity after the loss of $m^5C\,2278$ also suggests that the conformation of domain IV of 25S rRNA is crucial for anisomycin sensitivity as both $m^1A2142$ and $m^5C\,2278$ reside in the domain IV of the 25S rRNA [66].

To understand how 25S/28S rRNA cytosine methylation ($m^5C$) and its corresponding enzyme (Rcm1/NSUN5) impact biological functions, in a collaboration with Johannes Grillari's lab, we found, that reduced levels of the enzyme increase the life span and stress resistance in yeast, worms, and flies [69]. Loss of $m^5C$ alters the structural conformation of the ribosome and promotes translational reprogramming by favoring translation of a distinct subset of oxidative stress-responsive mRNAs [69]. Thus, rather than merely being a static molecular machine executing translation, the ribosome exhibits functional diversity by modification of just a single rRNA nucleotide, resulting in an alteration of organismal physiological behavior, and linking rRNA-mediated translational regulation to the modulation of life span, and differential stress response.

### 6.4 Bmt5 and Bmt6 Catalyze $m^3U2634$ and $m^3U2843$ Methylation

Bmt5 and Bmt6 catalyze the $m^3U$ methylations at positions 2634 and 2843 of the 25S rRNA [70]. Both enzymes belong to the Rossmann-like fold protein family. The substitution of highly conserved glycine residues in the SAM binding motif of both Bmt5 and Bmt6 with arginine abolished their catalytic activity. Surprisingly, $m^3U$ methylation in the 16S rRNA of E. coli is catalyzed by proteins of the SPOUT methyltransferase family which had led to the assumption that $m^3U$ methylation could only be performed by SPOUT methyltransferases [71]. With the identification of Bmt5 and Bmt6 this convention is no more valid.

Both Bmt5 and Bmt6 are highly conserved in lower eukaryotes including yeasts like Schizosaccharomyces pombe, Neurospora crassa, and Kluyveromyces lactis. The Bmt5 and Bmt6 homologs are likely performing the same function in these organisms.

### 6.5 25S rRNA of Yeast Does Not Contain any $m^5U$ Residues

Yeast 25S rRNA was predicted to contain two $m^5U$ residues at position 956 and 2924 [20, 72]. Using both RP-HPLC and mass spectrometry this was disproved [70]. Similarly, the 25S rRNA of C. albicans and S. pombe also did not contain any $m^5U$ residues [73]. This has been also confirmed for higher eukaryotes, whereas $m^5U$ residues have been only observed in tRNAs, which is in consent with the presence of only one $m^5U$ methyltransferase, Trm2 (in yeast and its homologs), responsible for $m^5U$ modification of tRNAs at position 54. Up till now, Trm2 has not been observed to display any interaction with the rRNA in yeast. Taken together, this would apparently suggest that during the course of evolution m$^5$U methylation have disappeared in rRNA of eukaryotes.

## Acknowledgments

We thank Jun Yang, Peter Kötter, and Britta Meyer for fruitful discussions and suggestions. We would also like to thank Deutsche Forschungsgemeinschaft (DFG), Goethe-University, Frankfurt/ M., and the state of Hesse for financial support.

## References

1. Boccaletto P, Machnicka MA, Purta E, Piatkowski P, Baginski B, Wirecki TK, de Crecy-Lagard V, Ross R, Limbach PA, Kotter A et al (2018) MODOMICS: a database of RNA modification pathways. 2017 update. Nucleic Acids Res 46:D303–D307

2. Woolford JL Jr, Baserga SJ (2013) Ribosome biogenesis in the yeast Saccharomyces cerevisiae. Genetics 195:643–681

3. Cech TR (2000) Structural biology. The ribosome is a ribozyme. Science 289:878–879

4. Klootwijk J, Planta RJ (1973) Analysis of the methylation sites in yeast ribosomal RNA. Eur J Biochem 39:325–333

5. Motorin Y, Helm M (2011) RNA nucleotide methylation. Wiley Interdiscip Rev RNA 2: 611–631

6. Sharma S, Lafontaine DLJ (2015) 'View from a Bridge': a new perspective on eukaryotic rRNA base modification. Trends Biochem Sci 40: 560–575

7. Armistead J, Khatkar S, Meyer B, Mark BL, Patel N, Coghlan G, Lamont RE, Liu S, Wiechert J, Cattini PA et al (2009) Mutation of a gene essential for ribosome biogenesis, EMG1, causes Bowen-Conradi syndrome. Am J Hum Genet 84:728–739

8. Meyer B, Wurm JP, Kotter P, Leisegang MS, Schilling V, Buchhaupt M, Held M, Bahr U, Karas M, Heckel A et al (2011) The Bowen-Conradi syndrome protein Nep1 (Emg1) has a dual role in eukaryotic ribosome biogenesis, as an essential assembly factor and in the methylation of Psi1191 in yeast 18S rRNA. Nucleic Acids Res 39:1526–1537

9. Wurm JP, Meyer B, Bahr U, Held M, Frolow O, Kotter P, Engels JW, Heckel A, Karas M, Entian KD et al (2010) The ribosome assembly factor Nep1 responsible for Bowen-Conradi syndrome is a pseudouridine-N1-specific methyltransferase. Nucleic Acids Res 38:2387–2398

10. Doll A, Grzeschik KH (2001) Characterization of two novel genes, WBSCR20 and WBSCR22, deleted in Williams-Beuren syndrome. Cytogenet Cell Genet 95:20–27

11. Knight SW, Heiss NS, Vulliamy TJ, Greschner S, Stavrides G, Pai GS, Lestringant G, Varma N, Mason PJ, Dokal I et al (1999) X-linked dyskeratosis congenita is predominantly caused by missense mutations in the DKC1 gene. Am J Hum Genet 65: 50–58

12. Nachmani D, Bothmer AH, Grisendi S, Mele A, Bothmer D, Lee JD, Monteleone E, Cheng K, Zhang Y, Bester AC et al (2019) Germline NPM1 mutations lead to altered rRNA 2′-O-methylation and cause dyskeratosis congenita. Nat Genet 51:1518–1529

13. Venturi G, Montanaro L (2020) How altered ribosome production can cause or contribute to human disease: the spectrum of ribosomopathies. Cell 9:2300

14. Buchhaupt M, Sharma S, Kellner S, Oswald S, Paetzold M, Peifer C, Watzinger P, Schrader J, Helm M, Entian KD (2014) Partial methylation at Am100 in 18S rRNA of baker's yeast reveals ribosome heterogeneity on the level of eukaryotic rRNA modification. PLoS One 9: e89640

15. Sloan KE, Warda AS, Sharma S, Entian KD, Lafontaine DLJ, Bohnsack MT (2017) Tuning the ribosome: the influence of rRNA modification on eukaryotic ribosome biogenesis and function. RNA Biol 14:1138–1152

16. Taoka M, Nobe Y, Yamaki Y, Yamauchi Y, Ishikawa H, Takahashi N, Nakayama H, Isobe T (2016) The complete chemical structure of Saccharomyces cerevisiae rRNA: partial pseudouridylation of U2345 in 25S rRNA by

snoRNA snR9. Nucleic Acids Res 44: 8951–8961

17. Vlachos A (2017) Acquired ribosomopathies in leukemia and solid tumors. Hematology Am Soc Hematol Educ Program 2017:716–719

18. Aspesi A, Ellis SR (2019) Rare ribosomopathies: insights into mechanisms of cancer. Nat Rev Cancer 19:228–238

19. Barbieri I, Kouzarides T (2020) Role of RNA modifications in cancer. Nat Rev Cancer 20: 303–322

20. Bakin A, Lane BG, Ofengand J (1994) Clustering of pseudouridine residues around the peptidyltransferase center of yeast cytoplasmic and mitochondrial ribosomes. Biochemistry 33: 13475–13483

21. Maden BE (1988) Locations of methyl groups in 28 S rRNA of Xenopus laevis and man. Clustering in the conserved core of molecule. J Mol Biol 201:289–314

22. Yang J, Sharma S, Watzinger P, Hartmann JD, Kotter P, Entian KD (2016) Mapping of complete set of ribose and base modifications of yeast rRNA by RP-HPLC and mung bean nuclease assay. PLoS One 11:e0168873

23. Yang J, Sharma S, Kotter P, Entian KD (2015) Identification of a new ribose methylation in the 18S rRNA of S. cerevisiae. Nucleic Acids Res 43:2342–2352

24. Sharma S, Marchand V, Motorin Y, Lafontaine DLJ (2017) Identification of sites of 2'-O-methylation vulnerability in human ribosomal RNAs by systematic mapping. Sci Rep 7:11490

25. Shi Z, Barna M (2015) Translating the genome in time and space: specialized ribosomes, RNA regulons, and RNA-binding proteins. Annu Rev Cell Dev Biol 31:31–54

26. Kiss L (1996) Site-specific ribose methylation of preribosomal RNA: a novel function for small nucleolar RNAs. Cell 85:1077–1088

27. Watkins NJ, Bohnsack MT (2012) The box C/D and H/ACA snoRNPs: key players in the modification, processing and the dynamic folding of ribosomal RNA. Wiley Interdiscip Rev RNA 3:397–414

28. Sharma S, Yang J, van Nues R, Watzinger P, Kotter P, Lafontaine DLJ, Granneman S, Entian KD (2017) Specialized box C/D snoRNPs act as antisense guides to target RNA base acetylation. PLoS Genet 13: e1006804

29. Noon KR, Guymon R, Crain PF, McCloskey JA, Thomm M, Lim J, Cavicchioli R (2003) Influence of temperature on tRNA modification in archaea: Methanococcoides burtonii (optimum growth temperature [Topt], 23 degrees C) and Stetteria hydrogenophila

(Topt, 95 degrees C). J Bacteriol 185: 5483–5490

30. Ganot P, Bortolin ML, Kiss T (1997) Site-specific pseudouridine formation in preribosomal RNA is guided by small nucleolar RNAs. Cell 89:799–809

31. Duan J, Li L, Lu J, Wang W, Ye K (2009) Structural mechanism of substrate RNA recruitment in H/ACA RNA-guided pseudouridine synthase. Mol Cell 34:427–439

32. Kozbial PZ, Mushegian AR (2005) Natural history of S-adenosylmethionine-binding proteins. BMC Struct Biol 5:19

33. Schubert HL, Blumenthal RM, Cheng X (2003) Many paths to methyltransfer: a chronicle of convergence. Trends Biochem Sci 28: 329–335

34. Anantharaman V, Koonin EV, Aravind L (2002) SPOUT: a class of methyltransferases that includes spoU and trmD RNA methylase superfamilies, and novel superfamilies of predicted prokaryotic RNA methylases. J Mol Microbiol Biotechnol 4:71–75

35. Thomas G, Gordon J, Rogg H (1978) N4-Acetylcytidine. A previously unidentified labile component of the small subunit of eukaryotic ribosomes. J Biol Chem 253: 1101–1105

36. Johansson MJ, Bystrom AS (2004) The Saccharomyces cerevisiae TAN1 gene is required for N4-acetylcytidine formation in tRNA. RNA 10:712–719

37. Kawai G, Hashizume T, Miyazawa T, McCloskey JA, Yokoyama S (1989) Conformational characteristics of 4-acetylcytidine found in tRNA. Nucleic Acids Symp Ser (21):61–62

38. Kumbhar BV, Kamble AD, Sonawane KD (2013) Conformational preferences of modified nucleoside N(4)-acetylcytidine, ac4C occur at "wobble" 34th position in the anticodon loop of tRNA. Cell Biochem Biophys 66: 797–816

39. Stern L, Schulman LH (1978) The role of the minor base N4-acetylcytidine in the function of the Escherichia coli noninitiator methionine transfer RNA. J Biol Chem 253:6132–6139

40. Ben-Shem A, Garreau de Loubresse N, Melnikov S, Jenner L, Yusupova G, Yusupov M (2011) The structure of the eukaryotic ribosome at 3.0 A resolution. Science 334: 1524–1529

41. Ikeuchi Y, Kitahara K, Suzuki T (2008) The RNA acetyltransferase driven by ATP hydrolysis synthesizes N4-acetylcytidine of tRNA anticodon. EMBO J 27:2194–2203

42. Chimnaronk S, Suzuki T, Manita T, Ikeuchi Y, Yao M, Suzuki T, Tanaka I (2009) RNA

helicase module in an acetyltransferase that modifies a specific tRNA anticodon. EMBO J 28:1362–1373

43. Ito S, Akamatsu Y, Noma A, Kimura S, Miyauchi K, Ikeuchi Y, Suzuki T, Suzuki T (2014) A single acetylation of 18 S rRNA is essential for biogenesis of the small ribosomal subunit in Saccharomyces cerevisiae. J Biol Chem 289:26201–26212

44. Sharma S, Langhendries JL, Watzinger P, Kotter P, Entian KD, Lafontaine DL (2015) Yeast Kre33 and human NAT10 are conserved 18S rRNA cytosine acetyltransferases that modify tRNAs assisted by the adaptor Tan1/THUMPD1. Nucleic Acids Res 43:2242–2258

45. Ohashi Z, Maeda M, McCloskey JA, Nishimura S (1974) 3-(3-Amino-3-carboxypropyl) uridine: a novel modified nucleoside isolated from Escherichia coli phenylalanine transfer ribonucleic acid. Biochemistry 13:2620–2625

46. Meyer B, Immer C, Kaiser S, Sharma S, Yang J, Watzinger P, Weiss L, Kotter A, Helm M, Seitz HM et al (2020) Identification of the 3-amino-3-carboxypropyl (acp) transferase enzyme responsible for acp3U formation at position 47 in Escherichia coli tRNAs. Nucleic Acids Res 48:1435–1450

47. Meyer B, Wurm JP, Sharma S, Immer C, Pogoryelov D, Kotter P, Lafontaine DL, Wohnert J, Entian KD (2016) Ribosome biogenesis factor Tsr3 is the aminocarboxypropyl transferase responsible for 18S rRNA hypermodification in yeast and humans. Nucleic Acids Res 44:4304–4316

48. Lafontaine DL, Preiss T, Tollervey D (1998) Yeast 18S rRNA dimethylase Dim1p: a quality control mechanism in ribosome synthesis? Mol Cell Biol 18:2360–2370

49. Lafontaine D, Delcour J, Glasser AL, Desgres J, Vandenhaute J (1994) The DIM1 gene responsible for the conserved m6(2)Am6 (2)A dimethylation in the 3′-terminal loop of 18 S rRNA is essential in yeast. J Mol Biol 241:492–497

50. White J, Li Z, Sardana R, Bujnicki JM, Marcotte EM, Johnson AW (2008) Bud23 methylates G1575 of 18S rRNA and is required for efficient nuclear export of pre-40S subunits. Mol Cell Biol 28:3151–3161

51. Figaro S, Wacheul L, Schillewaert S, Graille M, Huvelle E, Mongeard R, Zorbas C, Lafontaine DL, Heurgue-Hamard V (2012) Trm112 is required for Bud23-mediated methylation of the 18S rRNA at position G1575. Mol Cell Biol 32:2254–2267

52. Sardana R, White JP, Johnson AW (2013) The rRNA methyltransferase Bud23 shows functional interaction with components of the SSU processome and RNase MRP. RNA 19:828–840

53. Liang XH, Liu Q, Fournier MJ (2009) Loss of rRNA modifications in the decoding center of the ribosome impairs translation and strongly delays pre-rRNA processing. RNA 15:1716–1728

54. Taylor AB, Meyer B, Leal BZ, Kotter P, Schirf V, Demeler B, Hart PJ, Entian KD, Wohnert J (2008) The crystal structure of Nep1 reveals an extended SPOUT-class methyltransferase fold and a pre-organized SAM-binding site. Nucleic Acids Res 36:1542–1554

55. Wurm JP, Duchardt E, Meyer B, Leal BZ, Kotter P, Entian KD, Wohnert J (2009) Backbone resonance assignments of the 48 kDa dimeric putative 18S rRNA methyltransferase Nep1 from Methanocaldococcus jannaschii. Biomol NMR Assign 3:251-254. [Epub 2009, Sep 25, https://doi.org/10.1007/s12104-009-9187-z]

56. Buchhaupt M, Kotter P, Entian KD (2007) Mutations in the nucleolar proteins Tma23 and Nop6 suppress the malfunction of the Nep1 protein. FEMS Yeast Res 7:771–781

57. Eschrich D, Buchhaupt M, Kotter P, Entian KD (2002) Nep1p (Emg1p), a novel protein conserved in eukaryotes and archaea, is involved in ribosome biogenesis. Curr Genet 40:326–338

58. Buchhaupt M, Meyer B, Kotter P, Entian KD (2006) Genetic evidence for 18S rRNA binding and an Rps19p assembly function of yeast nucleolar protein Nep1p. Mol Gen Genomics 276:273–284

59. Strunk BS, Karbstein K (2009) Powering through ribosome assembly. RNA 15:2083–2104

60. Bousquet-Antonelli C, Vanrobays E, Gelugne JP, Caizergues-Ferrer M, Henry Y (2000) Rrp8p is a yeast nucleolar protein functionally linked to Gar1p and involved in pre-rRNA cleavage at site A2. RNA 6:826–843

61. Peifer C, Sharma S, Watzinger P, Lamberth S, Kotter P, Entian KD (2013) Yeast Rrp8p, a novel methyltransferase responsible for m1A 645 base modification of 25S rRNA. Nucleic Acids Res 41:1151–1163

62. Sharma S, Hartmann JD, Watzinger P, Klepper A, Peifer C, Kotter P, Lafontaine DLJ, Entian KD (2018) A single N(1)-methyladenosine on the large ribosomal

subunit rRNA impacts locally its structure and the translation of key metabolic enzymes. Sci Rep 8:11904

63. Sharma S, Watzinger P, Kotter P, Entian KD (2013) Identification of a novel methyltransferase, Bmt2, responsible for the N-1-methyladenosine base modification of 25S rRNA in Saccharomyces cerevisiae. Nucleic Acids Res 41:5428–5443

64. Postma L, Lehrach H, Ralser M (2009) Surviving in the cold: yeast mutants with extended hibernating lifespan are oxidant sensitive. Aging (Albany NY) 1:957–960

65. Motorin Y, Lyko F, Helm M (2010) 5-methylcytosine in RNA: detection, enzymatic formation and biological functions. Nucleic Acids Res 38:1415–1430

66. Sharma S, Yang J, Watzinger P, Kotter P, Entian KD (2013) Yeast Nop2 and Rcm1 methylate C2870 and C2278 of the 25S rRNA, respectively. Nucleic Acids Res 41:9062–9076

67. Foster PG, Nunes CR, Greene P, Moustakas D, Stroud RM (2003) The first structure of an RNA m5C methyltransferase, Fmu, provides insight into catalytic mechanism and specific binding of RNA substrate. Structure 11:1609–1620

68. Hong B, Brockenbrough JS, Wu P, Aris JP (1997) Nop2p is required for pre-rRNA processing and 60S ribosome subunit synthesis in yeast. Mol Cell Biol 17:378–388

69. Schosserer M, Minois N, Angerer TB, Amring M, Dellago H, Harreither E, Calle-Perez A, Pircher A, Gerstl MP, Pfeifenberger S et al (2015) Methylation of ribosomal RNA by NSUN5 is a conserved mechanism modulating organismal lifespan. Nat Commun 6:6158

70. Sharma S, Yang J, Duttmann S, Watzinger P, Kotter P, Entian KD (2014) Identification of novel methyltransferases, Bmt5 and Bmt6, responsible for the m3U methylations of 25S rRNA in Saccharomyces cerevisiae. Nucleic Acids Res 42:3246–3260

71. Basturea GN, Rudd KE, Deutscher MP (2006) Identification and characterization of RsmE, the founding member of a new RNA base methyltransferase family. RNA 12:426–434

72. Nordlund ME, Johansson JO, von Pawel-Rammingen U, Bystrom AS (2000) Identification of the TRM2 gene encoding the tRNA (m5U54)methyltransferase of Saccharomyces cerevisiae. RNA 6:844–860

73. Taoka M, Nobe Y, Hori M, Takeuchi A, Masaki S, Yamauchi Y, Nakayama H, Takahashi N, Isobe T (2015) A mass spectrometry-based method for comprehensive quantitative determination of post-transcriptional RNA modifications: the complete chemical structure of Schizosaccharomyces pombe ribosomal RNAs. Nucleic Acids Res 43:e115

# Chapter 10

# In Vitro Selection of Deoxyribozymes for the Detection of RNA Modifications

## Anam Liaqat, Maksim V. Sednev, and Claudia Höbartner

## Abstract

Deoxyribozymes are artificially evolved DNA molecules with catalytic abilities. RNA-cleaving deoxyribozymes have been recognized as an efficient tool for detection of modifications in target RNAs and provide an alternative to traditional and modern methods for detection of ribose or nucleobase methylation. However, there are only few examples of DNA enzymes that specifically reveal the presence of a certain type of modification, including $N^6$-methyladenosine, and the knowledge about how DNA enzymes recognize modified RNAs is still extremely limited. Therefore, DNA enzymes cannot be easily engineered for the analysis of desired RNA modifications, but are instead identified by in vitro selection from random DNA libraries using synthetic modified RNA substrates. This protocol describes a general in vitro selection stagtegy to evolve new RNA-cleaving DNA enzymes that can efficiently differentiate modified RNA substrates from their unmodified counterpart.

**Key words** RNA, Deoxyribozymes, Modified RNA nucleotides, Catalytic DNA, Epitranscriptomics, In vitro selection, RNA cleavage

---

## 1 Introduction

Cellular RNAs can be modified posttranscriptionally through chemical modifications on nucleobases or the ribose-phosphate backbone. The flourishing field of "epitranscriptomics" explores the modifications that are functionally relevant to RNA structure, stability, base pairing, and binding potential to proteins and other ligands [1, 2]. Besides the reversible chemical modifications of DNA and proteins, posttranscriptional RNA modifications provide another layer of regulation for gene expression [3]. Although modified nucleotides are found in many different types of coding and noncoding transcripts and the precise roles are far from being completely understood, several tRNA and rRNA modifications are expected to play specific structural and functional roles [4]. For example, since ribosomal rRNA modifications are installed early in rRNA processing, it is possible that they assist RNA folding

Karl-Dieter Entian (ed.), *Ribosome Biogenesis: Methods and Protocols*, Methods in Molecular Biology, vol. 2533, https://doi.org/10.1007/978-1-0716-2501-9_10, © The Author(s) 2022

or are involved in the recruitment of chaperone proteins [5]. Interestingly, many ribosomal RNA modifications are evolutionary conserved but individual modifications are often not essential, while a global lack of rRNA modifications diminishes viability. Recently it was found that some rRNA modifications are installed substoichiometrically, resulting in different subpopulations of ribosomes with altered fitness or fine-tuned activity for translation of specific mRNA [6, 7].

Although more than 120 different modifications in various types of RNAs are known for decades, the field is still lagging on technologies for transcriptome-wide mapping for most of these modifications. Several techniques such as two-dimensional thin layer chromatography (2D-TLC), high-resolution liquid chromatography coupled to mass spectrometry (HPLC-MS), methylated RNA immunoprecipitation, and reverse transcriptase–based signatures followed by deep sequencing have been used to map modifications in RNA [8–12]. These techniques, however, suffer from various limitations such as the loss of sequence information upon digestion into mononucleotides as required for TLC and MS approaches, and from low specificity and selectivity of antibodies used for immunoprecipitation. Therefore a combination of different methods is necessary to obtain reliable insights into presence, distribution and abundance of certain modified nucleotides, and simple analytical tools are needed for validation [13].

Deoxyribozymes (alternatively called DNA enzymes) are attractive tools to expand the repertoire of methods for detecting RNA modifications in a sequence-specific manner. Deoxyribozymes are in vitro selected DNA molecules that have the potential to catalyze various chemical reactions, including protein modifications, DNA/RNA ligation, and DNA/RNA cleavage [14–16]. Among these, DNA enzymes that catalyze a site-specific RNA cleavage reaction are the most prominent group [17, 18].

Deoxyribozymes have a catalytic core that originates from a random region of 20–40 nucleotides and that is flanked by two binding arms complementary to the RNA substrate. DNA enzymes require metal ions ($Mg^{2+}$, $Mn^{2+}$, $Zn^{2+}$) for their catalytic activity. RNA-cleaving deoxyribozymes catalyze the cleavage reaction by mediating the attack of the 2′-hydroxyl group onto the adjacent phosphodiester linkage, which results in the formation of 2′,3′-cyclic phosphate and 5′-hydroxyl termini [18, 19]. This reaction gives the possibility to detect modifications that directly block the functional group in the cleavage reaction, such as 2′-O-methylation. In fact, this resulted in the first application of DNA enzymes to analyze ribosomal RNA modifications [20]. Alternatively, deoxyribozymes have been used to detect RNA modifications on the 5′-terminus of the cleavage site. DNA enzymes 8–17 and 10–23 [21] oriented to cleave various dinucleotide junctions served as tool for cleavage of phosphodiester linkage followed by radioactive labeling and 2D TLC for site-specific analysis of pseudouridine [22], one of the most important ribonucleotide modifications in rRNA. Recently, deoxyribozymes have been explored to sense other modifications such as $N^6$-methyladenosine (m$^6$A) and $N^6$-isopentenyladenosine (i$^6$A) [23, 24]. The m$^6$A-sensitive DNA enzymes have been shown to be generally applicable to analyze the presence of m$^6$A in DGACH sequence motifs, as demonstrated for lncRNAs and a set of C/D box snoRNAs that function as guides for 2'-O ribose methylation of ribosomal RNA. These recent examples demonstrated that catalytic DNA can likely be developed for various modifications as a tool to differentiate modified from unmodified RNA in a sequence-specific manner.

Deoxyribozymes are identified through in vitro selection based on the systematic evolution of ligands by exponential enrichment (SELEX) technique from a random pool of DNA through repetitive cycles of selection and amplification as shown in Fig. 1.

This chapter gives a detailed protocol for the gel-based SELEX technique to evolve catalytically active DNA species from a random pool that is capable of specifically detecting RNA modification, thus leading to an enhanced/reduced cleavage of the target RNA depending on the modification state. The in vitro selection cycle begins with the ligation of the DNA pool to the RNA substrate containing the desired RNA modification by T4 DNA ligase using a

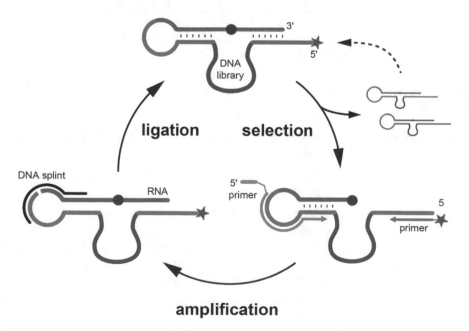

**Fig. 1** Overview of the in vitro selection scheme for the generation of modification-sensitive RNA cleaving deoxyribozymes. The red dot represents the modified nucleotide in the RNA substrate (green), in between Watson–Crick-base-paired regions. The constant regions of the DNA are shown in light blue, and the random region of the DNA library in dark blue. The yellow star represents a 5'-label on the DNA facilitating detection on PAGE

DNA splint. The ligated product is then incubated with $Mg^{2+}$ at 37 °C to initiate the cleavage reaction. The active fraction is isolated by PAGE due to the change in size. Active DNA enzymes are then amplified through PCR using a 5′-labeled forward primer (fluorescein or $^{32}P$-labeled for detection of bands on PAGE) and a tailed reverse primer containing a nonextendable ethylene glycol spacer to allow separation of sense and antisense strands. After isolation of the single-stranded PCR product through denaturing PAGE, the enriched active species are ligated to the RNA substrate to initiate the next round of selection. To increase the specificity of the resulting deoxyribozymes, negative selection rounds are introduced, in which the DNA library is challenged with the unmodified RNA. Other factors that can be adapted to enhance specificity are metal ion concentration, selection time and temperature. After several rounds of in vitro selection, the enriched pool is tested for its ability to discriminate modified from unmodified RNA. Finally, individual deoxyribozymes are identified by traditional cloning and Sanger sequencing and/or from Illumina NGS datasets that allow a deeper analysis of the enrichment of certain sequence motifs. New candidate DNA enzymes are characterized by analyzing cleavage kinetics for modified and unmodified RNA substrates and mutational analyses are performed to identify key sequence motifs responsible for recognition of the RNA modification. In exceptional cases, the modified nucleotide in the RNA may lead to switch in the cleavage site of the endonuclease deoxyribozyme, providing an additional opportunity for quantitative readout of the modification level [24].

## 2  Materials

### 2.1  Oligonucleotides

1. Use ultrapure water for all oligonucleotides, buffers, and reactions.

2. Purify oligonucleotides by denaturing PAGE before use and store all oligonucleotide solutions and buffers at −20 °C.

3. RNA substrates with and without modification (for counter selection), prepared by solid-phase synthesis on 0.5–1 μmol scale, using commercially available or in-house synthesized phosphoramidites of modified nucleotides. A fraction of RNA substrate is labeled at 3′-end or 5′-end for kinetic assays.

4. Deoxyribozyme library: 0.5 μmol synthesis scale, 100 μM stock solution.

5. Primers: 5′-fluorescein labeled forward primer and $PEG_3$-linked tailed reverse primer. 0.5 μmol synthesis scale, 100 μM solution.

6. Splint DNA for ligation of DNA library to RNA substrate. 0.5 μmol synthesis scale, 100 μM solution.

**2.2 Denaturing Polyacrylamide Gel Electrophoresis**

1. 10× TBE buffer: 89 mM Tris–HCl, pH 8.0 at 25 °C, 89 mM boric acid, 50 mM EDTA.

2. Acrylamide gel stock solution: acrylamide solution (10% and 20%), 7 M Urea, 1 × TBE (*see* **Note 1**).

3. 25% ammonium persulfate (APS). Store at 4 °C.

4. $N,N,N',N'$-tetramethyl ethylenediamine (TEMED). Store at 4 °C.

5. PAGE loading buffer: 70% formamide, 1× TBE buffer, 50 mM EDTA, 0.4 mM bromophenol blue, 0.4 mM xylene cyanol, pH 8.0.

6. Elution buffer: 10 mM Tris, 1 mM EDTA, 300 mM NaCl, pH 8.0.

7. Absolute ethanol and 70% ethanol. Store at −20 °C.

8. Glass plates (20 cm × 20 cm and 20 cm × 30 cm), combs, and spacers.

**2.3 In Vitro Selection**

**2.3.1 Phosphorylation of RNA Selection Substrates**

1. T4 PNK enzyme (10 U/μL).

2. T4 PNK buffer A: 500 mM Tris–HCl, 10 mM MgCl$_2$, 500 mM DTT, 1 mM spermidine.

3. 10 mM ATP.

4. Roti® phenol–chloroform–isoamyl alcohol for extraction of RNA.

5. Roti® chloroform.

**2.3.2 Splint Ligation**

1. T4 DNA ligase enzyme (5 U/μL). Store at −20 °C.

2. T4 DNA ligase buffer: (10×) 400 mM Tris–HCl, 100 mM MgCl$_2$, 100 mM DTT, 5 mM ATP, pH 7.8. Store at −20 °C.

3. 10× Annealing buffer: 40 mM Tris–HCl, 150 mM NaCl, 1 mM EDTA, pH 8.0.

**2.3.3 Selection Step**

1. 10× Selection buffer: 500 mM Tris–HCl, 1500 mM NaCl, pH 7.5.

2. 400 mM MgCl$_2$ (stock solution).

**2.3.4 PCR Amplification**

1. DreamTaq DNA polymerase. Store at −20 °C.

2. DreamTaq buffer®: (10×) 20 mM MgCl$_2$, KCl, (NH$_4$)$_2$SO$_4$). Store at −20 °C.

3. dNTPs mixture (20 mM each dNTP).

1. 10× Kinetic assay buffer: 500 mM Tris–HCl, 1500 mM NaCl, pH 7.5.

2. 400 mM $MgCl_2$ (stock solution).

3. Quench buffer: 70% formamide, 1× TBE buffer, 50 mM EDTA, pH 8.0.

# 3  Methods

### 3.1  DNA Library Design

1. Select RNA sequence with target modification, inspired by natural sequence context of the modification, for example, in tRNAs or rRNA (or conserved motifs such as DRACH for $m^6A$).

2. For DNA library, select a random region of about twenty nucleotides (*see* **Note 2**). Add flanking sequence complementary to RNA substrate upstream and downstream of the catalytic core, maintain two nucleotides in the vicinity of modified nucleotide unpaired, and add 3′-overhang for splinted ligation to RNA substrate (*see* Fig. 1).

3. Splint DNA should be complementary to 3′-end of deoxyribozyme library and 5′-end of RNA substrate (*see* **Note 3**).

4. Synthesize or custom order appropriately designed deoxyribozyme library (0.5 μmol scale), RNA substrate with and without desired modification, splint DNA and primers.

### 3.2  Denaturing Polyacrylamide Gel Electrophoresis

Purification of ligated DNA–RNA product, separation of active and inactive fraction of the DNA library, and separation of PCR products into single strands is performed by denaturing polyacrylamide gel electrophoresis.

1. Calculate the volume (×) of gel solution needed to pour gel of desired size, that is, 40 mL for 20 × 20 cm gel size.

2. Assemble the glass plates with spacer of 0.4 mm thickness.

3. Mix × mL of gel solution of desired percentage with ×/400 mL of 25% APS and ×/2000 mL of TEMED.

4. Pour the gel and insert the comb with well size of 3–4 cm.

5. Allow the gel to polymerize for 30 min.

6. Remove the comb and rinse wells thoroughly with ultrapure water.

7. Assemble the gel apparatus and prerun the gel for 30 min to equilibrate the temperature. Set the power to a constant value of 25–35 W depending on the size of the glass plates (25 W for 20 cm × 20 cm and 35 W for 20 cm × 30 cm).

8. Heat the sample for 2 min at 95 °C and then allow it to cool down to 25 °C for 5 min.

9. Switch off the power supply and wash the wells thoroughly with $1\times$ TBE buffer and load the samples to the gel.

10. Run the gel at the same setting as used for prerun for 1–2 h until bromophenol blue reaches the bottom of the gel.

11. Disassemble the gel and transfer the gel between two layers of Saran Wrap.

12. Visualize the bands using fluorescein gel documentation (Gel Doc) imager or UV-transilluminator.

13. Cut the bands with a scalpel and transfer the gel piece to a 1.5 mL test tube for recovery of DNA by crush and soak.

14. Crush the gel pieces by centrifugation at 21,000 rcf for 5 min.

15. Add elution buffer to completely immerse the gel and incubate it at 37 °C for 4 h at 700 rpm.

16. After incubation, transfer the elution buffer to another test tube.

17. Precipitate the oligonucleotide by adding 3 volumes of ethanol.

18. Mix properly by vortex and freeze the sample using liquid nitrogen.

19. Centrifuge for 30 min at 4 °C.

20. Carefully separate the supernatant and wash the pellet with 75 μL of 70% ethanol.

21. Centrifuge for 10 min at 4 °C and dry the pellet in vacuum.

22. Dissolve the pellet in an appropriate volume of ultrapure water.

**3.3  In Vitro Selection**

*3.3.1  Phosphorylation of RNA Selection Substrates*

In order to ligate RNA selection substrates with DNA library, RNA has to be phosphorylated at 5′-end.

1. Calculate the concentration of RNA and take 5 nmol of the RNA in 0.7-mL test tube.

2. Add 5 μL of $10\times$ PNK buffer A, 5 μL of ATP (10 mM), 4 μL of T4 PNK enzyme (10u/μL) and adjust the volume to 50 μL.

3. Incubate the reaction mixture at 37 °C for 5 h.

4. Afterward, dilute the reaction mixture to 300 μL with $1\times$ elution buffer.

5. Add equal volume of Roti® phenol–chloroform–isoamyl alcohol to the reaction mixture and vortex it for 1 min followed by centrifugation for 1 min.

6. Carefully separate the supernatant and transfer it to a new test tube.

7. Add equal volume of chloroform and vortex the sample for 1 min followed by centrifugation for 1 min.

8. Carefully separate the supernatant and add 3 volumes of chilled absolute ethanol.

9. Vortex to mix properly and freeze the sample using liquid nitrogen.

10. Centrifuge the sample for 30 min at 4 °C.

11. Carefully separate the supernatant and wash pellet with 75 μL of 70% ethanol.

12. Centrifuge the sample for 10 min at 4 °C and dry the pellet in vacuum.

13. Dissolve the pellet in an appropriate volume (50 μL) of ultrapure water.

*3.3.2 Splint Ligation of RNA Substrate to Deoxyribozyme Selection Pool*

Ligation of ssRNA substrate with ssDNA library is facilitated by complementary DNA splint in the presence of T4 DNA ligase.

1. Take 5′-phosphorylated RNA (2 nmol), DNA selection pool (1.6 nmol) and complementary DNA splint (1.8 nmol) in a total volume of 10 μL.

2. Add 1.5 μL of 10× annealing buffer and incubate the reaction mixture at 95 °C for 4 min. After denaturation, allow the solution to cool down to 25 °C for 15 min.

3. Add 1.5 μL of ligase buffer, 2 μL of T4 DNA ligase (5 U/μL) and incubate the sample at 37 °C for 16 h.

4. Add 15 μL of PAGE loading buffer to the reaction mixture.

5. Purify the ligated product (DNA–RNA hybrid) using denaturing PAGE as mentioned under Subheading 3.2.

*3.3.3 DNA-Catalyzed Cleavage of DNA–RNA Hybrids (Key Selection Step)*

Selection of active DNA enzymes is based on a change in size upon cleavage of the RNA substrate in the vicinity of the modified nucleotide.

1. Take 250 pmol (in a total volume of 7.5 μL) of DNA–RNA hybrid in the first round of selection, and approximately 10–30 pmol in further rounds.

2. Add 1 μL of 10× selection buffer and incubate at 95 °C for 4 min and at 25 °C for 15 min.

3. Add $MgCl_2$ to a final concentration of 5 mM in a final volume of 10 μL and incubate at 37 °C for 16 h.

4. Add 10 μL of PAGE loading dye to the reaction mixture.

5. Separate the active fraction of DNA enzymes using denaturing PAGE and determine the area corresponding to cleaved product by size marker (*see* **Note 4**).

6. Cut the bands and extract the DNA enzymes as mentioned under Subheading 3.2.

7. Dissolve the pellet in 30 μL of ultrapure water.

**3.3.4  PCR Amplification of Active DNA Enzymes**

The cleaved fraction of the DNA library containing active DNA enzymes is amplified through two subsequent asymmetric PCRs. To visualize the PCR product, the forward primer is labeled with fluorescein at 5′ end and reverse primer has a tail connected through PEG$_3$ linker to separate sense from antisense strand by denaturing PAGE. Forward primer and reverse primer are used in a ratio of 4:1 to preferentially amplify forward strand with fluorescein label.

**PCR-I**

1. Use 30 μL of the solution from the previous step (containing active DNA enzymes) as template.

2. Assemble the reaction: 30 μL of DNA template, forward primer (100 pmol), reverse primer (25 pmol), 0.625 μL of 20 mM dNTP mixture, 5 μL of 10× Dream taq buffer, 0.25 μL of Dream taq DNA polymerase (5 U/μL) and water up to 50 μL.

3. PCR conditions are: 95 °C for 4 min [10× (95 °C for 30 s, 60 °C for 30 s, 72 °C for 1 min), 72 °C for 5 min].

4. Use an aliquot of the sample for PCR-II and store the rest at −20 °C.

**PCR-II**

1. Take an aliquot of PCR-I product (2–5 μL) as the template.

2. Assemble the reaction: 5 μL of DNA template, forward primer (200 pmol), reverse primer (50 pmol), 1.25 μL of 20 mM dNTP mixture, 10 μL of 10× Dream taq buffer, 0.5 μL of Dream taq DNA polymerase (5 U/μL), and water up to 100 μL.

3. PCR conditions are: 95 °C for 4 min [30× (95 °C for 30 s, 60 °C for 30 s, 72 °C for 1 min), 72 °C for 5 min].

4. Purify the PCR product using denaturing PAGE.

5. Isolate the fluorescein labeled forward strand by extraction and precipitation as described under Subheading 3.2.

**3.3.5  Continuation of Selection and Identification of Deoxyribozyme Sequences**

Take the single-stranded PCR product from the previous step and ligate it to the RNA substrate using the DNA splint (*see* **Note 3**) and T4 DNA ligase, essentially as described under Subheading 3.3.2, but on a smaller scale (i.e., use only 100 pmol of RNA and 75 pmol of DNA splint in a final volume of 10 μL for the ligation reaction). The isolated ligation product is then subjected to the next round of incubation as described under Subheading 3.3.3.

After 6–8 rounds of in vitro selection, include negative selection rounds to enrich DNA enzymes having high selectivity toward modified RNA and eliminate DNA enzymes that can cleave both modified and unmodified RNA. For this purpose, ligate the DNA pool with the unmodified analog of the RNA substrate. During the selection step, perform all steps in identical manner and analyze the

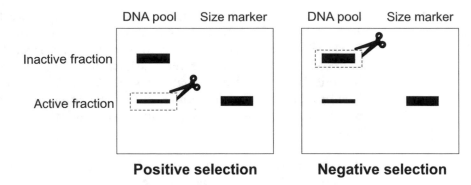

**Fig. 2** Schematic presentation of polyacrylamide gel electrophoresis (PAGE) for positive and negative selection rounds. The diagram presents the area of the gel from which the corresponding cleaved (positive selection round) or uncleaved fraction (negative selection round) is isolated

catalytic activity of the DNA pool by denaturing PAGE. Note that the uncleaved fraction on gel corresponds to the specific DNA enzymes that remain inactive toward unmodified substrate (*see* **Note 5**). The band signal observed at the height of the size marker corresponds to non-specific DNA enzymes that can cleave both modified and unmodified substrates. Therefore, in the negative selection round, the uncleaved fraction is isolated from the gel (Fig. 2) and amplified by PCR as described above. Each negative round is followed by a positive round (during these positive rounds, increase the stringency of the selection by decreasing the incubation time, i.e., 6 h, 3 h, and 1 h) and continue the cycle at least for four rounds of alternating negative and positive selections.

Afterward, amplify the active DNA pool through PCR. Due to non–template-dependent terminal transferase activity of *Taq* polymerase, the product will contain a 3′-A overhang that allows TOPO-TA cloning (commercially available kit). Select the individual clones and subject them to Sanger sequencing. Each sequence obtained from Sanger Sequencing data corresponds to individual deoxyribozyme candidates. These sequences are then synthesized by solid-phase syntheses and their catalytic potential and discrimination power for RNA modification are assessed by kinetic assays.

### 3.4 Kinetic Characterization of Deoxyribozymes

Kinetic characterization analyzes the *trans*-activity of individual deoxyribozyme to cleave modified and unmodified RNA (that are not ligated to the DNA library). Therefore, for each deoxyribozyme, the assay is performed in parallel with both, modified and unmodified RNA substrates of otherwise the same sequence. This allows to compare the cleavage rates and to determine calibration curves that are needed for quantitative estimation of modification levels.

1. Take 100 pmol of deoxyribozyme, 10 pmol of fluorescent labeled RNA substrate and adjust to a final volume of 7.5 μL.

2. Incubate at 95 °C for 4 min and 25 °C for 15 min.

3. Add 1 μL of 10× selection buffer and 0.5 μL of 400 mM MgCl$_2$ (final concentration 20 M) to start the reaction.

4. Incubate at 37 °C and take aliquots (1 μL) at different time points (e.g., 0, 10 min, 30 min, 60 min, 120 min, 180 min, 360 min).

5. Quench the reaction with 4 μL of quench buffer and analyze by denaturing PAGE. Take an image of the gel on a gel documentation system, determine the band intensities of cleaved and uncleaved RNA, and calculate cleavage yield and the observed rate constant ($k_{obs}$) (*see* **Note 6**).

# 4   Notes

1. For all in-vitro selection steps in this protocol use 10% acrylamide gel solution and for the analysis of *trans*-activity of individual DNA enzymes use 20% acrylamide stock solution.

2. For new selections, keep the catalytic core sequence completely random. The choice of 20 randomized positions allows a large fraction of the sequence space to be covered in one experiment. Larger random regions of 40 or more nucleotides have also be used successfully in earlier deoxyribozyme selections. To improve the selectivity of the obtained catalysts, reselection can be initiated from partially randomized DNA libraries. Also, the number and identity of the unpaired nucleotides around the desired cleavage site next to the modified nucleotide can be varied.

3. After PCR amplification, DNA library has 3′-A overhang due to the non-template dependent terminal transferase activity of *Taq* polymerase which reduces ligation efficiency. To overcome this problem, insert an extra T to the splint to base pair with 3′-A overhang and use it for all further rounds of selection starting from round 2, following a strategy introduced by [25].

4. Size marker is the oligonucleotide corresponding to the length of product size expected to be obtained after the selection round. It is prepared by ligating only the 5′-part of the RNA sequence without modification (corresponding to the expected cleavage product) to the DNA library. However, note that the selection strategy does not enforce a particular cleavage site, but due to the small number of 2–3 unpaired RNA nucleotides around the modification, cleavage usually happens near the modified base in RNA. The exact cleavage site then needs to be identified for each obtained deoxyribozyme by analyzing the size of the cleavage product next to an alkaline hydrolysis ladder.

5. As described in this protocol, the obtained DNA enzymes are trained to recognize the modified nucleotides in the positive selection round, that is, preferentially cleave the RNA substrate only when it contains the modification, but leaves unmodified RNA intact. However, the strategy can also be reversed, such that a modified nucleotide completely inhibits the DNA-catalyzed cleavage of the RNA target. For such a scenario, the positive selection is performed with unmodified RNA, and the modified RNA is used in the negative selection round. In this way, DNA enzymes were identified that are strongly inhibited by m$^6$A [23].

6. Analyze the cleavage yield by determining fluorescence intensities of the corresponding bands. Plot cleavage yield versus time (min). Determine k$_{obs}$ (observed cleavage rate) and, $\Upsilon_{max}$ (maximum yield) by using the first order kinetic equation: $\Upsilon = \Upsilon_{max} \times (1 - e^{-k_{obs} \times t})$.

## Acknowledgments

This work was supported by the European Research Council (ERC consolidator grant No. 682586) and by the German Academic Exchange Service (Deutscher Akademischer Austauschdienst, DAAD, PhD scholarship to A.L.). M.V.S. thanks the Graduate School of Life Sciences at the University of Würzburg for a Post-Doc Plus fellowship.

## References

1. Frye M, Jaffrey SR, Pan T et al (2016) RNA modifications: what have we learned and where are we headed? Nat Rev Genet 17:365–372

2. Lewis CJ, Pan T, Kalsotra A (2017) RNA modifications and structures cooperate to guide RNA-protein interactions. Nat Rev Mol Cell Biol 18:202–210

3. Zhao BS, Roundtree IA, He C (2017) Post-transcriptional gene regulation by mRNA modifications. Nat Rev Mol Cell Biol 18:31–42

4. Harcourt EM, Kietrys AM, Kool ET (2017) Chemical and structural effects of base modifications in messenger RNA. Nature 541:339–346

5. Bohnsack KE, Bohnsack MT (2019) Uncovering the assembly pathway of human ribosomes and its emerging links to disease. EMBO J 38(13):e100278. https://doi.org/10.15252/embj.2018100278

6. Buchhaupt M, Sharma S, Kellner S et al (2014) Partial methylation at Am100 in 18S rRNA of baker's yeast reveals ribosome heterogeneity on the level of eukaryotic rRNA modification. PLoS One 9:e89640

7. Sloan KE, Warda AS, Sharma S et al (2017) Tuning the ribosome: the influence of rRNA modification on eukaryotic ribosome biogenesis and function. RNA Biol 14:1138–1152

8. Grosjean H, Motorin Y, Morin A (1998) RNA-modifying and RNA-editing enzymes: methods for their identification. In: Modification and editing of RNA. American Society of Microbiology, pp 21–46

9. Li X, Xiong X, Yi C (2016) Epitranscriptome sequencing technologies: decoding RNA modifications. Nat Methods 14:23–31

10. Hartstock K, Rentmeister A (2019) Mapping $N^6$-Methyladenosine (m$^6$A) in RNA: established methods, remaining challenges, and emerging approaches. Chem Eur J 25:3455–3464

11. Aschenbrenner J, Werner S, Marchand V et al (2018) Engineering of a DNA polymerase for

direct m6A sequencing. Angew Chem Int Ed 57:417–421

12. Liu N, Parisien M, Dai Q et al (2013) Probing $N^6$-methyladenosine RNA modification status at single nucleotide resolution in mRNA and long noncoding RNA. RNA 19:1848–1856

13. Helm M, Motorin Y (2017) Detecting RNA modifications in the epitranscriptome: predict and validate. Nat Rev Genet 18:275

14. Silverman SK (2016) Catalytic DNA: scope, applications, and biochemistry of Deoxyribozymes. Trends Biochem Sci 41:595–609

15. Hollenstein M (2015) DNA catalysis: the chemical repertoire of DNAzymes. Molecules 20:20777–20804

16. Höbartner C, Silverman SK (2007) Recent advances in DNA catalysis. Biopolymers 87:279–292

17. Schlosser K, Li Y (2009) Biologically inspired synthetic enzymes made from DNA. Chem Biol 16:311–322

18. Silverman SK (2005) In vitro selection, characterization, and application of deoxyribozymes that cleave RNA. Nucleic Acids Res 33:6151–6163

19. Breaker RR, Joyce GF (1994) A DNA enzyme that cleaves RNA. Chem Biol 1:223–229

20. Buchhaupt M, Peifer C, Entian K-D (2007) Analysis of 2′-O-methylated nucleosides and pseudouridines in ribosomal RNAs using DNAzymes. Anal Biochem 361:102–108

21. Santoro SW, Joyce GF (1997) A general purpose RNA-cleaving DNA enzyme. Proc Natl Acad Sci U S A 94:4262–4266

22. Hengesbach M, Meusburger M, Lyko F et al (2008) Use of DNAzymes for site-specific analysis of ribonucleotide modifications. RNA 14:180–187

23. Sednev MV, Mykhailiuk V, Choudhury P et al (2018) $N^6$-Methyladenosine-sensitive RNA-cleaving Deoxyribozymes. Angew Chem Int Ed 57:15117–15121

24. Liaqat A, Stiller C, Michel M et al (2020) $N^6$-isopentenyladenosine in RNA determines the cleavage site of endonuclease deoxyribozymes. Angew Chem Int Ed 59:18627–18631

25. Brandsen BM, Velez TE, Sachdeva A et al (2014) DNA-catalyzed lysine side chain modification. Angew Chem Int Ed 53:9045–9050

# Chapter 11

# Mapping of the Chemical Modifications of rRNAs

## Jun Yang, Peter Watzinger, and Sunny Sharma

## Abstract

Cellular RNAs, both coding and noncoding, contain several chemical modifications. Both ribose sugars and nitrogenous bases are targeted for these chemical additions. These modifications are believed to expand the topological potential of RNA molecules by bringing chemical diversity to otherwise limited repertoire. Here, using ribosomal RNA of yeast as an example, a detailed protocol for systematically mapping various chemical modifications to a single nucleotide resolution by a combination of Mung bean nuclease protection assay and RP-HPLC is provided. Molar levels are also calculated for each modification using their UV (254 nm) molar response factors that can be used for determining the amount of modifications at different residues in other RNA molecules. The chemical nature, their precise location and quantification of modifications will facilitate understanding the precise role of these chemical modifications in cellular physiology.

Key words rRNA, Chemical modifications, Ribosomes, RP-HPLC, Mung bean nuclease assay

## 1 Introduction

Chemical modification of biomolecules is an impressive way of nature to expand their functional diversity. Like DNA and proteins, RNA molecules also undergo a variety of chemical modifications that allow them to enrich their topological potential and perform a variety of functions that go beyond their capacity to encode proteins [1, 2].

Around 163 different chemical modifications of RNA has been cataloged [3]. Both ribose sugar and the heterocyclic ring of the nucleobases are targeted for these chemical additions. Although the presence of these modifications was first acknowledged by some elegant studies in the middle of last century, it is only very recently that we have started compiling modification profiles for the cellular RNAs of model organisms, and explore the functions of few of these modifications [4]. This time lag has been primarily due to unavailability of advanced technology in studying these modifica-

Karl-Dieter Entian (ed.), *Ribosome Biogenesis: Methods and Protocols*, Methods in Molecular Biology, vol. 2533, https://doi.org/10.1007/978-1-0716-2501-9_11, © The Author(s) 2022

tions, which has been revolutionized in last two decades by introduction of both high-performance liquid chromatography (HPLC), mass spectrometry (MS), and RNA sequencing (RNA Seq) [5–8].

Ribosomes are highly conserved ribonucleoprotein complexes that synthesize cellular proteins. Eukaryotic ribosomes comprise of 4 ribosomal RNAs (rRNAs) and around 80 ribosomal proteins (r-proteins). Both enzymatic reactions of ribosomes, namely, peptidyl transfer and peptidyl hydrolysis are performed by rRNA [9]. In eukaryotes including *Saccharomyces cerevisiae*, a functional ribosome contains two asymmetric subunits, a small 40S and a large 60S. A small subunit (SSU) of the ribosome (the 40S) in yeast contains a single 18S rRNA of 1.8 kb together with 33 ribosomal proteins [10]. The 60S or the large subunit (LSU) of the yeast ribosome contains three rRNAs; 25S, 5.8S and 5S, and 46 ribosomal proteins. The 40S decodes the genetic information carried by mRNA, whereas the 60S catalyzes the joining of amino acids [11, 12]. Ribosomes have always been seen as homogeneous, constitutive protein-synthesizing machine, lacking any significant contribution in regulating gene expression. Typically, the efficiency of translation is suggested to be determined either by features intrinsic to the mRNAs or assisted by protein or RNA adaptors (translational factors). However, in contrast to this view, several recent studies have underscored the undeniable roles of ribosomes in gene regulation [13–17]. Emerging data have buttressed the notion that the ribosome population in cells is heterogeneous by virtue of its different components, including ribosomal proteins, rRNAs and their chemical modifications. It becomes more and more evident that this ribosomal heterogeneity provides a further regulatory level to the translation.

Ribosomal RNA contains three types of chemical modifications, 2′-O methylation of ribose sugars (Nm), base isomerization (pseudouridylation ($\Psi$)), and base modifications (methylation (mN) and acetylation (acN), aminocarboxypropylation (acpN)) [1, 2]. Methylated ribose sugars and pseudouridines represent the majority of rRNA modifications [18]. A methylated sugar is generated by the addition of one methyl group at the 2′-OH position of the ribose on the nucleoside and is independent of the nature of the base. Pseudouridylation results from uridine isomerization, involving a 180° rotation around the N3–C6 axis [19].

Box C/D snoRNPs (small nucleolar ribonucleoproteins) catalyzes site-directed methylation at the 2′-OH position on the sugar of the targeted nucleotide, whereas the box H/ACA snoRNPs isomerize targeted uridine to pseudouridine [20]. Remarkably, the substrate specificity for both ribose methylation and pseudouridylation is dictated by the RNA component of these snoRNP complexes [21, 22]. Here the complementary sequences in the guide RNA base pair with target RNAs to decide the nucleotide for modification [21, 22]. The catalytic activities are provided by the methyltransferase (Nop1 or Fibrillarin) or the pseudouridine synthase (Cbf5), respectively [23, 24]. In contrast, majority of base modifications are catalyzed by "protein only" enzymes with only exception being rRNA cytosine acetylation ($ac^4C$) [25].

To analyze and explore the significance of these modifications in ribosome biogenesis and ribosome function, a comprehensive analysis of their chemical nature and precise location on the ribosome is central. In this chapter, a detailed protocol for mapping these modifications on to the ribosomal RNA by mung bean nuclease (MBN) assay and RP-HPLC (reversed phase high-performance liquid chromatography) is provided [26].

MBN is a single strand specific nuclease, and can be used to isolate specific fragments of RNA by utilizing synthetic complementary DNA. These RNA fragments can then be subjected to RP-HPLC or LC-MS/MS analysis to identify the modification or modifications they harbor (Fig. 1) [26, 27]. This method also allows to achieve a single nucleotide resolution for mapping these modifications by isolating overlapping fragments [28, 29].

Although MBN assay and LC-MS/MS are work intensive, these are so far the only methods for a direct analysis of these chemical modifications. All other RNA sequencing based methods relies either on antibodies, which most of the time have issues with cross-reactivities or on the chemical reactivities of the modified residues, which are not very specific and are similar among many different modifications [30, 31]. The major limitation of the LC-MS/MS, on the other hand, is that it cannot be applied in a high throughput manner to reveal both the modification and the sequence context as in case of RNA Seq based methods. Oxford nanopore sequencing appears to be an ideal method of choice for the direct transcriptome-wide sequencing of these modifications [32].

## 2    Materials

### 2.1    Isolation of Intact 18S and 25S rRNA

1. Acid phenol–chloroform–isoamyl alcohol, pH 4.5 (25:24:1) (Invitrogen™, Catalog number: AM9720).

2. TEN buffer.

   100 mM Tris–HCl pH 7.8.

   1 mM EDTA.

   100 mM NaCl in nuclease-free water.

3. 5% and 25% sucrose solutions (w/v) in TEN buffer.

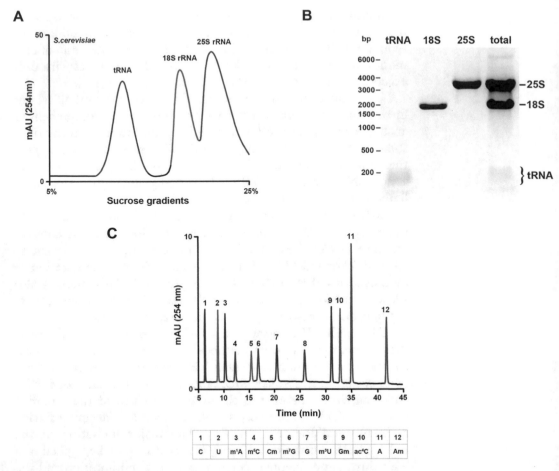

**Fig. 1** Reversed phase high-performance liquid chromatography (RP-HPLC) analysis. (**a**) Sucrose gradient sedimentation profile of yeast total RNA separated on 5% to 25% sucrose gradient. Fractions corresponding to tRNA (predominantly)), 18S rRNA, and 25S rRNA were collected and the rRNA was isolated using 95% ethanol precipitation at $-80\ ^{\circ}$C. (**b**) A representative 1.5% Agarose gel showing the rRNA recovered after ethanol precipitation. (**c**) RP-HPLC chromatogram of different commercially available nucleosides, showing peak corresponding to major nucleosides (adapted from [26])

**2.2 Mung Bean Nuclease Protection Assay**

1. Hybridization buffer.

   250 mM HEPES pH 7.0.

   500 mM KCl in nuclease-free water.

2. Mung bean nuclease (New England BioLabs (NEB), Catalog number: M0250L).

3. RNAse A DNase and protease free (Thermo Scientific™, Catalog number: EN0531).

4. 8M LiCl.

5. 3M sodium acetate (NaAc), pH 5.3.

6. GlycoBlue™ (Invitrogen™, Catalog number: AM9515).

7. UltraPureTM Formamide (Invitrogen™, Catalog number: 15515026).

8. 2× RNA loading buffer (Thermo Scientific™, Catalog number: R0641).

9. Novex™ TBE-Urea Gels, 10% (Invitrogen™, Catalog number: EC68755BOX).

**2.3 Quantitative Reversed Phase High-Performance Liquid Chromatography (qRP-HPLC)**

1. Millipore Water (18 MΩ·cm resistivity at 25°C).

2. Nuclease $P_1$ from *Penicillium citrinum* (Sigma-Aldrich, Catalog number: N8630) (200 units per mL in 30 mM sodium acetate, pH 5.4).

3. Phosphatase, Alkaline from *Escherichia coli* (Sigma-Aldrich, Catalog number: P4252).

4. 10mM $ZnSO_4$.

5. 0.5M Tris–HCl, pH 8.3.

6. HPLC grade Methanol (AppliChem, Catalog number: 361091).

7. HPLC Grade Acetonitrile (AppliChem, Catalog number: 221881).

8. Buffer A (10 mM of $NH_4H_2PO_4$, 2.5% of methanol, pH 5.3).

9. Buffer B (10 mM of $NH_4H_2PO_4$, 20% of methanol, pH 5.1).

10. Buffer C (66% acetonitrile).

11. All canonical and modified nucleosides standard—Carbosynth.

---

# 3  Methods

**3.1 Isolation of Intact 18S and 25S rRNA**

1. Harvest yeast cells at OD $_{600}$ 0.8 (*see* **Note 1**).

2. Extract the total RNA with hot acidic phenol exactly as described before [33].

3. To isolate intact 18S and 25S rRNA, layer 500 μg of total RNA onto a freshly prepared 5–25% sucrose gradient in TEN buffer (*see* **Note 2**). Prepare the sucrose gradients using Gradient Master 107 (Biocomp).

4. Centrifuge the samples at 67,000 × $g$ for 25 h at 4 °C in an SW40 rotor in an L-70 Beckman ultracentrifuge.

5. Fractionate the gradients by using a Teledyne Isco density gradient fraction collector. Collect 18S and 25S rRNA fractions in separate tubes and to each add 2.5 × volume of chilled ethanol. Incubate them overnight in a −20 freezer.

6. Next day, centrifuge the rRNA samples at 16,000 × $g$ for 30 min at 4 °C, air-dry the pellet, and resuspend it in nuclease-free water.

7. For the quantification of modified residues, it is very important to have intact rRNA. Since rRNA are abundant species, the quality (integrity) of purified 18S and 25S rRNA could be easily assesed by using 1.5% agarose gel stained with ethidium bromide.

### 3.2 Mung Bean Nuclease Protection assay (MBN Assay)

1. Mix the following components in a 1.5 mL Eppendorf tubes. DNA oligos listed in Table 4 have been used for mapping yeast rRNA modifications [26].

#### 3.2.1 Hybridization

| Components | Amount |
|---|---|
| 18S or 25S rRNA (*see* **Note 3**) | 100 pmoles |
| DNA oligo (Table 4) | 1000 pmoles |
| -DMSO | 3 µL |
| Nuclease-free water | Up to 100 µL |
| Hybridization buffer | 30 µL |

2. Heat the mixture to 90 °C for 5 min, and let it cool down to 45 °C on heating block (approximately 1.5 h). When the temperature drops down to 45 °C, move to the next step.

#### 3.2.2 Mung Bean Nuclease Digestion

1. Mung bean nuclease digestion are carried out by mixing following components.

| Components | Amount (µL) |
|---|---|
| RNA oligo mix | 130 |
| 10× MBN buffer | 20 |
| RNAse A (0.05 µg/µL) | 14 |
| Mung bean nuclease | 10 |
| Nuclease-free water | 26 |

2. Incubate the reaction at 35 °C for 1 h.

#### 3.2.3 Purification of the rRNA Fragments

1. After the MBN digestion, purify the rRNA fragment using phenol–chloroform extraction. Add 250 µL of acid phenol–chloroform–isoamyl alcohol, pH 4.5 (25:24:1) mixture to the 200 µL reaction mixture and vortex it for 1 min.

2. Centrifuge the Eppendorf tubes at $4000 \times g$ for 5 min at 4 °C.

3. Precipitate the rRNA fragments overnight at −20 °C by adding 350 µL of 8 M LiCl and 1 mL ethanol in 2 mL Eppendorf tubes.

4. Next day, centrifuge the tube at $16,000 \times g$ for 30 min at 4 °C, air-dry the pellet and resuspended the rRNA fragments in 30 µL nuclease-free water–formamide (1:2).

5. Add 30 µL of $2\times$ RNA loading buffer to the tubes and heat the samples to 70 °C for 10 min.

6. Load the samples on a Novex™ TBE-Urea Gels, 10% and run the gels as per manufacturer's instructions. Use DNA oligo and DNA oligo + total RNA as marker (*see* **Note 5**).

7. Slice out the gel containing the protected rRNA fragment using a fresh blade (*see* **Note 5**).

8. Wash gel slices with Millipore water 2–3 times with a pipette, do not crush the gel.

9. Add 450 µL nuclease-free water and 50 µL of 3 M NaAc pH 5.3 (final conc. = 0.3 M NaAc).

10. Elute the rRNA fragment from the gel slices by rotating on the rotor overnight at 4 °C (*see* **Note 6**).

11. Transfer the eluate into a 2 mL Eppendorf tube (Keep the gel slices in the old Eppendorf tube).

12. Add 1.25 mL ($2.5\times$ elution), 100% EtOH, and 0.5 µL Glyco-Blue™ to the eluate, and incubate the mix at −80 °C for at least 12 h for efficient precipitation.

13. Next day, centrifuge the tube at $16,000 \times g$ for 30 min at 4 °C, air-dry the pellet and resuspend in 45 µL of nuclease-free water. Store the samples at −20 °C.

14. Repeat the elution step. We get a better yield with two elution.

15. Quantify the rRNA fragment using a nanodrop.

*3.2.4 Mapping of Chemical Modifications to a Single Nucleotide Resolution*

As illustrated in Fig. 2, MBN assay could be easily used to achieve single nucleotide resolution by designing overlapping fragment around the modifications (*see* **Note 4**).

**3.3 Quantitative Reversed Phase High-Performance Liquid Chromatography (qRP-HPLC)**

Nucleosides for RP-HPLC are prepared as described by Gehrke and Kuo, and adapted for rRNA as described previously [7, 26].

*3.3.1 Preparation of Nucleosides*

1. Heat the rRNA fragments isolated after MBN assay as described above to 90 °C for 2 min on a heating block followed by rapid cooling on ice.

2. Add 5 µL of 10 mM $ZnSO_4$ and 10 µL of P1 nuclease. Incubate the samples for 16 h at 37 °C.

3. After 16 h, add 10 µL of 0.5 M Tris–HCl buffer, pH 8.3, and 10 µL of bacterial alkaline phosphatase and incubate the tubes at 37 °C for 2 h.

4. Next, before loading on the HPLC column clarify the nucleosides hydrolysates by centrifugation at $16,000 \times g$.

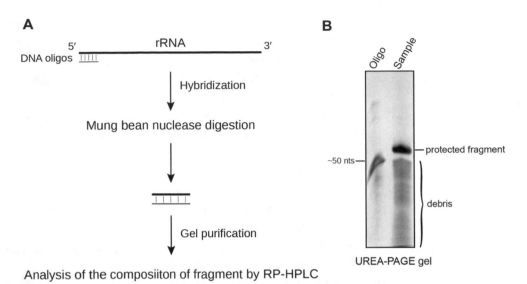

**Fig. 2** Mung bean nuclease protection assay. (**a**) Schematic illustration of mung bean nuclease protection assay (MBN). (**b**) Representative Urea PAGE gel for the MBN assay showing an intact protected fragment retrieved after the mung bean nuclease digestion. The synthetic antisense oligonucleotide used for the protection is used as a marker (*see* **Note 5**) (adapted from [26])

**Table 1**
**RP-HPLC elution protocol**

| Step no. | Step time (min) | Buffer composition (%) | | | Gradient type |
|----------|-----------------|------|------|------|---------------|
|          |                 | A    | B    | C    |               |
| 1        | 12              | 100  | 0    | 0    | Isocratic     |
| 2        | 8               | 90   | 10   | 0    | Linear        |
| 3        | 5               | 75   | 25   | 0    | Linear        |
| 4        | 7               | 40   | 60   | 0    | Linear        |
| 5        | 4               | 38   | 62   | 0    | Linear        |
| 6        | 9               | 0    | 100  | 0    | Linear        |
| 7        | 35              | 0    | 0    | 100  | Linear        |
| 8        | 10              | 0    | 0    | 100  | Isocratic     |

*3.3.2   RP-HPLC*

1. Load the nucleosides hydrolysates on Supelcosil LC-18-S HPLC column (25 cm × 4.6 mm, 5 mm) equipped with a precolumn (4.6 × 20 mm) at 30 °C on an Agilent 1200 HPLC system.

2. Use the following elution protocol (Table 1) described by Gehrke and Kuo for resolving majority of canonical and modified nucleosides in the rRNA (Fig. 1) [7]. For some

**Table 2**
**UV 254 nm Molar Response factors for canonical and modified nucleo-sides (*see* Note 8) [26]**

| Nucleosides | Molar response factors (area/nmole)—254 nm (Yang et al. 2016) |
|---|---|
| C | 209 |
| U | 278 |
| $m^1A$ | 387 |
| $m^5C$ | 163 |
| Cm | 199 |
| $m^7G$ | 333 |
| G | 461 |
| $m^3U$ | 306 |
| Gm | 490 |
| $ac^4C$ | 177 |
| A | 479 |
| Am | 348 |

modifications like $m^3U$ protocol has to be adjusted for better separation. In contrast to gradient elution for rest of the modified nucleosides, the elution conditions for $m^3U$ are changed to an isocratic mode using 50% buffer A and 50% buffer B.

*3.3.3 Quantification of the Modified Nucleosides*

Approximate modification levels for each ribose and base modifications can be calculated from HPLC peak areas ($UV_{254nm}$ absorption). For the quantification, the peak areas are divided by the standard molar response factors. Table 2 contains the $UV^{254nm}$ molar response factors calculated in our previous study. Similarly, mole % (Seq) for yeast (*S. cerevisiae*) are calculated assuming that 18S rRNA (1800 nts) contains 473 unmodified adenosines (A), 494 unmodified uridines (U), 453 unmodified guanosines (G), and 343 unmodified cytidines (C), and similarly for 25S rRNA (3396 nts) assuming that it contains 885 unmodified adenosines (A), 828 unmodified uridines (U), 956 unmodified guanosines (G), and 653 unmodified cytidines (C) Table 3. Likewise, for MBN protected fragments residues per moles or extent of modifications for each residue can be established using the sequence of the isolated fragment and its comparison to the residues/moles calculated from the 18S rRNA or 25S rRNA (*see* **Note 7**).

**Table 3**
**RP-HPLC quantification of Nucleosides in *S.cerevisiae* 18S and 25S rRNA [26]**

| Nucleosides | 18S rRNA | | 25S rRNA | |
|---|---|---|---|---|
| | Mole % (Seq) | Mole % (HPLC) | Mole % (Seq) | Mole %(HPLC) |
| C (cytidine) | 19.1 | 19.5 ± 0.48 | 19.2 | 19.4 ± 0.56 |
| U (uridine) | 27.4 | 27.1 ± 0.30 | 24.4 | 24.9 ± 0.39 |
| G (guanosine) | 25.2 | 25.7 ± 0.12 | 28.2 | 27.5 ± 0.17 |
| A (adenosine) | 26.3 | 26.6 ± 0.68 | 26.1 | 26.8 ± 0.64 |
| | Residues/ mole (predicted) | Residues/ mole (calculated) | Residues/ mole (predicted) | Residues/ mole (calculated) |
| $m^1A$ (N1-Methyladenosine) | 0 | 0 | 2 | 1.98 ± 0.10 |
| $m^5C$ (C5-Methylcytidine) | 0 | 0 | 2 | 1.81 ± 0.17 |
| Cm (2′-O-Methylcytidine) | 3 | 3.1 ± 0.26 | 7 | 6.74 ± 0.31 |
| $m^7G$ (N7-Methylguanosine | 1 | 0.72* ± 0.16 | 0 | 0 |
| $m^5U$ (C5-Methyluridine) | 0 | 0 | 0 | 0 |
| Um (2′-O-Methyluridine) | 2 | 1.89 ± 0.33 | 8 | 7.1 ± 0.31 |
| $m^3U$ (N3-Methyluridine) | 0 | 0 | 2 | 2.1 ± 0.17 |
| Gm (2′-O-Methylguanosine) | 5 | 4.91 ± 0.27 | 10 | 9.3 ± 0.39 |
| $ac^4C$ (N4-Acetylcytidine) | 2 | 2.12 ± 0.11 | 0 | 0 |
| Am (2′-O-Methyladenosine) | 8 | 7.33 ± 0.43 | 12 | 11.8 ± 0.48 |
| $m^6_2A$ (N6,N6-Dimethyladenosine) | 2 | nd | 0 | 0 |

*$m^7G$ has been shown to undergo partial-degradation during hydrolysis

## 4    Notes

1. Make sure that the yeast cells are grown for at least 6–7 generations.

2. Always prepare fresh TEN buffer and sucrose solutions. For isolation of rRNAs from higher eukaryotes including humans, the sucrose gradient should be adjusted—the one used here is optimized for both budding and fission yeast.

3. Instead of purified 18S and 25S rRNA, MBN assay can also be performed using total RNA, although the yield and efficiency was significantly higher with purified 18S and 25S rRNA.

4. Since several modifications impact the hydrogen bonding, isolation of fragment using MBN assay from highly modified regions of the rRNA is sometime challenging. The best oligo

**Table 4**
**List of oligonucleotides used for mapping base modifications (methylation and acetylation) and ribose methylation in *S. cerevisiae* rRNA using the MBN assay**

| No. | Sequence (5'-- > 3') |
| --- | --- |
| 18S-01 | -GGCTTAATCTTTGAGACAAGCATATGACTACTGGCAGGATCAACCAGATA |
| 18S-02 | -GCCATTCGCAGTTTCACTGTATAAATTGCTTATACTTAGACATGCATGGC |
| 18S-03 | TAGTAAAGGAACTATCAAATAAACGATAACTGATTTAATGAGCCATTCGC |
| 18S-04 | AAGCATGTATTAGCTCTAGAATTACCACAGTTATACCATGTAGTAAAGGA |
| 18S-05 | TTATCTAATAAATACATCTCTTCCAAAGGGTCGAGATTTTAAGCATGTAT |
| 18S-06 | GTTATTATGAATCATCAAAGAGTCCGAAGACATTGATTTTTTATCTAATA |
| 18S-07 | GAATGAACCATCGCCAGCACAAGGCCATGCGATTCGAAAAGTTATTATGA |
| 18S-08 | CACTATCCTACCATCGAAAGTTGATAGGGCAGAAATTTGAATGAACCATC |
| 18S-09 | CGAACCCTTATTCCCCGTTACCCGTTGAAACCATGGTAGGCCACTATCCT |
| 18S-10 | CTTGGATGTGGTAGCCGTTTCTCAGGCTCCCTCTCCGGAATCGAACCCTT |
| 18S-11 | CTGAATTAGGATTGGGTAATTTGCGCGCCTGCTGCCTTCCTTGGATGTGG |
| 18S-12 | CCGAATGGGCCCTGTATCGTTATTTATTGTCACTACCTCCCTGAATTAGG |
| 18S-13 | GTTAAGGTATTTACATTGTACTCATTCCAATTACAAGACCCGAATGGGCC |
| 18S-14 | CGCGGCTGCTGGCACCAGACTTGCCCTCCAATTGTTCCTCGTTAAGGTAT |
| 18S-15 | CTGCAACAACTTTAATATACGCTATTGGAGCTGGAATTACCGCGGCTGCT |
| 18S-16 | CCGGCCAACCGGGCCCAAAGTTCAACTACGAGCTTTTTAACTGCAACAAC |
| 18S-17 | GAAAGGCCCCGTTGGAAATCCAGTACACGAAAAAATCGGACCGGCCAACC |
| 18S-18 | GGTTCGCCAAGAGCCACAAGGACTCAAGGTTAGCCAGAAGGAAAGGCCCC |
| 18S-19 | GCCTGCTTTGAACACTCTAATTTTTTCAAAGTAAAAGTCCTGGTTCGCCA |
| 18S-20 | TCCTATTCTATTATTCCATGCTAATATATTCGAGCAATACGCCTGCTTTG |
| 18S-21 | CATTACGATGGTCCTAGAAACCAACAAAATAGAACCAAACGTCCTATTCT |
| 18S-22 | CAATTGAATACTGATGCCCCCGACCGTCCCTATTAATCATTACGATGGTC |
| 18S-23 | GTAGTTAGTCTTCAATAAATCCAAGAATTTCACCTCTGACAATTGAATAC |
| 18S-24 | TTCTTGATTAATGAAAACGTCCTTGGCAAATGCTTTCGCAGTAGTTAGTC |
| 18S-25 | CTACGACGGTATCTGATCATCTTCGATCCCCTAACTTTCGTTCTTGATTA |
| 18S-26 | CACCACCCGATCCCTAGTCGGCATAGTTTATGGTTAAGACTACGACGGTA |
| 18S-27 | CTTTGATTTCTCGTAAGGTGCCGAGTGGGTCATTAAAAAAACACCACCCG |
| 18S-28 | GTTTCAGCCTTGCGACCATACTCCCCCCAGAACCCAAAGACTTTGATTTC |
| 18S-29 | AGGCTCCACTCCTGGTGGTGCCCTTCCGTCAATTCCTTTAAGTTTCAGCC |
| 18S-30 | GACCTGGTGAGTTTCCCCGTGTTGAGTCAAATTAAGCCGCAGGCTCCACT |
| 18S-31 | CAAGAAAGAGCTCTCAATCTGTCAATCCTTATTGTGTCTGGACCTGGTGA |

(continued)

**Table 4**
**(continued)**

| No. | Sequence (5′-- > 3′) |
|---|---|
| 18S-32 | CACCAACTAAGAACGGCCATGCACCACCACCCACAAAATCAAGAAAGAGC |
| 18S-33 | GGTCTCGTTCGTTATCGCAATTAAGCAGACAAATCACTCCACCAACTAAG |
| 18S-34 | GATAACCAGCAAATGCTAGCACCACTATTTAGTAGGTTAAGGTCTCGTTC |
| 18S-35 | CTTCCATCGGCTTGAAACCGATAGTCCCTCTAAGAAGTGGATAACCAGCA |
| 18S-36 | GAACGTCTAAGGGCATCACAGACCTGTTATTGCCTCAAACTTCCATCGGC |
| 18S-37 | GACTCGCTGGCTCCGTCAGTGTAGCGCGCGTGCGGCCCAGAACGTCTAAG |
| 18S-38 | GGAGTTTCACAAGATTACCAAGACCTCTCGGCCAAGGTTAGACTCGCTGG |
| 18S-39 | TTGAAGAGCAATAATTACAATGCTCTATCCCCAGCACGACGGAGTTTCAC |
| 18S-40 | CAACGCAAGCTGATGACTTGCGCTTACTAGGAATTCCTCGTTGAAGAGCA |
| 18S-41 | ACTAGCGACGGGCGGTGTGTACAAAGGGCAGGGACGTAATCAACGCAAGC |
| 18S-42 | CTAAGCAGATCCTGAGGCCTCACTAAGCCATTCAATCGGTACTAGCGACG |
| 18S-43 | GTCCAAATTCTCCGCTCTGAGATGGAGTTGCCCCCTTCTCTAAGCAGATC |
| 18S-44 | CTTGTTACGACTTTTAGTTCCTCTAAATGACCAAGTTTGTCCAAATTCTC |
| 18S-45 | TAATGATCCTTCCGCAGGTTCACCTACGGAAACCTTGTTACGACTTTTAG |
| 25S-01 | CCTCCGCTTATTGATATGCTTAAGTTCAGCGGGTACTCCTACCTGATTTGAGG TCAAAC |
| 25S-02 | GCTTTTGCCGCTTCACTCGCCGTTACTAAGGCAATCCCGGTTGGTTTCTTTTCC TCCGC |
| 25S-03 | CCCTCTCCAAATTACAACTCGGGCACCGAAGGTACCAGATTTCAAATTTGAGC TTTTGCC |
| 25S-04 | CTCTATGACGTCCTGTTCCAAGGAACATAGACAAGGAACGGCCCCAAAG TTGCCCTCTCC |
| 25S-05 | CGAAGGCACTTTACAAAGAACCGCACTCCTCGCCACACGGGATTCTCACCCTC TATGACG |
| 25S-06 | GATGGAATTTACCACCCACTTAGAGCTGCATTCCCAAACAACTCGACTC TTCGAAGGCAC |
| 25S-07 | CATCACTGTACTTGTTCGCTATCGGTCTCTCGCCAATATTTAGCTTTAGATGGAA TTTAC |
| 25S-08 | CAATTTCACGTACTTTTTCACTCTCTTTTCAAAGTTCTTTTCATCTTTCCATCAC TGTAC |
| 25S-09 | GAGCAGAGGGCACAAAACACCATGTCTGATCAAATGCCCTTCCCTTTCAACAA TTTCACG |
| 25S-10 | CACCAAAACTGATGCTGGCCCAGTGAAATGCGAGATTCCCC TACCCACAAGGAGCAGAGG |

(continued)

**Table 4**
**(continued)**

| No. | Sequence (5'-- > 3') |
|---|---|
| 25S-11 | GGCTATAATACTTACCGAGGCAAGCTACATTCCTATGGATTTATCC TGCCACCAAAACTG |
| 25S-12 | CCTTGACTTACGTCGCAGTCCTCAGTCCCAGCTGGCAGTATTCCCACAGGCTA TAATAC |
| 25S-13 | CCTTGGTCCGTGTTTCAAGACGGGCGGCATATAACCATTATGCCAGCATCC TTGACTTAC |
| 25S-14 | CTTTCATTACGCGTATGGGTTTTACACCCAAACACTCGCATAGACGTTAGACTCC TTGGT |
| 25S-15 | CATCAGGATCGGTCGATTGTGCACCTCTTGCGAGGCCCCAACCTACGTTCAC TTTCATTAC |
| 25S-16 | CCATCTTTCGGGTCCCAACAGCTATGCTCTTACTCAAATCCATCCGAAGACA TCAGGATC |
| 25S-17 | GAGCCTCCACCAGAGTTTCCTCTGGCTTCACCCTATTCAGGCATAGTTCACCATC TTTCG |
| 25S-18 | CGCCCCTATACCCAAATTCGACGATCGATTTGCACGTCAGAACCGCTACGAGCC TCCACC |
| 25S-19 | GAGGGAAACTTCGGCAGGAACCAGCTACTAGATGGTTCGATTAGTC TTTCGCCCTATAC |
| 25S-20 | CTAATCATTCGCTTTACCTCATAAAACTGATACGAGCTTCTGCTATCC TGAGGGAAACTTC |
| 25S-21 | CATATTTAAAGTTTGAGAATAGGTCAAGGTCATTTCGACCCCGGAACCTCTAA TCATTCG |
| 25S-22 | GCTCTTCATTCAAATGTCCACGTTCAATTAAGTAACAAGGACTTCTTACATA TTTAAAG |
| 25S-23 | CGGTTCATCCCGCATCGCCAGTTCTGCTTACCAAAAATGGCCCACTAAAAGCTC TTCATTC |
| 25S-24 | CCTTTTGTGGTGTCTGATGAGCGTGTATTCCGGCACCTTAACTCTACGTTCGG TTCATCC |
| 25S-25 | GCGGATTCCGACTTCCATGGCCACCGTCCGGCTGTCTAGATGAACTAACACC TTTTGTGG |
| 25S-26 | CCATTTTCAGGGCTAGTTCATTCGGCCGGTGAGTTGTTACACACTCC TTAGCGGATTCCG |
| 25S-27 | CATCATATCAACCCTGACGGTAGAGTATAGGTAACACGCTTGAGCGCCATCCA TTTTCAG |
| 25S-28 | CTTACGGTCTAGGCTTCGTCACTGACCTCCACGCCTGCCTACTCGTCAGGGCA TCATATC |
| 25S-29 | GAATATTTGCTACTACCACCAAGATCTGCACTAGAGGCCGTTCGACCCGACC TTACGGTC |

(continued)

**Table 4**
**(continued)**

| No. | Sequence (5'-- > 3') |
|---|---|
| 25S-30 | CTGCTGTTGACGTGGAACCTTTCCCCACTTCAGTCTTCAAAGTTCTCATTTGAA TATTTGC |
| 25S-31 | CTTTGAAACGGAGCTTCCCCATCTCTTAGGATCGACTAACCCACGTCCAACTGC TGTTGAC |
| 25S-32 | CGGAATCTTAACCGGATTCCCTTTCGATGGTGGCCTGCATAAAATCAGGCC TTTGAAACG |
| 25S-33 | CGTCTCCACATTCAGTTACGTTACCGTGAAGAATCCATATCCAGGTTCCGGAATC TTAAC |
| 25S-34 | GGTGATAAGCTGTTAAGAAGAAAAGATAACTCCTCCCAGGGCTCGCGCCGACG TCTCCAC |
| 25S-35 | GTGCTGGCCTCTTCCAGCCATAAGACCCCATCTCCGGATAAACCAATTCCGGGG TGATAAG |
| 25S-36 | CTTCCTGTGGATTTTCACGGGCCGTCACAAGCGCACCGGAGCCAGCAAAGGTGC TGGCCTC |
| 25S-37 | CCTTGGAGACCTGCTGCGGTTATCAGTACGACCTGGCATGAAAACTATTCCTTCC TGTGG |
| 25S-38 | GCCGACTTCCCTTATCTACATTATTCTATCAACTAGAGGCTGTTCACC TTGGAGACC |
| 25S-39 | CTACCCGACCCTTAGAGCCAATCCTTATCCCGAAGTTACGGATCTA TTTTGCCGACTTCC |
| 25S-40 | CCCACCAAGCAGTCCACAAGCACGCCCGCTGCGTCTGACCAAGGCCCTCAC TACCCGACC |
| 25S-41 | CAAGGCCGTCTACAACAAGGCACGCAAGTAGTCCGCC TAGCAGAGCAAGCCCCACCAAGC |
| 25S-42 | GTTCTAAGTTGATCGTTAATTGTAGCAAGCGACGGTCTACAAGAGACC TACCAAGGCCGTC |
| 25S-43 | CGCAATGCTATGTTTTAATTAGACAGTCAGATTCCCCTTGTCCGTACCAGTTC TAAGTTG |
| 25S-44 | CAGAGCACTGGGCAGAAATCACATTGCGTCAACATCACTTTCTGACCATCGCAA TGCTATG |
| 25S-45 | GTTACTCCCGCCGTTTACCCGCGCTTGGTTGAATTTCTTCACTTTGACA TTCAGAGCACTG |
| 25S-46 | GCGCGTCACTAATTAGATGACGAGGCATTTGGCTACCTTAAGAGAGTCATAG TTACTCCC |
| 25S-47 | GTTTCGCTAGATAGTAGATAGGGACAGTGGGAATCTCGTTAATCCATTCA TGCGCGTCAC |
| 25S-48 | CAGGGTCTTCTTTCCCCGCTGATTCTGCCAAGCCCGTTCCCTTGGCTGTGG TTTCGCTAG |

(continued)

**Table 4**
**(continued)**

| No. | Sequence (5′-- > 3′) |
|---|---|
| 25S-49 | GAAGACCCTGTTGAGCTTGACTCTAGTTTGACATTGTGAAGAGACATAGAGGG TGTAG |
| 25S-50 | GAAACTATAAAGGTAGTGGTATTTCACTGGCGCCGAAGCTCCCACTTATTC TACACCCTC |
| 25S-51 | CTAGAACGTGGAAAATGAATTCCAGCTCCGCTTCATTGAATAAGTAAAGAAACTA TAAAG |
| 25S-52 | CCACCTGACAATGTCTTCAACCCGGATCAGCCCCGAATGGGACCTTGAATGC TAGAACGTG |
| 25S-53 | CTTAGGACATCTGCGTTATCGTTTAACAGATGTGCCGCCCCAGCCAAAC TCCCCACCTGAC |
| 25S-54 | GCTTTTACCCTTTTGTTCTACTGGAGATTTCTGTTCTCCATGAGCCCCCC TTAGGACATC |
| 25S-55 | GGCCACACTTTCATGGTTTGTATTCACACTGAAAATCAAAATCAAGGGGGC TTTTACCC |
| 25S-56 | GTAACTTTTCTGGCACCTCTAGCCTCAAATTCCGAGGGACTAAAGGATCGA TAGGCCACAC |
| 25S-57 | GCAATGTCGCTATGAACGCTTGACTGCCACAAGCCAGTTATCCCTGTGGTAAC TTTTCTG |
| 25S-58 | CGAATTCTGCTTCGGTATGATAGGAAGAGCCGACATCGAAGAATCAAAAAGCAA TGTCGC |
| 25S-59 | CCCAGCTCACGTTCCCTATTAGTGGGTGAACAATCCAACGCTTACCGAATTCTGC TTCGG |
| 25S-60 | GGTAACATTCATCAGTAGGGTAAAACTAACCTGTCTCACGACGGTC TAAACCCAGCTCAC |
| 25S-61 | CAATTATCCGAATGAACTGTTCCTCTCGTACTAAGTTCAATTACTATTGCGG TAACATTC |
| 25S-62 | CCAGCGGATGGTAGCTTCGCGGCAATGCCTGATCAGACAGCCGCAAAAACCAA TTATCCG |
| 25S-63 | GAAATCACCGCGTTCTAGCATGGATTCTGACTTAGAGGCGTTCAGCCATAA TCCAGCGGATG |
| 25S-64 | GACGCCACAAGGACGCCTTATTCGTATCCATCTATATTGTGTGGAGCAAAGAAA TCACCG |
| 25S-65 | CCCAAGGCCTTTCCGCCAAGTGCACCGTTGCTAGCCTGCTATGG TTCAGCGACGCCACAAG |
| 25S-66 | CAAATGATTTATCCCCACGCAAAATGACATTGCAA TTCGCCAGCAAGCACCCAAGGCC |
| 25S-67 | CAAGGCTACTCTACTGCTTACAATACCCCGTTGTACATCTAAGTCGTATACAAATG |
| 25S-68 | ACAAATCAGACAACAAAGGCTTAATCTCAGCAGATCGTAACAACAAGGCTACTC TACTGC |

set may have to be empirically determined by altering the Tm, either by increasing the length or sequence.

5. After MBN assay, fragments must be PAGE purified using appropriate marker—(DNA oligo used for the reaction can also be used). Often we see the protected fragment running a little higher than the expected size.

6. Instead of passive elution of the rRNA fragments, one can also use electro elution using Model 422 Electro-Eluter (BioRad).

7. MBN assay in combination with RP-HPLC is a valuable tool for both qualitative and quantitative of relatively abundant RNA species. For low abundant RNAs it is advised to use more sensitive methods like LC-MS/MS or upcoming Oxford nanopore base sequencing.

8. Molar response factors given here (Table 2) are calculated for $NH_4H_2PO_4$ buffer system. $NH_4H_2PO_4$ has a low UV absorption and higher solubility as compared to the potassium or sodium salts [7]. If other buffer system is used, the molar response factors should be recalculated.

## References

1. Sharma S, Lafontaine DLJ (2015) 'View from a bridge': a new perspective on eukaryotic rRNA base modification. Trends Biochem Sci 40: 560–575

2. Sloan KE, Warda AS, Sharma S, Entian K-D, Lafontaine DLJ, Bohnsack MT (2016) Tuning the ribosome: the influence of rRNA modification on eukaryotic ribosome biogenesis and function. RNA Biol 14(9):1138–1152. https://doi.org/10.1080/15476286.2016.1259781

3. Boccaletto P, Machnicka MA, Purta E, Piatkowski P, Baginski B, Wirecki TK, de Crécy-Lagard V, Ross R, Limbach PA, Kotter A et al (2018) MODOMICS: a database of RNA modification pathways. 2017 update. NAR 46:D303–D307

4. Klootwijk J, Planta RJ (1973) Analysis of the methylation sites in yeast ribosomal RNA. Eur J Biochem 39(2):325–333. https://doi.org/10.1111/j.1432-1033.1973.tb03130.x

5. Banoub JH, Limbach PA (2009) Mass spectrometry of nucleosides and nucleic acids. CRC Press

6. Gehrke CW, Kuo KCT (eds) (1989) Analytical methods for major and modified nucleosides - HPLC, GC, MS, NMR, UV and FT-IR. Elsevier

7. Gehrke CW, Kuo KC (1990) Chapter 1 Ribonucleoside analysis by reversed-phase high performance liquid chromatography. In: Chromatography and modification of nucleosides: analytical methods for major and modified nucleosides, HPLC, GC, MS, NMR, UV, and FT-IR, Journal of chromatography library, vol 45. Elsevier, pp A3–A71

8. Motorin Y, Helm M (2019) Methods for RNA modification mapping using deep sequencing: established and new emerging technologies. Genes 10:35

9. Woolford JL, Baserga SJ (2013) Ribosome biogenesis in the yeast Saccharomyces cerevisiae. Genetics 195:643–681

10. Henras AK, Plisson-Chastang C, O'Donohue M-F, Chakraborty A, Gleizes P-E (2015) An overview of pre-ribosomal RNA processing in eukaryotes. WIREs RNA 6:225–242

11. Ramakrishnan V (2002) Ribosome structure and the mechanism of translation. Cell 108: 557–572

12. Lilley DM (2001) The ribosome functions as a ribozyme. Chembiochem 2:31–35

13. Shi Z, Fujii K, Kovary KM, Genuth NR, Röst HL, Teruel MN, Barna M (2017) Heterogeneous ribosomes preferentially translate distinct subpools of mRNAs genome-wide. Mol Cell 67:71–83.e7

14. Simsek D, Tiu GC, Flynn RA, Byeon GW, Leppek K, Xu AF, Chang HY, Barna M (2017) The mammalian Ribo-interactome reveals ribosome functional diversity and heterogeneity. Cell 169:1051–1057.e18

15. Xue S, Barna M (2012) Specialized ribosomes: a new frontier in gene regulation and organismal biology. Nat Rev Mol Cell Biol 13: 355–369

16. Schosserer M, Minois N, Angerer TB, Amring M, Dellago H, Harreither E, Calle-Perez A, Pircher A, Gerstl MP, Pfeifenberger S et al (2015) Methylation of ribosomal RNA by NSUN5 is a conserved mechanism modulating organismal lifespan. Nat Commun 6: 6158

17. Sharma S, Hartmann JD, Watzinger P, Klepper A, Peifer C, Kötter P, Lafontaine DLJ, Entian K-D (2018) A single N1-methyladenosine on the large ribosomal subunit rRNA impacts locally its structure and the translation of key metabolic enzymes. Sci Rep 8:11904

18. Piekna-Przybylska D, Decatur WA, Fournier MJ (2008) The 3D rRNA modification maps database: with interactive tools for ribosome analysis. NAR 36:D178–D183

19. Gray MCMW (2000) Pseudouridine in RNA: what, where, how, and why. IUBMB Life 49: 341–351

20. Kiss T (2002) Small nucleolar RNAs: an abundant group of noncoding RNAs with diverse cellular functions. Cell 109:145–148

21. Kiss-László Z, Henry Y, Bachellerie JP, Caizergues-Ferrer M, KISS, T. (1996) Site-specific ribose methylation of preribosomal RNA: a novel function for small nucleolar RNAs. Cell 85:1077–1088

22. Ganot P, Bortolin ML, KISS, T. (1997) Site-specific pseudouridine formation in preribosomal RNA is guided by small nucleolar RNAs. Cell 89:799–809

23. Zebarjadian Y, King T, Fournier MJ, Clarke L, Carbon J (1999) Point mutations in yeast CBF5 can abolish in vivo pseudouridylation of rRNA. Mol Cell Biol 19:7461–7472

24. Tollervey D, Lehtonen H, Jansen R, Kern H, Hurt EC (1993) Temperature-sensitive mutations demonstrate roles for yeast fibrillarin in pre-rRNA processing, pre-rRNA methylation, and ribosome assembly. Cell 72:443–457

25. Sharma S, Yang J, van Nues R, Watzinger P, Kötter P, Lafontaine DLJ, Granneman S, Entian K-D (2017) Specialized box C/D snoRNPs act as antisense guides to target RNA base acetylation. PLoS Genet 13: e1006804

26. Yang J, Sharma S, Watzinger P, Hartmann JD, Kötter P, Entian K-D (2016) Mapping of complete set of ribose and base modifications of yeast rRNA by RP-HPLC and mung bean nuclease assay. PLoS One 11:e0168873

27. Buchhaupt M, Sharma S, Kellner S, Oswald S (2014) Partial methylation at Am100 in 18S rRNA of baker's yeast reveals ribosome heterogeneity on the level of eukaryotic rRNA modification. PLoS One 9(2):e89640. https://doi.org/10.1016/j.ab.2006.11.001

28. Sharma S, Yang J, Watzinger P, Kötter P, Entian K-D (2013) Yeast Nop2 and Rcm1 methylate C2870 and C2278 of the 25S rRNA, respectively. Nucleic Acids Res 41: 9062–9076

29. Sharma S, Langhendries J-L, Watzinger P, Kötter P, Entian K-D, Lafontaine DLJ (2015) Yeast Kre33 and human NAT10 are conserved 18S rRNA cytosine acetyltransferases that modify tRNAs assisted by the adaptor Tan1/THUMPD1. Nucleic Acids Res 43: 2242–2258

30. Helm M, Lyko F, Motorin Y (2019) Limited antibody specificity compromises epitranscriptomic analyses. Nat Commun 10:5669

31. Helm M, Motorin Y (2017) Detecting RNA modifications in the epitranscriptome: predict and validate. Nat Publ Group 18:275–291

32. Smith AM, Jain M, Mulroney L, Garalde DR, Akeson M (2019) Reading canonical and modified nucleobases in 16S ribosomal RNA using nanopore native RNA sequencing. PLoS One 14:e0216709

33. Collart MA, Oliviero S (2001) Preparation of yeast RNA. Curr Protoc Mol Biol Chapter 13: Unit13.12

# Chapter 12

# Non-radioactive In Vivo Labeling of RNA with 4-Thiouracil

## Christina Braun, Robert Knüppel, Jorge Perez-Fernandez ⓘ, and Sébastien Ferreira-Cerca ⓘ

## Abstract

RNA molecules and their expression dynamics play essential roles in the establishment of complex cellular phenotypes and/or in the rapid cellular adaption to environmental changes. Accordingly, analyzing RNA expression remains an important step to understand the molecular basis controlling the formation of cellular phenotypes, cellular homeostasis or disease progression. Steady-state RNA levels in the cells are controlled by the sum of highly dynamic molecular processes contributing to RNA expression and can be classified in transcription, maturation and degradation. The main goal of analyzing RNA dynamics is to disentangle the individual contribution of these molecular processes to the life cycle of a given RNA under different physiological conditions. In the recent years, the use of nonradioactive nucleotide/nucleoside analogs and improved chemistry, in combination with time-dependent and high-throughput analysis, have greatly expanded our understanding of RNA metabolism across various cell types, organisms, and growth conditions.

In this chapter, we describe a step-by-step protocol allowing pulse labeling of RNA with the nonradioactive nucleotide analog, 4-thiouracil, in the eukaryotic model organism *Saccharomyces cerevisiae* and the model archaeon *Haloferax volcanii*.

**Key words** 4-thiouracil, RNA, Pulse labeling, RNA tagging, *Haloferax volcanii*, *Saccharomyces cerevisiae*

## 1 Introduction

RNA homeostasis is a fundamental process for the regulation of gene expression and therefore for the physiology of living organisms [1, 2]. Several methods enable the characterization of the cellular RNA composition in a quantitative (relative amount) and qualitative manner (specific molecule identity) [1–3]. Classically, the presence and the relative amount of an RNA of interest can be easily assessed by northern blot or quantitative RT-PCR analyses

---

Christina Braun and Robert Knüppel contributed equally to this work.

Karl-Dieter Entian (ed.), *Ribosome Biogenesis: Methods and Protocols*, Methods in Molecular Biology, vol. 2533, https://doi.org/10.1007/978-1-0716-2501-9_12, © The Author(s) 2022

[1–3]. More recently, the emergence of high-throughput technologies, like DNA microarrays [4–6] or next generation sequencing analysis [7, 8], have leveraged our capacity to obtain a faithful qualitative and quantitative overview of the ensemble of RNA molecules present at equilibrium in varying conditions. However, all these methods are inherently lacking temporal resolution and hardly permit in depth systematic analysis of the relative contribution of the individual molecular processes underlying the life cycle of an RNA [9, 10].

This problem was recognized very early in the history of molecular biology. Pioneering studies have ingeniously taken advantage of metabolic labeling to reveal the importance of RNA dynamic for gene expression. For example, the seminal work of Brenner, Jacob, and Meselson in 1961 enabled the discovery of mRNA as a dynamic intermediate molecule required for protein synthesis [11]. Metabolic labeling of RNA using radioactively labeled molecules, like nucleotides/nucleosides, has been the method of choice to explore RNA dynamics. However, country-dependent administrative regulations of radioactive isotopes constrain the use of metabolic labeling using radioactive-labeled nucleotides. In addition, the inherent difficulty of this technique to analyze dynamics of individual RNAs in a global and systematic fashion, has often confined this methodology to assess global transcription output or production and maturation of abundant cellular RNA (like ribosomal RNA maturation [12–19]). Alternative methods using nonradioactive nucleotide analogs for the metabolic labeling of RNA were explored early on [20]. However, it is only recently, thanks to improvement of chemistry, labeled-RNA enrichment and detection methods, that the full potential of this approach is unfolding [9, 21–24].

Several nonradioactive nucleotide analogs providing different advantages/disadvantages have been described in the literature [9, 21]. Among them, uracil derivatives have been widely used [9]. Due to their versatile chemical properties, thiouracil/uridine and uracil/uridine derivatives compatible with click-chemistry have emerged as molecules of choice to perform RNA dynamic analysis [9]. These uracil/uridine derivatives allow for orthogonal chemistry with a large battery of reagents to facilitate downstream visualization, isolation and system-wide characterization of labeled RNA, thereby providing an unprecedented time and resolution depth of RNA metabolism [9, 10, 21–28].

Furthermore, the chemical properties of the uracil/uridine derivatives can be further harnessed in combination with other methodologies (e.g., UV cross-linking, structure probing, mass spectrometry, next-generation sequencing) to investigate the dynamics of structure and composition of ribonucleoprotein particle (RNP) [23, 24, 28–34]. Overall, the potential of using chemical biology strategies and their combinations is still emerging and will undoubtedly provide new molecular insights into the life cycle of RNA molecules.

In this chapter, we describe step-by-step conditions to successfully perform 4-thiouracil labeling in two model organisms, *Saccharomyces cerevisiae* and *Haloferax volcanii*, and provide general technical advice, which should facilitate application of this methodology (Fig. 1).

## 2   Materials

There are no specific preferences of sources of chemical reagents or materials, unless stated otherwise. Use ultrapure water with 18 MΩ·cm resistivity at 25 °C, unless stated otherwise.

### 2.1   Microbiological Cultures

#### 2.1.1   Strains

1. *Haloferax volcanii* H26 [35].

2. *Saccharomyces cerevisiae* (any genetic background prototroph for uracil).

#### 2.1.2   Haloferax Volcanii Enhanced Casamino Acids (Hv-Ca⁺)

1. 1 M Tris–HCl pH 7.0.

2. 1 M Tris–HCl pH 7.5.

3. 1 M KOH.

4. 30% (w/v) salt water: 4.1 M NaCl; 147.5 mM $MgCl_2$; 142 mM $MgSO_4$; 94 mM KCl; 20 M Tris–HCl pH 7.5.

5. 10× casamino acids solution: 10 g/L casamino acids.

6. *Haloferax volcanii* minimal carbon source: 10% sodium-DL-lactate; 9% succinic acid; 1% glycerol; pH 7.5. Sterilize by filtration.

7. *Haloferax volcanii* minimal salts: 417 mM $NH_4Cl$; 250 mM $CaCl_2$; 152 µM $MnCl_2$; 127 µM $ZnSO_4$; 689 µM $FeSO_4$; 16.7 µM $CuSO_4$. Sterilize by filtration.

8. Hv-Trace elements solution: 1.8 mM $MnCl_2$; 1.53 mM $ZnSO_4$; 8.27 mM $FeSO_4$; 0.2 mM $CuSO_4$.

9. 0.5 M $KPO_4$ buffer, pH 7.0.

10. 1 mg/L thiamine solution. Sterilize by filtration.

11. 1 mg/L biotin solution. Sterilize by filtration.

12. Uracil stock solution (500 mM in DMSO).

13. 4-thiouracil stock solution (500 mM in DMSO).

14. Sterile filters (0.22 µm) and syringes.

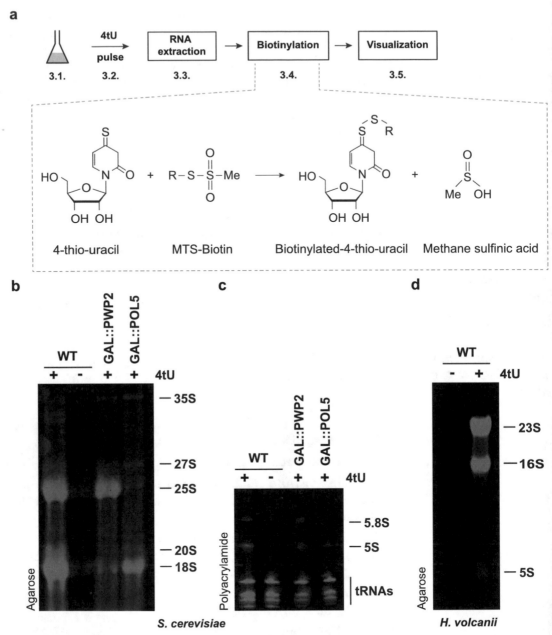

**Fig. 1** Exemplary 4-thiouracil (4-TU) labeling of total RNA in *S. cerevisiae* and *H. volcanii*: (**a**) Workflow summary of 4-TU labeling. 4-thiouracil labeling and biotinylation workflow is briefly depicted. Growing cells (*see* Subheading 3.1.) are pulse labeled with 4-thiouracil as described in Subheading 3.2. After RNA extraction (*see* Subheading 3.3), sulfhydryl groups are specifically biotinylated in the presence of methylthiosulfonate activated Biotin derivate (MTS-Biotin) (*see* Subheading 3.4). After biotinylation RNA are separated by gel electrophoresis and visualized as described in Subheading 3.5 and below. (**b** and **c**) Exemplary 4-TU labeling applied on the eukaryotic model organism *S. cerevisiae*. The indicated yeast cells, wild-type (WT), cells depleted for the small and large ribosomal subunit biogenesis factors Pwp2 (*GAL::PWP2*) and Pol5 (*GAL:: POL5*), respectively [39, 40] were labeled for 20 min with 4-thiouracil as indicated in Subheading 3.2. Labeled total RNA were separated by denaturing agarose (**b**) or polyacrylamide (**c**) gel electrophoresis, respectively. Biotinylated RNA was detected as described in Subheading 3.5. Ribosomal RNA precursors (35S, 27S, and

*2.1.3* Saccharomyces cerevisiae *Minimal Medium* (See **Note 1**)

1. 0.65 g/L Complete Supplement Mixture w/o histidine, leucine, uracil (CSM −His -Leu -Ura).

2. 6.7 g/L yeast nitrogen base containing ammonium sulfate as a nitrogen source (5 g/L) (YNB).

   (a)  20 g/L glucose (D) or galactose (G).

   (b)  0.1 g/L histidine.

   (c)  0.1 g/L leucine.

   (d)  Uracil stock solution (500 mM in DMSO).

   (e)  4-thiouracil stock solution (500 mM in DMSO).

**2.2 Chemical Reagents and Materials for RNA Extraction**

1. AE buffer (50 mM Na-acetate pH 5.3; 10 mM EDTA pH 8).

2. AE buffer-saturated phenol (*see* **Note 2**).

3. 10% sodium dodecyl sulfate (SDS) solution.

4. 3 M Na-acetate pH 5.3 solution.

5. RNA Precipitation mix (96% ethanol; 120 mM Na-acetate pH 5.3).

6. RNA sample solubilization buffer (95% deionized formamide, 20 mM EDTA, 0.05% bromophenol blue) (*see* **Note 3**).

7. Chloroform p.a.

8. Thermomixer.

9. 1.5 mL Safe-Lock tubes.

**2.3 Chemical Reagents for Biotinylation of 4TU-Labeled RNA**

1. MTSEA-Biotin-XX (Biotium—Cat Number:90066) (1 mg/mL solved in $N,N$-dimethylformamide).

2. 10× biotinylation buffer (100 mM Tris–HCl 7.4; 10 mM EDTA pH 8).

3. RNase-free $H_2O$.

4. Dark box.

---

**Fig. 1** (continued) 20S rRNA) and mature ribosomal RNA (25S, 18S, 5.8 and 5S rRNA) are indicated. Please note that depletion of the small ribosomal subunit biogenesis factor, Pwp2, for 14 h leads to the reduction of small ribosomal subunit pre- and mature rRNAs (20S and 18S rRNA, respectively) [39]. In contrast depletion of the large ribosomal subunit biogenesis factor, Pol5, for 9 h leads to the reduction of the common large ribosomal subunit precursor and corresponding mature rRNA (27S, 25S, and 5.8S, respectively) [39–41]. Additional application examples using this protocol and *S. cerevisiae* is described in [41]. (**d**) Exemplary 4-TU labeling applied on the archaeal model organism *H. volcanii. Haloferax volcanii* wildtype cells were labeled for 3 h with 4-thiouracil as indicated in Subheading 3.2. Labeled total RNA was separated by denaturing agarose electrophoresis. Biotinylated RNA was detected as described in Subheading 3.5. Mature ribosomal RNA (23S, 16S, and 5S rRNA) observed in these conditions are indicated. Additional application examples using this protocol and *H. volcanii* has been described previously [36]

**2.4  Separation and Immobilization of RNA**

*2.4.1  Agarose Gel Electrophoresis and Capillary Transfer*

1. RNase-free agarose.

2. 10× MOPS buffer (0.2 M MOPS, 20 mM Na-acetate, 10 mM EDTA, pH 7).

3. 37% formaldehyde p.a.

4. Running buffer (20 mM MOPS, 2 mM Na-acetate, 1 mM EDTA, 2% formaldehyde, pH 7).

5. Power pack.

6. Gel Chamber (20 × 25 cm gel tray).

7. 0.05 M NaOH.

8. 10× SSC (1.5 M NaCl, 0.15 M sodium citrate, pH 7).

9. Whatman paper.

10. Positively charged Nylon membrane.

11. UV cross-linking device.

*2.4.2  Polyacrylamide Gel Electrophoresis and Electro Transfer*

1. Urea.

2. 5× TBE buffer (445 mM Tris, 445 mM boric acid, 10 mM EDTA pH 8).

3. 30% acrylamide mix (acrylamide–bisacrylamide 37.5:1).

4. $N,N,N',N'$-tetramethyl ethylenediamine (TEMED).

5. 10% ammonium persulfate (APS) solved in $H_2O$.

6. Gel system apparatus including glass plates (20 × 10 cm), comb, spacers.

7. Power pack.

8. Whatman paper.

9. Positively charged nylon membrane.

10. Wet blot transfer cell with cassette clamping system.

11. Magnetic stirrer.

12. Magnetic stir bar.

13. UV cross-linking device.

**2.5  Detection of 4-TU Labeled RNA**

1. Blocking solution: 1× PBS pH 7.5, 1 mM EDTA pH 8; 10% SDS.

2. IR-dye conjugated Streptavidin (1 mg/mL).

3. Wash solution I: 1× PBS pH 7.5, 1 mM EDTA pH 8; 1% SDS.

4. Wash solution II: 1× PBS pH 7.5, 1 mM EDTA pH 8; 0.1% SDS.

5. Infrared detection system.

# 3    Methods (*See* Notes 4 and 5)

1. Prepare 30% (w/v) Salt water by dissolving in 4 L of Millipore water 1200 g NaCl; 150 g $MgCl_2 \cdot 6H_2O$; 175 g $MgSO_4 \cdot 7H_2O$; 35 g KCl; 100 mL 1 M Tris–HCl, pH 7.5. Fill up with $H_2O$ to 5 L. Autoclave and store at room temperature.

2. Prepare Hv-Min carbon source by dissolving in 150 mL $H_2O$: 41.7 mL 60% sodium-DL-lactate, 37.5 g succinic acid $Na_2$ salt- $\cdot 6H_2O$; 3.15 mL 80% glycerol. Carefully adjust to pH 7.5 with first 5 M NaOH and then 1 M NaOH. Fill up with $H_2O$ to a final volume of 250 mL and sterilized by filtration. Aliquot in 50 mL and store at 4 °C.

3. Prepare Hv-Trace elements solution by adding to 100 mL water a few drops of 37% concentrated HCl. Dissolve the following salts one by one in the following order: 36 mg $MnCl_2 \cdot 4H_2O$; 44 mg $ZnSO_4 \cdot 7H_2O$; 230 mg $FeSO_4 \cdot 7H_2O$; 5 mg $CuSO_4 \cdot 5H_2O$. Sterilize by filtration and store at 4 °C (*see* **Note 7**).

4. Prepare Hv-minimal salts by mixing 30 mL 1 M $NH_4Cl$; 36 mL 0.5 M $CaCl_2$ and 6 mL Hv-Trace elements solution (*see* **step 3**). Sterilize by filtration and store at 4 °C.

5. Prepare 0.5 M $KPO_4$ buffer (pH 7.0). Mix 61.5 mL 1 M $K_2HPO_4$ and 38.5 mL 1 M $KH_2PO_4$. Check pH and adjust to pH 7.0, if required. Add an equal volume of $H_2O$ (100 mL). Autoclave and store at room temperature.

6. Prepare thiamine–biotin mix by combining 9.5 mL thiamine (1 mg/mL) and 1.2 mL biotin (1 mg/mL).

7. Prepare 10× casamino acids solution. For 100 mL dissolve 5.1 g casamino acids in ~75 mL $H_2O$. Add 2.4 mL 1 M KOH. Fill up to 100 mL with $H_2O$. Sterilize by filtration.

8. Prepare Hv-$Ca^+$ medium. For 1 L medium mix 600 mL 30% salt water, 225 mL $H_2O$ and 30 mL Tris–HCl pH 7.0. Autoclave. When cooled down add 100 mL 10× casamino acids solution (*see* **step 7**), 25.5 mL Hv-Min Carbon Source (*see* **step 2**), 12 mL Hv-Min Salts (*see* **step 4**), 1.95 mL 0.5 M $KPO_4$ buffer pH 7.0 (*see* **step 5**), 900 μL thiamine–biotin mix (*see* step **6**). Store at room temperature in a dark cupboard.

9. Scratch the surface of an *Haloferax volcanii* glycerol cryo-stock with a sterile inoculating loop and inoculate 5 to 10 mL Hv-$Ca^+$ medium supplemented with Uracil (end concentration = 400 μM) as a start culture. Incubate at 42 °C under agitation. Dilute with prewarmed medium or let grow until the culture has reached the desired cell density ($OD_{600nm} = 0.5$–0.8).

**3.1.2 Saccharomyces cerevisiae *Medium and Cultivation***

1. Prepare SCG-Ura medium for precultures (*see* **Note 8**). For 300 mL medium dissolve 0.195 g CSM-His-Leu-Ura, 2.01 g YNB, 6 g galactose, 0.03 g histidine, and 0.03 g leucine in 250 mL $H_2O$. Fill up to 300 mL with $H_2O$. Aliquot in 50 mL, autoclave, and store at room temperature.

2. Prepare SCD-Ura medium for main cultures. For 800 mL medium dissolve 0.52 g CSM-His-Leu-Ura, 5.36 g YNB, 16 g glucose, 0.08 g histidine, and 0.08 g Leucine in 700 mL $H_2O$. Fill up to 800 mL with $H_2O$. Aliquot in 200 mL, autoclave, and store at room temperature.

3. Inoculate uracil prototroph yeast strains in 50 mL SCG-Ura medium with a sterile inoculating loop by picking one single colony from agar plate and grow yeast cells overnight at 30 °C under shaking.

4. Measure absorbance at 600 nm ($OD_{600nm}$) of overnight cultures and dilute them to $OD_{600nm} = 0.2$ in 50 mL SCG-Ura medium. Let cells grow to exponential phase to $OD_{600nm} = 0.5$–$0.8$.

5. Inoculate main cultures in 200 mL SCD-Ura medium to the appropriate cell density using exponentially growing precultures (*see* above **step 4**). Incubate yeast cells until the culture has reached the desired cell density.

**3.2 In Vivo Pulse Labeling with 4-TU (See Note 9)**

**3.2.1 *Uracil and 4-Thiouracil Stocks***

1. Prepare 500 mM uracil stock solution. For 5 mL, dissolve 280.2 mg uracil powder in 3 mL DMSO. Fill up to 5 mL with DMSO. Store aliquots at −20 °C.

2. Prepare 500 mM 4-thiouracil stock solution. For 5 mL, dissolve 320.4 mg 4-thiouracil powder in 3 mL DMSO. Fill up to 5 mL with DMSO. Store aliquots at −20 °C.

**3.2.2 *Haloferax volcanii Labeling***

1. Grow *H. volcanii* cells in Hv-Ca$^+$ medium containing 400 μM uracil.

2. Centrifuge cells for 8 min at $4,500 \times g$.

3. Resuspend cell pellet in prewarmed Hv-Ca$^+$ supplemented with 100 μM uracil.

4. Split the cells in an appropriate number of cultures.

5. Add 300 μM uracil (mock control) or add 300 μM 4-thiouracil (pulse).

6. Incubate at 42 °C under agitation.

7. Centrifuge cells (~2 $OD_{600nm}$ equivalent) 5 min at $10,000 \times g$.

8. Discard supernatant.

9. Freeze the cells in liquid nitrogen.

10. Proceeds with RNA extraction (*see* Subheading 3.3).

*3.2.3* Saccharomyces
cerevisiae *Labeling*

1. Take a volume corresponding to 30 $OD_{600nm}$ of exponentially growing yeast culture and centrifuge for 3 min at $1,700 \times g$.

2. Discard supernatant and resuspend cell pellets in 40 mL SCD-Ura medium and transfer to 100 mL Erlenmeyer flasks.

3. Add either 100 μM uracil (mock control) or 100 μM 4-thiouracil (pulse).

4. Incubate for 20 min at 30 °C under agitation.

5. Centrifuge cells for 5 min at $3,000 \times g$.

6. Discard supernatant.

7. Freeze the cells in liquid nitrogen.

8. Proceed with RNA extraction (*see* Subheading 3.3).

**3.3 RNA Extraction
[36]**

Perform all RNA extractions as fast as possible in a controlled RNase-free environment (*see* **Note 10**).

1. Label a total of four 1.5 mL safe-seal tubes (1–4) for each sample condition.

2. Prewarm Thermomixer to 65 °C.

3. Add reagents as described in Table 1.

4. Dissolve cell pellets in 500 μL AE buffer and keep on ice.

5. Add the dissolved pellet to the corresponding prepared Tube 1 (*see* Table 1).
   Close the tube properly and vortex briefly. Keep at room temperature until all the Tube 1 series is completed.

6. Incubate at 65 °C (Thermomixer) for 5 min with full speed agitation.

7. Vortex all the samples and keep on ice for 1 min.

8. Centrifuge 2 min at $18,000 \times g$, room temperature (*see* **Note 11**).

9. Transfer ~450 μL aqueous phase (upper phase) (*see* **Note 12**) to the corresponding prepared Tube. Vortex briefly. Keep at room temperature until all the Tube 2 series is completed.

**Table 1**
**Tube series required for RNA extraction (*see* Subheading 2.2)**

|  | Sample X |
| --- | --- |
| Tube 1 | 500 μL AE buffer-saturated phenol<br>50 μL 10% SDS |
| Tube 2 | 500 μL AE buffer-saturated phenol |
| Tube 3 | 500 μL chloroform |
| Tube 4 | 780 μL RNA precipitation mix |

10. Centrifuge for 1 min at $18,000 \times g$, room temperature.

11. Transfer ~360 μL aqueous phase (upper phase) (*see* **Note 12**) to the corresponding prepared Tube 3. Vortex briefly. Keep at room temperature until all the Tube 3 series is completed.

12. Centrifuge 1 min at $18,000 \times g$, room temperature.

13. Transfer ~300 μL aqueous phase (upper phase) (*see* **Note 12**) to the corresponding prepared Tube 4. Invert to mix and precipitate the RNA at least 60 min at −20 °C.

14. Centrifuge for 20 min at $18,000 \times g$ at 4 °C.

15. Discard supernatants.

16. Optional recommended step: wash pellets with cold (−20 °C) 75% Ethanol. Centrifuge if necessary and discard supernatants.

17. Let the pellet dry at room temperature.

18. Dissolve RNA pellet in 20–40 μL RNase-free water. Store at −20 °C or −80 °C.

19. Measure RNA concentration.

### 3.4 4-TU–Labeled RNA Biotinylation

1. Mix 25–50 μg extracted RNA, 5 μL MTSEA-Biotin-XX (5 μg), 25 μL 10× biotinylation buffer in a total volume of 250 μL.

2. Incubate for 30 min in the dark at room temperature.

3. Add 250 μL AE buffer (*see* **item 1** Subheading 2.2).

4. Proceed with RNA extraction by adding the sample to a prepared tube containing 500 μL AE buffer-saturated phenol and 50 μL 10% SDS (*see* Subheading 3.3).

5. Dissolved RNA pellet in RNA loading buffer (*see* **item 6** Subheading 2.2).

### 3.5 Separation and Immobilization of RNA (See Note 11)

#### 3.5.1 Preparation of Denaturing Agarose Gel

1. Mix 1.3% agarose in 0.85 final volume of $H_2O$.

2. Dissolve the agarose by heating the mixture in the microwave.

3. Let cool down under agitation (~50 °C) and add 0.1 volume of 10× MOPS running buffer and 0.054 volume of 37% Formaldehyde (final concentration 2%).

4. Cast the gel.

5. Prepare running buffer (1× MOPS, 2% formaldehyde).

6. Load the RNA samples (obtained in Subheading 3.4).

7. Run the gel overnight at 40 V and room temperature.

#### 3.5.2 Preparation of Denaturing Polyacrylamide Gel

1. Prepare urea–polyacrylamide gel solution (6% acrylamide, 7 M urea solved in 0.5× TBE). Mix by stirring at room temperature until urea is properly dissolved.

2. Add 0.001% (v/v) TEMED and 0.1% (v/v) APS.

3. Cast gel immediately and store it after polymerization at 4 °C overnight.

4. Prepare running buffer ($0.5\times$ TBE).

5. Load the RNA samples (obtained in Subheading 3.4). Prior to sample loading, flush pockets very well with $0.5\times$ TBE using an hollow needle to remove urea.

6. Run the gel for 1 h and 15 min at 150 V.

*3.5.3 Northern Blotting (Agarose Gel)*

1. Rinse gel in 5 gel volumes of $H_2O$ for 5 min.

2. Hydrolyzed RNA in 5 gel volumes of 0.05 M NaOH for 20 min under mild agitation.

3. Rinse twice with 5 gel volumes of $10\times$ SSC for 20 min under mild agitation.

4. Prepare nylon membrane, Whatman paper, and soaking paper.

5. Transfer RNA overnight onto the Nylon membrane by capillary transfer.

6. Cross-link RNA to the membrane by exposing the membrane twice with 0.5 $J/cm^2$.

*3.5.4 Northern Blotting (Polyacrylamide Gel)*

1. Rinse gel in 5 gel volumes of $0.5\times$ TBE for 5 min.

2. Equilibrate Nylon membrane, Whatman paper, and clamping nets in $0.5\times$ TBE.

3. Set up blotting sandwich and fill transfer tank with blotting buffer ($0.5\times$ TBE).

4. Transfer RNA at room temperature for 1 h and 20 min at 50 V. Blotting buffer should be stirring constantly with the help of a magnetic stir device.

5. Cross-link RNA to the membrane by exposing the membrane twice with 0.5 $J/cm^2$.

*3.5.5 Detection of Biotinylated RNA*

1. Incubate membrane for 20 min in blocking buffer under mild agitation.

2. Add IR-dye conjugated Streptavidin (0.1 µg/mL) and incubate for 20 min under mild agitation in the dark.

3. Wash the membrane twice 10 min with blocking buffer under mild agitation in the dark.

4. Wash the membrane twice 10 min with washing buffer I under mild agitation in the dark.

5. Wash the membrane twice 10 min with washing buffer II under mild agitation in the dark.

6. Visualized biotinylated RNA with an infrared detection system (Fig. 1b–d).

## 4    Notes

1. Increased labeling is obtained when using a prototroph yeast strain. When using an uracil prototroph yeast strains, all used media lack uracil.

2. AE buffer-saturated phenol is obtained by equilibrating phenol water 3 times with 1/10th volume of AE buffer (50 mM Na-acetate pH 5.3; 10 mM EDTA pH 8). The equilibrated phenol solution should be stored at 4 °C in the dark in a safety cabinet. Phenol can cause severe burns. Always work with phenol in a fume hood and wear safety glasses, gloves, and a lab coat. Avoid direct contact.

3. Deionized formamide is essential to resolve RNA correctly on polyacrylamide gel and can be purchased from most providers. For agarose gel deionized formamide is not required. Formamide is a moderate irritant and is hazardous for health. Handle using the necessary safety precautions.

4. Use ultrapure water with 18 MΩ cm resistivity at 25 °C unless stated otherwise.

5. All solutions/media should be autoclaved, unless stated otherwise.

6. Use standard microbiological practices required for the cultivation of noninfectious or low-risk microorganisms (Risk Group 1 applies for *H. volcanii* and *S. cerevisiae*). In other cases, apply specific additional safety measures related to the organism used and according to biological safety law. In case of doubt, contact your local biology safety officer. Ensure that glassware used for the cultivation of *H. volcanii* are well cleaned and do not contain residual traces of detergents/chemicals.

7. Order is critical to ensure proper solubility of the chemicals.

8. In this example, precultures must necessarily be cultivated in galactose containing medium to avoid premature depletion of proteins of interest in glucose containing medium. Otherwise, SCD medium containing 2% dextrose instead of galactose can be used.

9. 4-thiouracil is toxic at different concentrations depending on the organism used [36–38]. Make sure to determine the optimal amounts of uracil analog for the organism used. *H. volcanii* cells can tolerate up to 75% of thiouracil as uracil source (total concentration of uracil and analog 400 µM) [36]. In absence of uracil, uracil prototroph *S. cerevisiae* cells can tolerate up to 200 µM of thiouracil in 24 h cultures with only a 15% decrease on cell growth.

10. For best results keep all reagents free of RNases. If possible, keep glassware and materials separated and, set up a dedicated area for RNA work only. Keep the working place tidy.

11. Temperature is critical to allow correct phase separation. Do not use a cooled centrifuge since SDS will tend to precipitate.

12. For best results avoid phase contamination by collecting the upper phase using 3 fractions of equal volumes ($3\times 150$ µL, $3\times 120$ µL, and $3\times 100$ µL, respectively).

13. To avoid high level of autofluorescence background, avoid staining the gel with staining reagents like ethidium bromide and SYBR Safe.

## Acknowledgments

We are grateful to Prof. Dr. Karl-Dieter Entian (University of Frankfurt) for comments and suggestions, to Corinna Reglin for early contribution to this project. We would like to thank our colleagues from the chair of Biochemistry III and Biochemistry I for sharing protocols, materials, equipment, and discussion. Thanks to Prof. Dr. Thorsten Allers (University of Nottingham), Prof. Dr. Anita Marchfelder (University of Ulm) for kindly sharing strains and protocols. Work in the Perez-Fernandez and Ferreira-Cerca laboratories are supported by the chair of Biochemistry III "House of the Ribosome"—University of Regensburg, by the DFG-funded collaborative research center CRC/SFB960 "RNP biogenesis: assembly of ribosomes and nonribosomal RNPs and control of their function" (project AP2 and project AP1/B13, respectively) and by an individual DFG grant to S.F.-C. (FE1622/2-1; Project Nr. 409198929). This work is dedicated to the memory of Prof. Dr. Jonathan Warner who has among other important contributions, pioneered pulse labeling of pre-rRNAs.

## References

1. Elliott D, Ladomery M (2016) Molecular biology of RNA. Oxford University Press, Oxford

2. Cech T, Steitz JA, Atkins JF (2019) RNA worlds: new tools for deep exploration. Cold Spring Harbor Laboratory Press, New York

3. Hartmann RK, Bindereif A, Schön A, Westhof E (2015) Handbook of RNA biochemistry. Wiley, Hoboken, New Jersey

4. Duggan DJ, Bittner M, Chen Y et al (1999) Expression profiling using cDNA microarrays. Nat Genet 21:10–14. https://doi.org/10.1038/4434

5. Southern E, Mir K, Shchepinov M (1999) Molecular interactions on microarrays. Nat Genet 21:5–9. https://doi.org/10.1038/4429

6. Lennon GG, Lehrach H (1991) Hybridization analyses of arrayed cDNA libraries. Trends Genet 7:314–317. https://doi.org/10.1016/0168-9525(91)90420-U

7. McGettigan PA (2013) Transcriptomics in the RNA-seq era. Curr Opin Chem Biol 17:4–11. https://doi.org/10.1016/j.cbpa.2012.12.008

8. Wang Z, Gerstein M, Snyder M (2009) RNA-Seq: a revolutionary tool for transcriptomics. Nat Rev Genet 10:57–63. https://doi.org/10.1038/nrg2484

9. Duffy EE, Schofield JA, Simon MD (2019) Gaining insight into transcriptome-wide RNA population dynamics through the chemistry of 4-thiouridine. Wiley Interdiscip Rev RNA 10: e1513. https://doi.org/10.1002/wrna.1513

10. Barrass JD, Reid JEA, Huang Y et al (2015) Transcriptome-wide RNA processing kinetics revealed using extremely short 4tU labeling. Genome Biol 16:282. https://doi.org/10.1186/s13059-015-0848-1

11. Brenner S, Jacob F, Meselson M (1961) An unstable intermediate carrying information from genes to ribosomes for protein synthesis. Nature 190:576–581. https://doi.org/10.1038/190576a0

12. Kos M, Tollervey D (2010) Yeast pre-rRNA processing and modification occur cotranscriptionally. Mol Cell 37:809–820. https://doi.org/10.1016/j.molcel.2010.02.024

13. Udem SA, Warner JR (1972) Ribosomal RNA synthesis in Saccharomyces cerevisiae. J Mol Biol 65:227–242. https://doi.org/10.1016/0022-2836(72)90279-3

14. Udem SA, Warner JR (1973) The cytoplasmic maturation of a ribosomal precursor ribonucleic acid in yeast. J Biol Chem 248:1412–1416

15. Retèl J, Planta RJ (1967) Ribosomal precursor RNA in Saccharomyces carlsbergensis. Eur J Biochem 3:248–258. https://doi.org/10.1111/j.1432-1033.1967.tb19524.x

16. Smitt WWS, Vlak JM, Schiphof R, Rozijn TH (1972) Precursors of ribosomal RNA in yeast nucleus: biosynthesis and relation to cytoplasmic ribosomal RNA. Exp Cell Res 71:33–40. https://doi.org/10.1016/0014-4827(72)90259-5

17. Trapman J, Retèl J, Planta RJ (1975) Ribosomal precursor particles from yeast. Exp Cell Res 90:95–104. https://doi.org/10.1016/0014-4827(75)90361-4

18. Trapman J, Planta RJ (1975) Detailed analysis of the ribosomal RNA synthesis in yeast. Biochim Biophys Acta 414:115–125. https://doi.org/10.1016/0005-2787(75)90214-2

19. Hadjiolov AA (1985) The nucleolus and ribosome biogenesis. Springer-Verlag Wien, Wien

20. Melvin WT, Milne HB, Slater AA et al (1978) Incorporation of 6-Thioguanosine and 4-Thiouridine into RNA. Eur J Biochem 92:373–379. https://doi.org/10.1111/j.1432-1033.1978.tb12756.x

21. Muthmann N, Hartstock K, Rentmeister A (2019) Chemo-enzymatic treatment of RNA to facilitate analyses. Wiley Interdiscip Rev RNA 0:e1561. https://doi.org/10.1002/wrna.1561

22. Hendriks G-J, Jung LA, Larsson AJM et al (2019) NASC-seq monitors RNA synthesis in single cells. Nat Commun 10:3138–3138. https://doi.org/10.1038/s41467-019-11028-9

23. Bao X, Guo X, Yin M et al (2018) Capturing the interactome of newly transcribed RNA. Nat Methods 15:213

24. Huang R, Han M, Meng L, Chen X (2018) Transcriptome-wide discovery of coding and noncoding RNA-binding proteins. Proc Natl Acad Sci U S A 115:E3879. https://doi.org/10.1073/pnas.1718406115

25. Kiefer L, Schofield JA, Simon MD (2018) Expanding the nucleoside recoding toolkit: revealing RNA population dynamics with 6-Thioguanosine. J Am Chem Soc 140:14567–14570. https://doi.org/10.1021/jacs.8b08554

26. Schofield JA, Duffy EE, Kiefer L et al (2018) TimeLapse-seq: adding a temporal dimension to RNA sequencing through nucleoside recoding. Nat Methods 15:221–225. https://doi.org/10.1038/nmeth.4582

27. Herzog VA, Reichholf B, Neumann T et al (2017) Thiol-linked alkylation of RNA to assess expression dynamics. Nat Methods 14:1198

28. Hafner M, Landthaler M, Burger L et al (2010) Transcriptome-wide identification of RNA-binding protein and MicroRNA target sites by PAR-CLIP. Cell 141:129–141. https://doi.org/10.1016/j.cell.2010.03.009

29. Swiatkowska A, Wlotzka W, Tuck A et al (2012) Kinetic analysis of pre-ribosome structure in vivo. RNA 18:2187–2200. https://doi.org/10.1261/rna.034751.112

30. Hulscher RM, Bohon J, Rappé MC et al (2016) Probing the structure of ribosome assembly intermediates in vivo using DMS and hydroxyl radical footprinting. Methods 103:49–56. https://doi.org/10.1016/j.ymeth.2016.03.012

31. Granneman S, Petfalski E, Swiatkowska A, Tollervey D (2010) Cracking pre-40S ribosomal subunit structure by systematic analyses of RNA–protein cross-linking. EMBO J 29:2026–2036. https://doi.org/10.1038/emboj.2010.86

32. Duffy EE, Rutenberg-Schoenberg M, Stark CD et al (2015) Tracking distinct RNA

populations using efficient and reversible covalent chemistry. Mol Cell 59:858–866. https://doi.org/10.1016/j.molcel.2015.07.023

33. Ascano M, Hafner M, Cekan P et al (2012) Identification of RNA–protein interaction networks using PAR-CLIP. WIREs RNA 3:159–177. https://doi.org/10.1002/wrna.1103

34. Trendel J, Schwarzl T, Horos R et al (2019) The human RNA-binding proteome and its dynamics during translational arrest. Cell 176: 391–403.e19. https://doi.org/10.1016/j.cell.2018.11.004

35. Allers T, Ngo H-P, Mevarech M, Lloyd RG (2004) Development of additional selectable markers for the halophilic archaeon Haloferax volcanii based on the leuB and trpA genes. Appl Environ Microbiol 70:943–953. https://doi.org/10.1128/AEM.70.2.943-953.2004

36. Knüppel R, Kuttenberger C, Ferreira-Cerca S (2017) Towards time-resolved analysis of RNA metabolism in archaea using 4-thiouracil. Front Microbiol 8:286. https://doi.org/10.3389/fmicb.2017.00286

37. Barrass JD, Beggs JD (2019) Extremely rapid and specific metabolic labelling of RNA in vivo with 4-Thiouracil (Ers4tU). J Vis Exp. https://doi.org/10.3791/59952

38. Burger K, Mühl B, Kellner M et al (2013) 4-thiouridine inhibits rRNA synthesis and causes a nucleolar stress response. RNA Biol 10:1623–1630. https://doi.org/10.4161/rna.26214

39. Boissier F, Schmidt CM, Linnemann J et al (2017) Pwp2 mediates UTP-B assembly via two structurally independent domains. Sci Rep 7:3169–3169. https://doi.org/10.1038/s41598-017-03034-y

40. Ramos-Sáenz A, González-Álvarez D, Rodríguez-Galán O et al (2019) Pol5 is an essential ribosome biogenesis factor required for 60S ribosomal subunit maturation in Saccharomyces cerevisiae. RNA 25:1561–1575. https://doi.org/10.1261/rna.072116.119

41. Braun CM, Hackert P, Schmid CE et al (2020) Pol5 is required for recycling of small subunit biogenesis factors and for formation of the peptide exit tunnel of the large ribosomal subunit. Nucleic Acids Res 48:405–420. https://doi.org/10.1093/nar/gkz1079

# Part VI

## Translation

# Chapter 13

# Translation Phases in Eukaryotes

## Sandra Blanchet and Namit Ranjan

## Abstract

Protein synthesis in eukaryotes is carried out by 80S ribosomes with the help of many specific translation factors. Translation comprises four major steps: initiation, elongation, termination, and ribosome recycling. In this review, we provide a comprehensive list of translation factors required for protein synthesis in yeast and higher eukaryotes and summarize the mechanisms of each individual phase of eukaryotic translation.

**Key words** Translation, Ribosome, mRNA, tRNA, Yeast

## 1 Introduction

In all domains of life, information encoded in mRNA is translated to protein by a supramolecular machine called ribosome. Eukaryotic ribosome consists of a small subunit (40S) and a large subunit (60S) that together form the 80S ribosome. The ribosome reads the information one codon (three nucleotides) at a time using aminoacyl-tRNAs as adaptor molecules that recognize each codon to insert the appropriate amino acid. Ribosomes from bacteria, archaea, and eukarya share a high degree of sequence and structure conservation, indicating a common evolutionary origin. Furthermore, they share a similar central core where mRNA decoding, peptidyl transfer, and translocation of tRNA and mRNA by one codon take place. The process of translation can be divided into four main phases: initiation, elongation, termination, and ribosome recycling. During the initiation phase, eukaryotic translation initiation factors (eIFs) promote the assembly of 80S ribosomes at the AUG start codon with an initiator methionyl-tRNA bound to the P site (Table 1). During elongation, 80S ribosomes move processively along the mRNA, synthesizing the encoded protein through the coordinated actions of aminoacyl-tRNAs and the eukaryotic translation elongation factors (eEFs) (Table 2). At the end of the open reading frame, the ribosome encounters a termination codon recognized by eukaryotic release factors (eRFs) (Table 2), which

Karl-Dieter Entian (ed.), *Ribosome Biogenesis: Methods and Protocols*, Methods in Molecular Biology, vol. 2533, https://doi.org/10.1007/978-1-0716-2501-9_13, © The Author(s) 2022

**Table 1**
**Eukaryotic translation initiation factors**

| Name | Number of subunits and their molecular mass (kDa) | | Function |
|------|-------|-------------------|----------|
| | **Yeast** | **Higher eukayotes** | |
| *Initiation factors* | | | |
| eIF1 | 1 (12.3) | 1 (12.7) | Facilitates recognition of the initiator codon, modulates translation accuracy at the initiation phase |
| eIF1A | 1 (17.4) | 1 (16.5) | Stimulates eIF2–GTP–Met-tRNA$_i$$^{Met}$ binding to 40S subunits and promotes ribosome scanning and initiation codon selection together with eIF1 |
| eIF2 | α (34.7)<br>β (31.5)<br>γ (57.8) | α (36.1)<br>β (38.4)<br>γ (51.1) | Forms an eIF2–GTP–Met-tRNA$_i$$^{Met}$ ternary complex and delivers Met-tRNA$_i$$^{Met}$ to the 40S subunit |
| eIF3 | a (110.3)<br>b (88.1)<br>c (93.2)<br>g (30.5)<br>i (38.7) | a (166.6), b (92.5)<br>c (105.3), d (64)<br>e (52.2), f (37.6)<br>g (35.6), h (39.9)<br>i (36.5)<br>j (29.1)<br>k (25.1), l (66.7)<br>m (42.5) | Is involved in the preinitiation complex assembly and start codon selection, stimulates the binding of mRNA and Met-tRNA$_i$$^{Met}$ to the ribosome |
| eIF4A | 1 (44.6) | 1 (46.1) | DEAD-box ATPase and ATP-dependent RNA helicase |
| eIF4B | 1 (48.5) | 1 (69.3) | RNA-binding protein that enhances eIF4A helicase activity |
| eIF4E | 1 (24.2) | 1 (24.5) | mRNA cap-binding protein |
| eIF4F | A (24.2)<br>E (44.6)<br>G (103.9) | A (24.5)<br>E (46.1)<br>G (175.5) | Cap-binding complex that unwinds the 5′ UTR of mRNA, mediates the binding of 43S complexes and assists the ribosomal complexes during scanning |
| eIF4G | 1 (103.9) | 1 (175.5) | Platform protein that binds eIF4E, A, 3; PABP; and mRNA, and enhances the helicase activity of eIF4A |
| eIF4H | None | 1 (27.4) | RNA-binding protein that enhances eIF4A helicase activity; is homologous to a fragment of eIF4B |
| eIF5 | 1 (45.2) | 1 (49.2) | GTPase-activating protein that induces hydrolysis of eIF2-bound GTP upon initiation codon recognition |
| eIF5B | 1 (112.2) | 1 (138.9) | Mediates ribosomal subunit joining in a GTP-dependent manner |

(continued)

**Table 1**
**(continued)**

| Name | Number of subunits and their molecular mass (kDa) | | Function |
|------|-------|-------|----------|
| | Yeast | Higher eukayotes | |
| eIF2B | α (34) | α (33.7) | Guanosine nucleotide exchange factor |
| | β (42.5) | β (39) | that promotes GDP–GTP exchange |
| | γ (65.6) | γ (50.2) | on eIF2 |
| | δ (70.8) | δ (59.7) | |
| | ε (81.1) | ε (80.3) | |

**Table 2**
**Eukaryotic translation elongation and termination factors**

| Name | Number of subunits and their molecular mass (kDa) | | Function |
|------|-------|-------|----------|
| | Yeast | Higher eukayotes | |
| *Elongation factors* | | | |
| eEF1A | 1 (50) | 1 (50.1) | Forms an eEF1A–GTP–aa-tRNA ternary complex that delivers aa-tRNA to the 80S ribosomes during elongation |
| eEF2 | 1 (93.3) | 1 (95.3) | Ribosome-dependent GTPase that facilitates tRNA–mRNA translocation |
| eIF5A | 1 (17.1) | 1 (16) | Is involved in translation elongation, promotes the translation of stalling sequences |
| eEF3 | 1 (115.9) | Not known | Ribosome-dependent ATPase involved in elongation |
| *Termination factors* | | | |
| eRF1 | 1 (48.9) | 1 (49) | Directs the termination of nascent peptide synthesis and the release of polypeptide upon eRF3 GTP hydrolysis |
| eRF3 | 1 (76.5) | 1 (68.8) | GTPase that stimulates eRF1 activity and polypeptide release |
| *Recycling factors* | | | |
| ABCE1 | Rli1 (68.3) | 1 (67.3) | Promotes peptide release and is involved in ribosomal subunits recycling |
| eIF2D | 1 (64) | 1 (64.7) | Potentially promotes dissociation of deacylated tRNA and mRNA from post-termination complexes |

promote the release of the nascent protein from the ribosome. Finally, during the recycling phase, the ribosome complex is recycled to the 40S and 60S subunits to begin a new round of translation. In this review, we describe the four phases of eukaryotic translation and function of translation factors (Tables 1 and 2). In the accompanying methods chapter, we focus on in vitro reconstitution of initiation and elongation phases of translation. Detailed aspects of translation termination and recycling are discussed in recent reviews [1, 2].

## 2    Initiation

The initiation phase leads to the formation of 80S ribosomes where the initiator tRNA (Met-tRNA$_i$$^{Met}$) and the start codon are positioned in the P site. This process requires at least ten eukaryotic initiation factors, eIFs (Table 1), and comprises two major steps. In the first step, Met-tRNA$_i$$^{Met}$ binds to the start codon in the P site of the 40S subunit to form the 48S initiation complex. In the second step, the 60S subunit joins the 48S complex to form the 80S initiation complex that is ready for elongation (Fig. 1) [3, 4].

*Formation of 48S preinitiation complex.* During this step, eIF3, eIF1, and eIF1A are recruited to 40S subunits, followed by subsequent attachment of eIF5 and eIF2–GTP–Met-tRNA$_i$$^{Met}$ to form 43S complexes. eIF3 binds to the 40S subunit side that faces the solvent in the 80S ribosome [5], whereas eIF1 binds between the platform of the 40S subunit and Met-tRNA$_i$$^{Met}$ to the 40S side that will form the interface to the 60S subunit [6]. The structured domain of eIF1A resides in the A site, forming a bridge over the mRNA channel, and its N- and C-terminal tails extend into the P site. Binding of eIF1 and eIF1A to the 40S subunit induces conformational changes [7, 8], which result in the opening of the mRNA entry channel and the establishment of a new connection between the head and body domains of the 40S subunit on the solvent side between helix 16 of 18S rRNA and the ribosomal protein uS3. Although 43S complexes can bind model mRNAs with completely unstructured 5′ UTRs in the absence of eIFs [9], attachment of natural mRNAs requires a coordinated activity of eIF4F protein complex, which unwinds the 5′ cap-proximal region of mRNA. Following mRNA attachment, the 43S complex scans the mRNA downstream of the cap in search for the initiation codon. During the scanning process, the secondary structures in the 5′ UTR unwind and the 43S complex moves until the initiation codon is recognized. eIF1 and eIF1A play key roles in the 43S complex formation and scanning; omission of either or both reduces or suppresses the scanning ability, indicating that the movement of 43S complexes requires the scanning-competent conformation induced by eIF1 and eIF1A [7]. eIF3, which is indispensable for

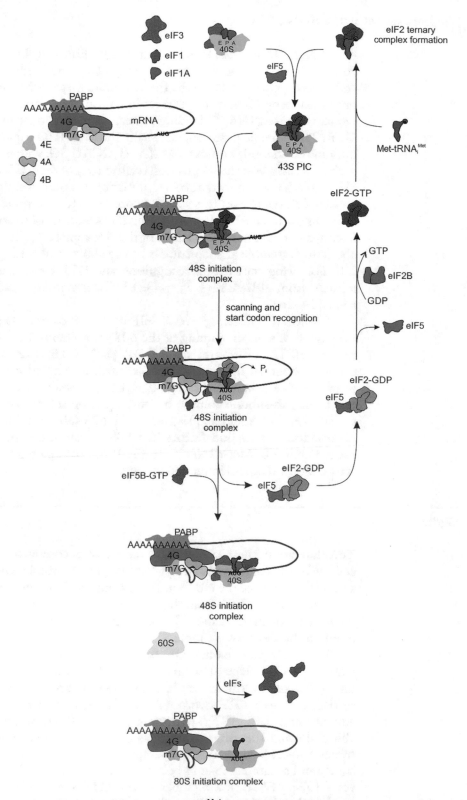

**Fig. 1** Translation initiation. eIF2–GTP–Met-tRNA$_i^{Met}$ binds to the 40S ribosomes in presence of eIF1, eIF1A, eIF3, and eIF5 to form 43S PIC. Then mRNA is recruited with the help of eIF4F complex to form the 48S PIC. After mRNA scanning and recognition of the start codon, the 60S subunit joins with the help of eIF5B to form the 80S IC [4, 59, 60]

48S complex formation, forms an extension of the mRNA-binding channel that might contribute to scanning [10]. The fidelity of start codon recognition is ensured by the discriminatory mechanism that promotes recognition of the correct initiation codon and prevents premature Met-tRNA$_i^{Met}$ landing at near-cognate triplets in the 5′ UTR. The bona fide start site is usually the first AUG triplet in an optimum nucleotide context GCC(A/G)CCAUGG, with a purine at the −3 and a G at the +4 position relative to A of the AUG codon [11]. eIF1 has an important role in initiation codon recognition: it enables 43S complexes to select the correct AUG in a poor initiation context or an AUG located within 8 nucleotides of the mRNA 5′ end, and promotes dissociation of the ribosomal complexes that aberrantly assemble at such triplets in the absence of eIF1 [9, 12, 13]. Following start codon recognition and GTP hydrolysis, P$_i$ is released from eIF2–GTP + P$_i$ and eIF1 dissociates from the ribosome [14–16].

*Ribosomal subunit joining.* eIF5B, a ribosome-associated GTPase, facilitates the joining of the 60S subunit and the dissociation of eIF1A, eIF5, and eIF2–GDP [17]. GTP hydrolysis by eIF5B is essential for its own release from assembled 80S ribosomes. eIF5B occupies the region in the intersubunit cleft [18] and promotes subunit joining by burying large solvent-accessible surfaces on both subunits [19]. After the 60S subunit joining and dissociation of initiation factors, the 80S initiation complex with the anticodon of Met-tRNA$_i^{Met}$ in the P site base-paired with the start codon becomes elongation competent.

# 3 Elongation

The elongation phase comprises three steps: decoding of mRNA codons by the cognate aminoacyl-tRNAs, peptide bond formation, and translocation of the tRNA–mRNA complex, resulting in movement of peptidyl-tRNA from the A site to the P site and presenting the next codon in the A site [1] (Fig. 2). Four elongation factors are required the three steps (Table 2).

The eukaryotic elongation factor eEF1A binds aminoacyl-tRNA in a GTP-dependent manner and delivers the aa-tRNA to the A site of the ribosome (Fig. 2). Codon recognition by the aa-tRNA triggers GTP hydrolysis by eEF1A, releasing the factor and enabling the aa-tRNA to accommodate in the A site, presumably following the same pathway as described for bacterial ribosomes [20–24]. However, decoding appears to take place more slowly and accurately than in bacteria, particularly in higher eukaryotes [25]. eEF1A is a member of the GTPase superfamily that binds and hydrolyzes GTP. The dissociation of GDP from eEF1A is accelerated by a guanine nucleotide exchange factor (GEF), eEF1B, which is composed of two subunits, eEF1Bα and eEF1Bγ in yeast,

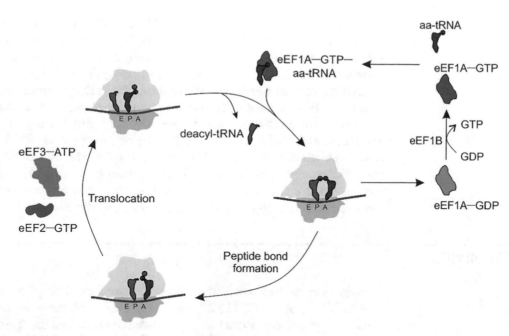

**Fig. 2** Translation elongation. During decoding, eEF1A delivers aa-tRNA to the A site. After peptide bond formation, the A-site peptidyl-tRNA and P-site tRNA are translocated to the P and E sites, respectively, with the help of eEF2. Deacylated tRNA is released from the E site and the elongation cycle repeats until a stop codon is reached. In yeast, an additional factor eEF3 is required during elongation [1]

the first one containing the catalytic domain necessary for nucleotide exchange. eIF5A, which was originally identified as initiation factor, functions globally in translation elongation, especially when ribosome encounter polyproline sequences [2].

Following the accommodation of the aminoacyl-tRNA into the A site, the peptide bond formation with the P-site peptidyl-tRNA occurs rapidly in the peptidyl transferase center (PTC). The PTC consists mainly of conserved rRNA elements of the 60S subunit that position the substrates for catalysis. Structural studies have revealed that the rRNA structure of the PTC is nearly superimposable between the eukaryotic and bacterial ribosomes [26–28], supporting the notion that the mechanism of peptide bond formation is universally conserved.

The pretranslocation complex formed as a result of peptide bond formation is dynamic and can spontaneously fluctuate between several conformations, in prokaryotes and eukaryotes alike [29, 30]. The ribosomal subunits undergo a ratchet-like motion from the so-called classical to rotated state triggering movement of the tRNAs to adopt hybrid states. In this state, the anticodon ends of the tRNAs remain positioned in the P and A sites of the 40S subunit, while the tRNA acceptor ends are positioned in the E site and P site of the 60S subunit (P/E and E/P states, respectively) [31–33]. Translocation of the mRNA–tRNA in the ribosome requires elongation factor eEF2, which facilitates the return of hybrid tRNAs to the classical state, E/E and P/P (canonical E and P sites). eEF2 in its GTP-bound state facilitates and stabilizes the hybrid rotated state. Conformational changes in eEF2 upon GTP hydrolysis and Pi release unlock the ribosome allowing tRNA and mRNA movement and then lock the subunits in the posttranslocation state. In that state of the ribosome, a deacylated tRNA occupies the E site and the peptidyl-tRNA is in the P site, leaving the A site vacant and available for binding of the next aminoacyl-tRNA in complex with eEF1A [34, 35]. In addition to eEF1A and eEF2, a third factor, eEF3, is essential for elongation in fungi [36]. The elongation cycle is repeated until a complete protein has been synthesized and a stop codon is encountered by the ribosome.

## 4   Termination

Termination occurs when the ribosome reaches a stop codon (UAA, UGA, or UAG) [1, 37–39] (Fig. 3). Termination is catalyzed by two protein factors, eRF1, which recognizes all three stop codons, and the GTPase eRF3, which facilitates termination at a cost of GTP hydrolysis [39–41]. eRF1 contains a structural Asn-Ile-Lys-Ser (NIKS) motif and several other conserved elements, including the Gly-Thr-Ser (GTS) and YxCxxxF motifs, which are involved in the recognition of the termination codons [42–46]. In addition, the central domain of eRF1 contains a Gly-Gly-Gln (GGQ) motif that extends into the peptidyl-transferase center to promote peptidyl-tRNA hydrolysis and the release of nascent peptide [47–50]. eRF1 requires eRF3 (a specialized GTPase) for proper function (Table 2). eRF1 and eRF3 bind to one another with very high affinity and probably enter the

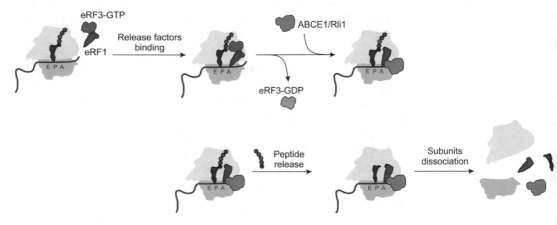

**Fig. 3** Translation termination and recycling. Termination occurs when a stop codon enters the A site of the ribosome and is catalyzed by eRF1 and eRF3. Peptide release is promoted by ABCE1 which also induces subunits dissociation [1]

ribosome as a complex [51]. GTP hydrolysis positions the GGQ region of eRF1 in the peptidyl transferase center and triggers peptidyl-tRNA hydrolysis. eRF3 strongly enhances peptide release by eRF1 in the presence of GTP, but not GDP or nonhydrolyzable GTP analogs [39]. Moreover, other *trans*-acting factors are known to affect translation termination. ABCE1 (Rli1 in yeast) interacts with eRF1 to stimulate its catalytic activity by stabilizing the active conformation of eRF1 [52–55].

# 5    Ribosome Recycling

During recycling the ribosomal subunits dissociate and the mRNA together with the deacylated tRNA are released to regenerate the necessary components for subsequent rounds of translation. Recycling of ribosomal subunits is achieved by the ATPase ABCE1 (Rli1 in yeast), an essential protein which contains two nucleotide-binding domains and an amino-terminal iron–sulfur cluster (Fe-S) and induces subunits dissociation at the cost of ATP hydrolysis [53, 54, 56]. Upon binding and hydrolysis of ATP, the Fe-S cluster undergoes a conformational change that drives eRF1 into the ribosomal intersubunit space, leading to dissociation of posttermination ribosomes into 40S and 60S subunits. Deacylated tRNA and mRNA are then released from the 40S subunits, which may be additionally promoted by Ligatin (eIF2D) [57] (Table 2). Initiation factors eIF1, eIF1A, and eIF3j can also promote tRNA and mRNA dissociation from the 40S subunit in vitro [54]. Following termination, in some cases full dissociation of the ribosomal complex will occur, whereas in other cases partial dissolution of the complex will allow for reinitiation, a term used to describe a process wherein ribosome translates two or more ORFs in a transcript without undergoing complete recycling between these events [58]. However, the mechanism of reinitiation is not fully understood.

# Acknowledgments

We thank Prof. Marina Rodnina for critical reading of the manuscript. This work is supported by the Deutsche Forschungsgemeinschaft (DFG) in the framework of the Schwerpunktprogram (SPP1784), and by the Max Planck Society.

# References

1. Dever TE, Green R (2012) The elongation, termination, and recycling phases of translation in eukaryotes. Cold Spring Harb Perspect Biol 4:a013706

2. Schuller AP, Wu CC, Dever TE, Buskirk AR, Green R (2017) eIF5A functions globally in translation elongation and termination. Mol Cell 66:194–205 e5

3. Hinnebusch AG, Lorsch JR (2012) The mechanism of eukaryotic translation initiation: new insights and challenges. Cold Spring Harb Perspect Biol 4:a011544

4. Jackson RJ, Hellen CU, Pestova TV (2010) The mechanism of eukaryotic translation initiation and principles of its regulation. Nat Rev Mol Cell Biol 11:113–127

5. Siridechadilok B, Fraser CS, Hall RJ, Doudna JA, Nogales E (2005) Structural roles for human translation factor eIF3 in initiation of protein synthesis. Science 310:1513–1515

6. Lomakin IB, Kolupaeva VG, Marintchev A, Wagner G, Pestova TV (2003) Position of eukaryotic initiation factor eIF1 on the 40S ribosomal subunit determined by directed hydroxyl radical probing. Genes Dev 17:2786–2797

7. Passmore LA, Schmeing TM, Maag D, Applefield DJ, Acker MG, Algire MA, Lorsch JR, Ramakrishnan V (2007) The eukaryotic translation initiation factors eIF1 and eIF1A induce an open conformation of the 40S ribosome. Mol Cell 26:41–50

8. Llacer JL, Hussain T, Marler L, Aitken CE, Thakur A, Lorsch JR, Hinnebusch AG, Ramakrishnan V (2015) Conformational differences between open and closed states of the eukaryotic translation initiation complex. Mol Cell 59:399–412

9. Pestova TV, Kolupaeva VG (2002) The roles of individual eukaryotic translation initiation factors in ribosomal scanning and initiation codon selection. Genes Dev 16:2906–2922

10. Pisarev AV, Kolupaeva VG, Yusupov MM, Hellen CU, Pestova TV (2008) Ribosomal position and contacts of mRNA in eukaryotic translation initiation complexes. EMBO J 27:1609–1621

11. Kozak M (1991) Structural features in eukaryotic mRNAs that modulate the initiation of translation. J Biol Chem 266:19867–19870

12. Pestova TV, Borukhov SI, Hellen CU (1998) Eukaryotic ribosomes require initiation factors 1 and 1A to locate initiation codons. Nature 394:854–859

13. Pisarev AV, Kolupaeva VG, Pisareva VP, Merrick WC, Hellen CU, Pestova TV (2006) Specific functional interactions of nucleotides at key −3 and +4 positions flanking the initiation codon with components of the mammalian 48S translation initiation complex. Genes Dev 20:624–636

14. Cheung YN, Maag D, Mitchell SF, Fekete CA, Algire MA, Takacs JE, Shirokikh N, Pestova T, Lorsch JR, Hinnebusch AG (2007) Dissociation of eIF1 from the 40S ribosomal subunit is a key step in start codon selection in vivo. Genes Dev 21:1217–1230

15. Martin-Marcos P, Nanda J, Luna RE, Wagner G, Lorsch JR, Hinnebusch AG (2013) Beta-hairpin loop of eukaryotic initiation factor 1 (eIF1) mediates 40 S ribosome binding to regulate initiator tRNA(met) recruitment and accuracy of AUG selection in vivo. J Biol Chem 288:27546–27562

16. Nanda JS, Saini AK, Munoz AM, Hinnebusch AG, Lorsch JR (2013) Coordinated movements of eukaryotic translation initiation factors eIF1, eIF1A, and eIF5 trigger phosphate release from eIF2 in response to start codon recognition by the ribosomal preinitiation complex. J Biol Chem 288:5316–5329

17. Pestova TV, Lomakin IB, Lee JH, Choi SK, Dever TE, Hellen CU (2000) The joining of ribosomal subunits in eukaryotes requires eIF5B. Nature 403:332–335

18. Unbehaun A, Marintchev A, Lomakin IB, Didenko T, Wagner G, Hellen CU, Pestova TV (2007) Position of eukaryotic initiation factor eIF5B on the 80S ribosome mapped by directed hydroxyl radical probing. EMBO J 26:3109–3123

19. Allen GS, Zavialov A, Gursky R, Ehrenberg M, Frank J (2005) The cryo-EM structure of a translation initiation complex from Escherichia coli. Cell 121:703–712

20. Diaconu M, Kothe U, Schlunzen F, Fischer N, Harms JM, Tonevitsky AG, Stark H, Rodnina MV, Wahl MC (2005) Structural basis for the function of the ribosomal L7/12 stalk in factor binding and GTPase activation. Cell 121:991–1004

21. Ogle JM, Ramakrishnan V (2005) Structural insights into translational fidelity. Annu Rev Biochem 74:129–177

22. Rodnina MV, Wintermeyer W (2001) Fidelity of aminoacyl-tRNA selection on the ribosome: kinetic and structural mechanisms. Annu Rev Biochem 70:415–435

23. Daviter T, Gromadski KB, Rodnina MV (2006) The ribosome's response to codon-anticodon mismatches. Biochimie 88:1001–1011

24. Zaher HS, Green R (2009) Fidelity at the molecular level: lessons from protein synthesis. Cell 136:746–762

25. Rodnina MV, Wintermeyer W (2009) Recent mechanistic insights into eukaryotic ribosomes. Curr Opin Cell Biol 21:435–443

26. Ben-Shem A, Jenner L, Yusupova G, Yusupov M (2010) Crystal structure of the eukaryotic ribosome. Science 330:1203–1209

27. Ben-Shem A, Garreau de Loubresse N, Melnikov S, Jenner L, Yusupova G, Yusupov M (2011) The structure of the eukaryotic ribosome at 3.0 A resolution. Science 334: 1524–1529

28. Klinge S, Voigts-Hoffmann F, Leibundgut M, Arpagaus S, Ban N (2011) Crystal structure of the eukaryotic 60S ribosomal subunit in complex with initiation factor 6. Science 334: 941–948

29. Fischer N, Konevega AL, Wintermeyer W, Rodnina MV, Stark H (2010) Ribosome dynamics and tRNA movement by time-resolved electron cryomicroscopy. Nature 466:329–333

30. Munro JB, Altman RB, Tung CS, Cate JH, Sanbonmatsu KY, Blanchard SC (2010) Spontaneous formation of the unlocked state of the ribosome is a multistep process. Proc Natl Acad Sci U S A 107:709–714

31. Behrmann E, Loerke J, Budkevich TV, Yamamoto K, Schmidt A, Penczek PA, Vos MR, Burger J, Mielke T, Scheerer P, Spahn CM (2015) Structural snapshots of actively translating human ribosomes. Cell 161: 845–857

32. Budkevich T, Giesebrecht J, Altman RB, Munro JB, Mielke T, Nierhaus KH, Blanchard SC, Spahn CM (2011) Structure and dynamics of the mammalian ribosomal pretranslocation complex. Mol Cell 44:214–224

33. Moazed D, Noller HF (1989) Intermediate states in the movement of transfer RNA in the ribosome. Nature 342:142–148

34. Ferguson A, Wang L, Altman RB, Terry DS, Juette MF, Burnett BJ, Alejo JL, Dass RA, Parks MM, Vincent CT, Blanchard SC (2015) Functional dynamics within the human ribosome regulate the rate of active protein synthesis. Mol Cell 60:475–486

35. Taylor DJ, Nilsson J, Merrill AR, Andersen GR, Nissen P, Frank J (2007) Structures of modified eEF2 80S ribosome complexes reveal the role of GTP hydrolysis in translocation. EMBO J 26:2421–2431

36. Andersen CB, Becker T, Blau M, Anand M, Halic M, Balar B, Mielke T, Boesen T, Pedersen JS, Spahn CM, Kinzy TG, Andersen GR, Beckmann R (2006) Structure of eEF3 and the mechanism of transfer RNA release from the E-site. Nature 443:663–668

37. Stansfield I, Jones KM, Kushnirov VV, Dagkesamanskaya AR, Poznyakovski AI, Paushkin SV, Nierras CR, Cox BS, Ter-Avanesyan MD, Tuite MF (1995) The products of the SUP45 (eRF1) and SUP35 genes interact to mediate translation termination in Saccharomyces cerevisiae. EMBO J 14:4365–4373

38. Zhouravleva G, Frolova L, Le Goff X, Le Guellec R, Inge-Vechtomov S, Kisselev L, Philippe M (1995) Termination of translation in eukaryotes is governed by two interacting polypeptide chain release factors, eRF1 and eRF3. EMBO J 14:4065–4072

39. Alkalaeva EZ, Pisarev AV, Frolova LY, Kisselev LL, Pestova TV (2006) In vitro reconstitution of eukaryotic translation reveals cooperativity between release factors eRF1 and eRF3. Cell 125:1125–1136

40. Fan-Minogue H, Du M, Pisarev AV, Kallmeyer AK, Salas-Marco J, Keeling KM, Thompson SR, Pestova TV, Bedwell DM (2008) Distinct eRF3 requirements suggest alternate eRF1 conformations mediate peptide release during eukaryotic translation termination. Mol Cell 30:599–609

41. Salas-Marco J, Bedwell DM (2004) GTP hydrolysis by eRF3 facilitates stop codon decoding during eukaryotic translation termination. Mol Cell Biol 24:7769–7778

42. Song H, Mugnier P, Das AK, Webb HM, Evans DR, Tuite MF, Hemmings BA, Barford D (2000) The crystal structure of human eukaryotic release factor eRF1--mechanism of stop codon recognition and peptidyl-tRNA hydrolysis. Cell 100:311–321

43. Frolova L, Le Goff X, Rasmussen HH, Cheperegin S, Drugeon G, Kress M, Arman I, Haenni AL, Celis JE, Philippe M et al (1994) A highly conserved eukaryotic protein family possessing properties of polypeptide chain release factor. Nature 372:701–703

44. Brown A, Shao S, Murray J, Hegde RS, Ramakrishnan V (2015) Structural basis for stop codon recognition in eukaryotes. Nature 524:493–496

45. Matheisl S, Berninghausen O, Becker T, Beckmann R (2015) Structure of a human translation termination complex. Nucleic Acids Res 43:8615–8626

46. des Georges A, Hashem Y, Unbehaun A, Grassucci RA, Taylor D, Hellen CU, Pestova TV, Frank J (2014) Structure of the mammalian ribosomal pre-termination complex associated with eRF1.eRF3.GDPNP. Nucleic Acids Res 42:3409–3418

47. Bertram G, Bell HA, Ritchie DW, Fullerton G, Stansfield I (2000) Terminating eukaryote translation: domain 1 of release factor eRF1 functions in stop codon recognition. RNA 6: 1236–1247

48. Frolova LY, Tsivkovskii RY, Sivolobova GF, Oparina NY, Serpinsky OI, Blinov VM, Tatkov SI, Kisselev LL (1999) Mutations in the highly conserved GGQ motif of class 1 polypeptide release factors abolish ability of human eRF1 to trigger peptidyl-tRNA hydrolysis. RNA 5:1014–1020

49. Merkulova TI, Frolova LY, Lazar M, Camonis J, Kisselev LL (1999) C-terminal domains of human translation termination factors eRF1 and eRF3 mediate their in vivo interaction. FEBS Lett 443:41–47

50. Cheng Z, Saito K, Pisarev AV, Wada M, Pisareva VP, Pestova TV, Gajda M, Round A, Kong C, Lim M, Nakamura Y, Svergun DI, Ito K, Song H (2009) Structural insights into eRF3 and stop codon recognition by eRF1. Genes Dev 23:1106–1118

51. Pisareva VP, Pisarev AV, Hellen CU, Rodnina MV, Pestova TV (2006) Kinetic analysis of interaction of eukaryotic release factor 3 with guanine nucleotides. J Biol Chem 281:40224–40235

52. Khoshnevis S, Gross T, Rotte C, Baierlein C, Ficner R, Krebber H (2010) The iron-Sulphur protein RNase L inhibitor functions in translation termination. EMBO Rep 11:214–219

53. Shoemaker CJ, Green R (2011) Kinetic analysis reveals the ordered coupling of translation termination and ribosome recycling in yeast. Proc Natl Acad Sci U S A 108:E1392–E1398

54. Pisarev AV, Skabkin MA, Pisareva VP, Skabkina OV, Rakotondrafara AM, Hentze MW, Hellen CU, Pestova TV (2010) The role of ABCE1 in eukaryotic posttermination ribosomal recycling. Mol Cell 37:196–210

55. Preis A, Heuer A, Barrio-Garcia C, Hauser A, Eyler DE, Berninghausen O, Green R, Becker T, Beckmann R (2014) Cryoelectron microscopic structures of eukaryotic translation termination complexes containing eRF1-eRF3 or eRF1-ABCE1. Cell Rep 8:59–65

56. Pisareva VP, Skabkin MA, Hellen CU, Pestova TV, Pisarev AV (2011) Dissociation by Pelota, Hbs1 and ABCE1 of mammalian vacant 80S ribosomes and stalled elongation complexes. EMBO J 30:1804–1817

57. Skabkin MA, Skabkina OV, Dhote V, Komar AA, Hellen CU, Pestova TV (2010) Activities of Ligatin and MCT-1/DENR in eukaryotic translation initiation and ribosomal recycling. Genes Dev 24:1787–1801

58. Kozak M (1984) Selection of initiation sites by eucaryotic ribosomes: effect of inserting AUG triplets upstream from the coding sequence for preproinsulin. Nucleic Acids Res 12:3873–3893

59. Dever TE, Kinzy TG, Pavitt GD (2016) Mechanism and regulation of protein synthesis in Saccharomyces cerevisiae. Genetics 203:65–107

60. Jennings MD, Pavitt GD (2010) eIF5 is a dual function GAP and GDI for eukaryotic translational control. Small GTPases 1:118–123

# Chapter 14

# Differential Translation Activity Analysis Using Bioorthogonal Noncanonical Amino Acid Tagging (BONCAT) in Archaea

## Michael Kern and Sébastien Ferreira-Cerca ⓘ

## Abstract

The study of protein production and degradation in a quantitative and time-dependent manner is a major challenge to better understand cellular physiological response. Among available technologies **bioorthogo-nal noncanonical amino acid tagging** (BONCAT) is an efficient approach allowing for time-dependent labeling of proteins through the incorporation of chemically reactive noncanonical amino acids like L-azidohomoalanine (L-AHA). The azide-containing amino-acid derivative enables a highly efficient and specific reaction termed click chemistry, whereby the azide group of the L-AHA reacts with a reactive alkyne derivate, like dibenzocyclooctyne (DBCO) derivatives, using strain-promoted alkyne–azide cycloaddition (SPAAC). Moreover, available DBCO containing reagents are versatile and can be coupled to fluorophore (e.g., Cy7) or affinity tag (e.g., biotin) derivatives, for easy visualization and affinity purification, respectively.

Here, we describe a step-by-step BONCAT protocol optimized for the model archaeon *Haloferax volcanii*, but which is also suitable to harness other biological systems. Finally, we also describe examples of downstream visualization, affinity purification of L-AHA-labeled proteins and differential expression analysis.

In conclusion, the following BONCAT protocol expands the available toolkit to explore proteostasis using time-resolved semiquantitative proteomic analysis in archaea.

**Key words** BONCAT, L-Azidohomoalanine, L-AHA, Archaea, Time-dependent, Translation, Trans-latome, Proteostasis, *Haloferax volcanii*, *Sulfolobus acidocaldarius*, *Escherichia coli*, Click chemistry

## 1 Introduction

Cellular adaptation depends on efficient and timely controlled variation of the cellular protein synthesis and degradation capacity [1–3]. Accordingly, the resulting qualitative and quantitative ensemble of proteins present at a given time, in a given cell or tissue, or in a given environmental condition is instrumental for proper cell fate determination. Hence, proteome plasticity is a key feature in enabling suitable gene expression modulation.

Karl-Dieter Entian (ed.), *Ribosome Biogenesis: Methods and Protocols*, Methods in Molecular Biology, vol. 2533,
https://doi.org/10.1007/978-1-0716-2501-9_14, © The Author(s) 2022

Depending on the nature of intra- and extracellular cues, changes in the protein repertoire and individual protein levels may occur at different time-scales, and need to be experimentally captured with accuracy to understand the underlying cellular and physiological mechanisms [1–3].

Over the last decade(s) various approaches have been used to explore protein synthesis and degradation dynamics [1–3]. Among these methods, *ribosome profiling*, which takes advantage of high-throughput sequencing of ribosome associated mRNA, has emerged as the method of choice to assess the translational capacity and properties of various cellular systems across different conditions [1–3]. Even though extremely powerful, this method remains an indirect measurement of protein synthesis, as it fails to directly measure the product of translation itself. Moreover, protein degradation is not monitored using this experimental setup. An alternative, but still emerging method, is the use of time-dependent semiquantitative proteomic approaches, which allow for analysis of both protein synthesis and degradation [1]. While less popular, and still technically challenging, various mass spectrometry–based approaches have been developed and significantly improved over the years and are now able to provide semiquantitative and direct analysis of cellular protein composition in a time-dependent manner [1, 4–8]. To achieve such in-depth analysis various experimental setups can be used depending on the time resolution and desired extensiveness of the analyses [1, 3]. Early on, time-dependent proteomics have relied on isotope labeling (e.g., SILAC), whereby differential incorporation of heavy and light isotope metabolites like amino acids are used over a specified time to sort protein populations [1, 3, 9–11]. However, isotope labeling strategies have different drawbacks: (1) some labeled metabolites can be rather expensive, (2) efficiency of labeling is highly dependent on cellular uptake and metabolism capacity, and usually requires defined synthetic growth medium, (3) multiplexing is limited due to the lack of different reagents, (4) short kinetic pulse, low-abundant or proteins with a high turnover rate are difficult to be properly analyzed due to the lack of a specific enrichment step of the isotopically labeled peptides [1, 3, 9–11].

An emerging complementary strategy allowing to circumvent some of these limitations and facilitating time-dependent proteomic analysis is **bio**orthogonal **n**oncanonical **a**mino acids **t**agging (BONCAT) [12, 13]. In brief, BONCAT exploits the power of in vivo incorporation of bioorthogonal molecules into polypeptides and of click chemistry which enables enrichment and/or visualization of the labeled proteins synthesized over a defined time window [4, 5, 8, 13–18]. Most importantly, BONCAT can be easily combined with isotope labeling and/or multiplexing (e.g., [4, 5, 8, 17]), thereby allowing to fully harness the potential of time-dependent proteomic analysis.

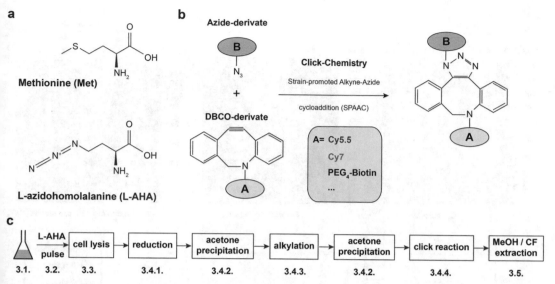

**Fig. 1** Optimized BONCAT workflow in *H. volcanii*. (**a**) Chemical structures of L-methionine and L-azidoho-moalanine (**b**) Click chemistry: Strain Promoted Alkyne–Azide Cycloaddition (SPAAC) reaction. Azide-containing polypeptide, DBCO derivate, and the results of click chemistry reaction are schematically depicted (**c**). Workflow summary of BONCAT in *H. volcanii*. Typical workflow as described in this protocol. The numbering below the different steps refers to the corresponding protocol steps described in the Methods section (*see* Subheading 3)

Most commonly BONCAT experiments utilize, L-azidoho-moalanine (L-AHA), a methionine analogue containing a functional azide group (Fig. 1a). L-AHA is recognized, albeit with less efficiency, by the methionyl-tRNA^Met acyl transferase, and is charged onto tRNA^Met, thereby allowing for incorporation of L-AHA into polypeptides instead of methionine during protein synthesis [19]. The resulting L-AHA-modified polypeptides can be further altered using strain-promoted alkyne–azide cycloaddition (SPAAC) as outlined in Fig. 1b [20]. Alkyne derivative of biotin or various fluorophores can be efficiently and quantitatively coupled to the azide-containing proteins, thereby facilitating their further visualization and/or subsequent specific enrichment for downstream analysis (Fig. 1b) and exemplary results shown in Figs. 2, 3 and 4).

Interestingly, BONCAT has been successfully applied in a wide variety of organisms and/or tissues across the tree of life, thereby highlighting its potential [4, 5, 8, 13–19]. However, despite its broad application potential, proteomics analysis in general and time-dependent analysis of protein synthesis and degradation in particular, remains in its early days in archaea.

*Haloferax volcanii,* an extreme halophile Euryarchaeota, has emerged as a very powerful model organism to perform genetic and functional analysis in archaea [21, 22]. Its handling simplicity has attracted several scientists who aim to push the

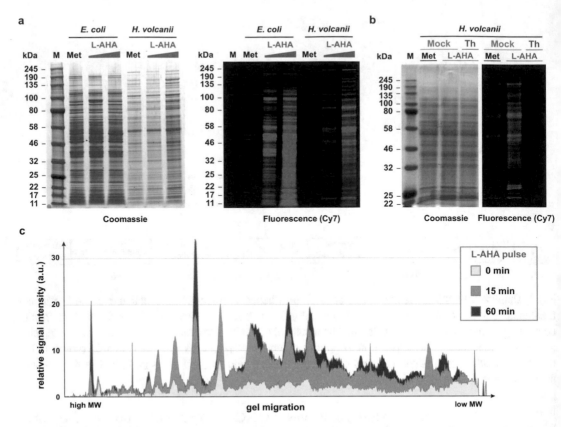

**Fig. 2** Exemplary BONCAT of prokaryotic cells. (**a**) L-AHA-based labeling of proteins in *E. coli* and *H. volcanii*. The corresponding cells (*E. coli* K12 and *H. volcanii* H26) were grown in synthetic medium lacking methionine (M9 and Hv-min, respectively) and pulse labeled with increasing amounts of L-AHA (0.1 mM and 1 mM) or 1 mM Methionine for 3 h. Cells were lysed, proteins were extracted and subjected to SPAAC click chemistry with DBCO-Cy7 as described in Subheading 3. Around 150 µg of proteins were subsequently fractionated on a 4–12% polyacrylamide gradient gel and the fluorescence signal was acquired with an Odyssey Infrared Imager (right panel). Coomassie staining (loading control) is depicted in the left panel (**b**) Inhibition of L-AHA-based labeling in presence of translation inhibitor in *H. volcanii*. Same as in (**a**) except that cells (*H. volcanii* H26) were grown in synthetic medium lacking methionine and supplemented with 0.1 mM methionine or 0.1 mM of L-AHA with or without 2.5 µM of the translation inhibitor Thiostrepton (Th) [31] for 1 h. (**c**) Short-time L-AHA labeling in *H. volcanii*. Same as in (**a**) except that cells (*H. volcanii* H26) were grown in synthetic medium lacking methionine and supplemented with 1 mM L-AHA for the indicated time. The depicted fluorescence signal intensities across single lanes were quantified using Fiji [32] and visualized in Microsoft Excel. Adapted from [33] under CC-BY License

experimentational limits of this organism and crack open its molecular biology. Efforts in proteomics analysis do not escape this trend. In fact, proteomics analyses in *H. volcanii* have been making significant progress over the last years [23–27], and are currently being improved by a concerted action of several groups working on *H. volcanii* (see Archaeal Proteome Project—ArcPP—https://archaealproteomeproject.org and https://github.com/arcpp/ArcPP—[28]). Finally, recent methodological breakthroughs using isotope labeling, SILAC reagents or [15]N-labeled nitrogen

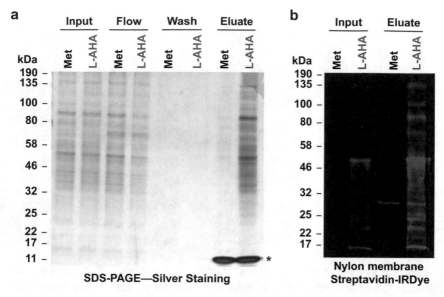

**Fig. 3** Enrichment of L-AHA-containing protein by affinity purification. H26 cells were grown in synthetic medium lacking methionine and supplemented with 0.1 mM of L-AHA or methionine (Met) for 5 h. Cells were lysed and proteins were extracted and subjected to click chemistry with 1 μM DBCO-PEG4-Biotin as described in Subheading 3.4. Affinity purification was performed as described in Subheading 3.6. Sample aliquots for input, unbound fraction (Flow), wash fraction and elution were taken at each step of the AP. Elution was performed as described in Subheading 3.6.4. 0.5% of the input, unbound (Flow) and 0.25% of the wash fraction and 20% of the eluate were loaded on two SDS-PAGE gels respectively. The fractionated proteins were visualized by silver staining (**a**) and transferred onto a nylon membrane (**b**). Membrane was incubated with IRDye-coupled streptavidin to visualize the biotinylated proteins. Images were acquired either with the Epson Scanner (silver staining) (**a**) or the Li-COR Odyssey Infrared Imager (IRDye signal) (**b**). Asterisk indicates streptavidin monomers that are coeluted

source, in *H. volcanii* [24, 27] offer a unique opportunity to perform cutting-edge time-dependent proteomics analysis in this model archaeon.

Here we expand the *H. volcanii* proteomics toolkit and describe a step-by-step BONCAT protocol and downstream visualization/enrichment procedures of labeled proteins optimized for *H. volcanii* (summarized in Fig. 1c). In addition, this protocol has been validated in another model archaeon (i.e., *Sulfolobus acidocaldarius*—Ferreira-Cerca lab *unpublished*), another model bacterium (i.e., *Escherichia coli*—see below) and is likely to be suitable for various additional biological systems [4, 5, 8, 13–19].

Together with the isotope-labeling strategy mentioned above and additional multiplexing [4, 5, 8], the following BONCAT protocol allows for global inspection of protein synthesis capacity in *Haloferax volcanii* and paves the way to time-dependent proteomics analysis in this ever more versatile model archaeon [21, 22]. Moreover, these additional experimental possibilities position *H. volcanii* as a unique experimental system to explore the molecular principles of proteostasis in archaea.

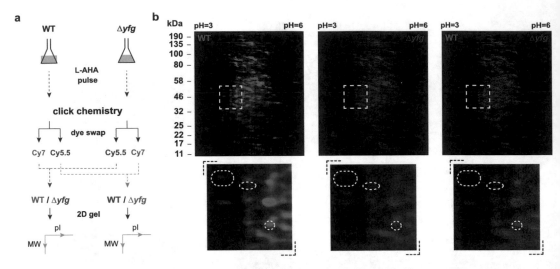

**Fig. 4** Differential 2D gel analysis of L-AHA-labeled proteins. (**a**) Differential 2D gel experimental workflow. Exponentially growing wildtype (WT) and △*yfg* (your favorite gene mutant/or perturbation) cells grown in Hv-min lacking methionine were pulse-labeled with 1 mM L-AHA for 45 min (representing approx. 20% of the *H. volcanii* doubling time in these growth conditions). Cells were lysed, protein were extracted and subjected to click chemistry with DBCO-Cy7 and DBCO-Cy5.5 as described in Subheading 3.4. Equal protein amounts of WT cells labeled with DBCO-Cy7 and △*yfg* cells labeled with DBCO-Cy5.5 and vice versa (dye swap to control fluorescence bias) were mixed cells with DBCO-Cy5.5 and vice versa to control fluorescence bias. Sample mixtures were used to rehydrate immobilized pH stripe and isoelectric focusing as describe in Subheading 3.7.2. Second dimension was resolved using 4–12% polyacrylamide gradient gel and the fluorescence signals were acquired with the Li-COR Odyssey Infrared Imager. (**b**) Exemplary results of differentially expressed proteins. Full gel scan (upper part) for the 2D gel analysis obtained for the wild-type (Cy7-red channel) and mutant *H. volcanii* cells (Cy5.5-green channel) mixture are provided. Zoom in of the 2D gel (boxing) showing representative differential expression between wildtype and exemplary mutant cell used in this study is provided in the lower part. Note that the dye-swap experiment (WT-Cy5.5/△*yfg*-Cy7) provided very similar results (data not shown). (Adapted from [33] under CC-BY License)

## 2    Materials

There are no specific preferences of sources of chemical reagents or materials, unless stated otherwise. Use ultrapure water with 18 MΩ·cm resistivity at 25 °C.

**2.1   Microbiological Cultures**

**2.1.1   Strains**

1. *Haloferax volcanii* H26 [29].
2. *Escherichia coli* K12 [30].

**2.2   Haloferax volcanii *Minimal Medium (Hv-min)***

1. 1 M Tris–HCl pH 7.0.
2. 1 M Tris–HCl pH 7.5.
3. 30% (w/v) Salt Water: 4.1 M NaCl; 147.5 mM MgCl$_2$; 142 mM MgSO$_4$; 94 mM KCl; 20 mM Tris–HCl pH 7.5.
4. *Haloferax volcanii* minimal carbon source: 10% sodium DL-lactate; 9% succinic acid; 1% glycerol; pH 7.5. Sterilize by filtration.

5. *Haloferax volcanii* minimal salts: 417 mM $NH_4Cl$; 250 mM $CaCl_2$; 152 µM $MnCl_2$; 127 µM $ZnSO_4$; 689 µM $FeSO_4$; 16.7 µM $CuSO_4$. Sterilize by filtration.

6. Hv-Trace elements solution: 1.8 mM $MnCl_2$; 1.53 mM $ZnSO_4$; 8.27 mM $FeSO_4$; 0.2 mM $CuSO_4$ (*see* **step 4** Subheading 3.1).

7. 0.5 M $KPO_4$ buffer, pH 7.0.

8. 1 mg/L thiamine solution. Sterilize by filtration.

9. 1 mg/L biotin solution. Sterilize by filtration.

10. 1,000× uracil stock solution (50 mg/mL in DMSO).

11. 200× methionine stock solution (10 mg/mL in $H_2O$).

12. Sterile filters (0.22 µm) and syringes.

**2.3 Noncanonical Amino Acid Pulse Reagents**

1. L-azidohomoalanine (L-AHA) stock solution (100 mM).

2. 200× methionine stock solution (10 mg/mL in $H_2O$).

3. *Haloferax volcanii* methionine free minimal medium (*see* **Note 1**).

**2.4 Cell Lysis**

1. Extraction Buffer (EB) + 1% SDS: 150 mM NaCl, 100 mM EDTA, 50 mM Tris–HCl pH 8.5, 1 mM $MgCl_2$, 1% SDS.

2. Extraction Buffer (EB) without detergent: 150 mM NaCl, 100 mM EDTA, 50 mM Tris–HCl pH 8.5, 1 mM $MgCl_2$.

3. Thermoblock.

4. Benchtop centrifuge.

**2.5 Protein Reduction**

1. β-mercaptoethanol.

2. Dark box.

**2.6 Acetone Precipitation of Total Proteins**

1. Precooled (−20 °C) Acetone p.a.

2. 2 mL reagent tubes.

3. Precooled benchtop centrifuge.

**2.7 Protein Alkylation**

1. Extraction Buffer (EB) + 1% SDS: 150 mM NaCl, 100 mM EDTA, 50 mM Tris–HCl pH 8.5, 1 mM $MgCl_2$, 1% SDS.

2. Extraction Buffer (EB) without detergent: 150 mM NaCl, 100 mM EDTA, 50 mM Tris–HCl pH 8.5, 1 mM $MgCl_2$.

3. 10× Alkylation buffer: 10× PBS, 2 M 2-chloroacetamide.

4. Thermoblock.

5. Benchtop centrifuge.

6. Black 1.5 mL reagent tubes.

7. Rotating wheel.

**2.8 Click-Chemistry Reagents—Strain-Promoted Alkyne–Azide Cycloaddition (SPAAC)**

1. Extraction Buffer (EB) + 1% SDS: 150 mM NaCl, 100 mM EDTA, 50 mM Tris–HCl pH 8.5, 1 mM $MgCl_2$, 1% SDS.

2. Extraction Buffer (EB) without detergent: 150 mM NaCl, 100 mM EDTA, 50 mM Tris–HCl pH 8.5, 1 mM $MgCl_2$.

3. Stock solution (100 µM) DBCO-reagents for strain-promoted alkyne–azide cycloaddition (e.g., DBCO-Cy5, DBCO-Cy7, DBCO-PEG4-Biotin) (*see* **Note 2**).

4. L-Azidohomoalanine (L-AHA) stock solution (100 mM).

**2.9 Methanol–Chloroform Extraction of Proteins**

1. Methanol p.a.

2. Chloroform p.a.

3. Benchtop cooled centrifuge.

**2.10 Affinity Purification**

1. AP buffer: 300 mM NaCl, 10 mM $MgCl_2$, 50 mM Tris–HCl pH 8.4.

2. AP buffer + 2% SDS: 300 mM NaCl, 10 mM $MgCl_2$, 50 mM Tris–HCl pH 8.4, 2% SDS.

3. AP buffer + 1% SDS: 300 mM NaCl, 10 mM $MgCl_2$, 50 mM Tris–HCl pH 8.4, 1% SDS.

4. HiAP buffer + 1% SDS: 1 M NaCl, 10 mM $MgCl_2$, 50 mM Tris–HCl pH 8.4, 1% SDS.

5. HiAP buffer + 0.1% SDS: 1 M NaCl, 10 mM $MgCl_2$, 50 mM Tris–HCl pH 8.4, 0.1% SDS.

6. BSA Fraction V.

7. Streptavidin-bound agarose beads.

8. Gravity flow chromatography column.

9. DBCO-PEG4-Biotin.

10. 2× HU-buffer: 100 mM Tris–HCl pH 6.8, 0.5 mM EDTA pH 8, 4 M urea, 0.75% β-mercaptoethanol, 2.5% SDS, bromophenol blue.

11. 1 M DTT.

12. 2× HU-buffer + DTT: 100 mM Tris–HCl pH 6.8, 0.5 mM EDTA pH 8, 4 M Urea, 200 mM DTT, 2.5% SDS.

13. 0.1 mM $NH_4OAc$, 0.1 mM $MgCl_2$.

14. Competitive elution buffer: 1 mM biotin, 1% $NH_4OH$.

**2.11 1D/2D Gel Electrophoresis and Detection**

1. 2× HU buffer (*see* **item 10** Subheading 2.10).

2. Immobilized pH strip and 2D gel reagents (*see* **Note 3**).

3. Low-melting agarose.

4. Gel fixation solution: 40% methanol, 10% acetic acid.

5. Blocking buffer + 10% SDS: 1× PBS, 1 mM EDTA pH 8, 10% SDS.

6. Blocking buffer + 1% SDS: 1× PBS, 1 mM EDTA pH 8, 1% SDS.

7. Blocking buffer + 0.1% SDS: 1× PBS, 1 mM EDTA pH 8, 0.1% SDS.

8. IRDye-coupled streptavidin (1 mg/mL).

---

# 3 Methods (Workflow Is Summarized in Fig. 1c)

Use ultra-pure water with 18 MΩ·cm resistivity at 25 °C.

## 3.1 Microbiological Methods

All solutions/media should be autoclaved, unless stated otherwise.

### 3.1.1 Haloferax volcanii Media and Cultivation

1. Prepare 30% (w/v) salt water by dissolving in 4 L of Millipore water 1,200 g NaCl; 150 g MgCl$_2$·6H$_2$O; 175 g MgSO$_4$·7H$_2$O; 35 g KCl; 100 mL 1 M Tris–HCl pH 7.5. Fill up with H$_2$O to 5 L. Autoclave and store at room temperature.

2. Prepare Hv-Min Carbon Source by dissolving in 150 mL H$_2$O: 41.7 mL 60% Sodium DL-lactate, 37.5 g Succinic acid Na$_2$ salt·6H$_2$O; 3.15 mL 80% Glycerol. Carefully adjust to pH 7.5 with first 5 M NaOH and then 1 M NaOH. Fill up with H$_2$O to a final volume of 250 mL and sterilized by filtration. Aliquot in 50 mL and store at 4 °C.

3. Prepare Tris–HCl pH 7.0.

4. Prepare Hv-Trace elements solution by adding to 100 mL water a few drops of 37% concentrated HCl. Dissolve the following salts one by one in the following order: 36 mg MnCl$_2$·4H$_2$O; 44 mg ZnSO$_4$·7H$_2$O; 230 mg FeSO$_4$·7H$_2$O; 5 mg CuSO$_4$·5H$_2$O. Sterilize by filtration and store at 4 °C.

5. Prepare Hv-minimal salts by mixing 30 mL 1 M NH$_4$Cl; 36 mL 0.5 M CaCl$_2$ and 6 mL Hv-Trace elements solution (*see* **step 4**). Sterilize by filtration and store at 4 °C.

6. Prepare 0.5 M KPO$_4$ buffer (pH 7.0). Mix 61.5 mL 1 M K$_2$HPO$_4$ and 38.5 mL 1 M KH$_2$PO$_4$. Check pH and adjust to pH 7.0, if required. Add an equal volume of H$_2$O (100 mL). Autoclave and store at room temperature.

7. Prepare Thiamine/Biotin mix by combining 9.5 mL Thiamine (1 mg/mL) and 1.2 mL Biotin (1 mg/mL).

8. Prepare Hv-minimal medium (Hv-min). For 1 L medium mix: 600 mL 30% salt water, 330 mL H$_2$O and 30 mL Tris–HCl pH 7.0. Autoclave. When cooled down add 25.5 mL Hv-Min Carbon Source (*see* **step 2**), 12 mL Hv-Min Salts (*see* **step 5**), 1.95 mL 0.5 M KPO$_4$ buffer pH 7.0 (*see* **step 6**), 900 μL Thiamine/Biotin mix (*see* **step 7**), 1 mL 1,000× Uracil stock solution (*see* **item 10** Subheading 2.2). Store at room temperature in a dark cupboard.

9. Scratch the surface of an *Haloferax volcanii* glycerol cryo-stock with a sterile inoculation loop and inoculate 5 to 10 mL medium as a start culture. Incubate at 42 °C under agitation. Dilute with prewarmed medium or let grow until the culture has reached the desired cell density/volume ($OD_{600nm} = 0.6$).

**3.2 In Vivo Pulse Labeling with L-AHA**

1. Prepare a fresh stock solution of L-AHA (*see* **item 1** Subheading 2.3).

2. Pulse label 5 mL of cells at $OD_{600nm} = 0.6$ with 0.1–1 mM L-AHA (or methionine as negative control) at the desired temperature and time (*see* **Note 4**).

3. Fractionate cells in two 2 mL aliquots and centrifuge for 3 min at 6,000 × *g*.

4. Discard supernatant.

5. Snap-freeze cell pellet in liquid nitrogen.

**3.3 Protein Extraction**

1. Resuspend cell pellet in 500 µL Extraction Buffer (EB) supplemented with 1% SDS (*see* **item 1** Subheading 2.4 and **Note 5**).

2. Boil the samples for 13 min at 95 °C.

3. Cool for 5 min at RT.

4. Centrifuge at 16,000 × *g* for 5–10 min RT.

5. Transfer supernatant into a fresh cup.

6. Optional: Freeze supernatant at −20 °C or proceed with click chemistry (*see* Subheading 3.4).

**3.4 Click-Chemistry**

*3.4.1 Reduction*

1. Add 10 µL of β-Mercaptoethanol (final concentration 2%).

2. Incubate the lysate for 1 h in the dark (RT).

*3.4.2 Acetone Precipitation*

1. Afterward, split the 500 µL of cell lysate into two cups.

2. Add 4 Volume (1 mL) of acetone precooled at −20 °C (acetone end concentration = 80%).

3. Vortex and let proteins precipitate for 1 h at −20 °C.

4. Centrifuge for 10 min at 16,000 × *g* at 4 °C.

5. Discard the supernatant without disturbing the protein pellet.

6. Wash the pellet with 1 mL of acetone precooled at −20 °C.

7. Centrifuge for 10 min at 16,000 × *g* at 4 °C.

8. Discard the supernatant and air-dry the protein pellet (*see* **Note 6**).

*3.4.3 Alkylation*

1. Resuspend pellet in 25 µL of EB + 1% SDS (*see* **item 1** Subheading 2.7).

2. Add 225 µL EB without detergent (*see* **item 2** Subheading 2.7).

3. Vortex and denature proteins for 5 min at 95 °C.

4. Let cool down at RT.

5. Merge the corresponding supernatant together in a fresh cup.

6. Measure protein concentration with a NanoDrop or equivalent (vortex samples before measuring).

7. Prepare 200 µL of extracted protein at a protein concentration 1–2 µg/µL.

8. **Optional**: use black tubes to keep the samples in the dark.

9. Depending on protein concentration and the L-AHA pulse, aim for 200–400 µg of proteins.

10. Equalize the volumes of added protein with EB without detergent (*see* **item 2** Subheading 2.7).

11. Add 20 µL of freshly prepared 10× concentrated alkylation solution (10× PBS, 2 M 2-chloroacetamide) (*see* **item 3** Subheading 2.7 and **Note 7**).

12. Incubate for 1 h on a rotating wheel in the dark.

13. Afterward, precipitate the proteins via acetone precipitation as described above (*see* Subheading 3.4.2).

*3.4.4   Click-Chemistry: Strain Promoted Alkyne– Azide Cycloaddition (SPAAC)*

1. Resuspend the pellet in 20 µL of EB containing 1% SDS (**item 1** Subheading 2.8).

2. Add 180 µL of EB without detergent (**item 2** Subheading 2.8).

3. Denature samples for 5 min at 95 °C.

4. Let cool down to room temperature.

5. Add 2 µL of 100 µM solution DBCO reagent (1 µM final concentration) to allow for strain-promoted cycloaddition to the L-AHA azide group (e.g., DBCO-Cy5, DBCO-Cy7, DBCO-PEG4-Biotin) (*see* **Note 8**).

6. Incubate on a rotating wheel for 30 min at room temperature in the dark.

7. Eliminate unreacted DBCO reagent by adding excess of L-AHA to 0.1–1 mM.

*3.5   Methanol– Chloroform Extraction*

1. Add 480 µL methanol, 160 µL chloroform to the sample (~200 µL).

2. Vortex vigorously and add 640 µL $H_2O$.

3. Vortex and centrifuge for 5 min at 16,000 × $g$ RT.

4. Suck off and discard the aqueous phase (upper phase).

5. Add 300 µL methanol.

6. Vortex and centrifuge for 30 min at 16,000 × $g$ 4 °C.

7. Discard supernatant and shortly air-dry the protein pellet.

8. Proceed with the desired step.

**3.6  Affinity Purification of Biotinylated Protein**

*3.6.1  Sample Preparation*

1. Performed PEG4-Biotin cycloaddition of 400 µg protein as described in Subheading 3.4.4.

2. After the final methanol–chloroform extraction (*see* Subheading 3.5) resuspend protein pellet in 100 µL of AP buffer + 2% SDS (*see* **item 2** Subheading 2.10).

3. Denature for 5 min at 95 °C.

4. Add 900 µL AP buffer without SDS (*see* **item 1** Subheading 2.10).

5. Take and store an aliquot as Input (5% of total volume).

*3.6.2  Streptavidin Beads Preparation*

1. For each purification prepare 100 µL of slurry streptavidin-bound agarose beads. Centrifuge for 1 min at 100 × *g* to discard the supernatant.

2. Wash the beads twice with 1 mL AP buffer + 1% SDS (*see* **item 3** Subheading 2.10) for 5 min on a rotating wheel. Centrifuge for 1 min at 100 × *g* to discard the supernatant.

3. Block the beads twice with 500 µL AP buffer + 1% SDS (*see* **item 3** Subheading 2.10) and 1 mg/mL BSA for 5 min on a rotating wheel. Centrifuge for 1 min at 100 × *g* to discard the supernatant.

4. Wash the beads with 1 mL AP buffer + 1% SDS (*see* **item 3** Subheading 2.10) for 5 min on a rotating wheel. Centrifuge for 1 min at 100 × *g* to discard the supernatant.

*3.6.3  Affinity Purification*

1. Mix the sample (*see* **step 4** Subheading 3.6.1) with the prepared streptavidin beads (*see* Subheading 3.6.2).

2. Incubate for 30 min on a rotating wheel at room temperature.

3. Transfer the material onto a gravity flow column. Collect and store the flow-through (= unbound fraction) (5% of total volume).

4. Wash the beads 3 times with 2 mL HiAP buffer + 1% SDS (*see* **item 4** Subheading 2.10). Collect all the wash in a single 15 mL tube and store 10% of the resulting pooled wash fractions.

5. Wash the beads twice 1 mL AP buffer + 0.1% SDS (*see* **item 5** Subheading 2.10).

6. Beads were collected with 1 mL AP buffer + 0.1% SDS (*see* **item 5** Subheading 2.10) and transfer to a fresh cup.

7. Centrifuge for 1 min at 100 × *g* and discard as much of the supernatant as possible.

**3.6.4   Elution (See Note 9) (an Exemplary Result Is Provided in Fig. 3)**

1. Add 50–100 μL 2× HU buffer + DTT (*see* **item 12** Subheading 2.10) to the beads.

2. Incubate for 10 min at 95 °C.

3. Collect supernatant.

**Fast-Elution for Gel Electrophoresis**

**Competitive Elution for Downstream Processing**

1. Wash twice the beads with 0.1 M $NH_4OAc$, 0.1 mM $MgCl_2$ solution.

2. Centrifuge for 1 min at $100 \times g$ and discard as much of the supernatant as possible.

3. Elute bound material twice with 500 μL Competitive elution buffer (*see* **item 14** Subheading 2.10) for 10 min at 95 °C.

4. Collect and pool the supernatants.

5. Split the collected supernatant into 2 unequal fractions (80–90%) and (10–20%).

6. Fill up the splitter eluate with competitive elution buffer.

7. Lyophilized overnight using a speed-vac.

8. Resuspend the 10–20% eluate fraction in 40 μL 2× HU buffer + DTT (*see* **item 12** Subheading 2.10). Denature sample and check pull-down efficiency (*see* Subheading 3.9).

9. If desired, proceed with the 80–90% eluate fraction with desired downstream analysis.

**3.7   Gel Electrophoresis and Detection**

1. Resuspend pellet in 2× HU buffer + DTT (*see* **item 12** Subheading 2.10).

2. Denature samples for 5 min at 60 °C.

**3.7.1   SDS-PAGE**

3. Vortex firmly before loading 15–25 μL on an SDS-polyacrylamide gradient gel.

4. Separate samples for around 1 h at constant 170–190 V.

**3.7.2   2D Gel Electrophoresis (an Exemplary Result Is Provided in Fig. 4)**

1. Sample (*see* Subheading 3.5) are solubilized in sample buffer containing 7 M urea, 2 M thiourea, 4% CHAPS, 40 mM DTT, and 0.4% ampholytes (pH 3–10) as suggested by the manufacturer.

**Isoelectric Focusing (*See* Note 2)**

2. Isoelectric focusing is performed overnight using an immobilized pH gradient strip (pH 3–6) using the run parameters described below (Table 1).

**Second Dimension SDS-PAGE**

1. Immobilized pH gradient strip is incubated in equilibration solution 1 (6 M urea, 30% glycerol, 2% SDS, and 0.05 M Tris–HCl pH 8.5) for 10 min.

2. The strip is incubated for 10 min in equilibration solution base mix.

**Table 1**
**Parameters for isoelectric focusing**

| Voltage | Ramp | Time |
|---------|------|------|
| 250 V | Hold | 15 min |
| 4,000 V | Gradient | 1 h |
| 4,000 V | Hold | 20,000 VHr |
| 500 V | Hold | ∞ |

3. The strip is shortly immersed in SDS-PAGE running buffer.

4. Load the strip on a 4–12% polyacrylamide gradient gel (keep the strip in place by adding 40 °C warm low-melting agarose).

5. The gel was run for 15 min at 80 V followed by 1 h at 160 V.

6. Proceed with gel fixation (*see* Subheading 3.8).

***3.8 In-Gel Detection (Exemplary Results Are Provided in Figs. 2 and 4)***

1. Incubate the gel in gel fixation solution (*see* **item 4** Subheading 2.11) for at least 20 min under agitation.

2. Wash the gel 3 times with $H_2O$ for 5 min under agitation.

3. Scan the gel using a compatible fluorescence imager.

***3.9 Detection of Affinity Purified L-AHA-Labeled Proteins***

(an exemplary result is provided in Fig. 3).

1. Proceed with gel electrophoresis as described in Subheading 3.7.1.

2. Transfer and immobilized proteins on Nylon-Immobilon membrane using your favorite transfer protocol.

3. Incubate the membrane for 20 min in blocking buffer + 10% SDS (*see* **item 5** Subheading 2.11) under agitation.

4. Incubate with 0.1 μg/mL IRDye-conjugated Streptavidin in blocking buffer + 10% SDS for 20 min under agitation (*see* **Note 10**).

5. Wash twice the membrane with blocking buffer + 10% SDS (*see* **item 5** Subheading 2.11) for 20 min under agitation.

6. Wash twice the membrane with blocking buffer + 1% SDS (*see* **item 6** Subheading 2.11) for 20 min under agitation.

7. Wash twice the membrane with blocking buffer + 0.1% SDS (*see* **item 7** Subheading 2.11) for 20 min under agitation.

8. Use compatible imaging system to record fluorescent (chemiluminescent) signals (*see* **Note 10**).

## 4   Notes

1. Culture in methionine-free medium is critical for the efficiency of L-AHA labeling.

2. There is a multitude of DBCO reagents available which offer various advantages for downstream analysis. The DBCO reagents should be wisely selected depending on the experimental goals.

3. Use commercial immobilized strips and follow the protocol recommended by the manufacturer.

4. Depending of the doubling time of your experimental system and the time of labeling use concentration of 0.1–1 mM L-AHA. At this point $^{15}NH_4$-salt or SILAC based labeling (*see* [24, 27], respectively, for procedure suitable for *H. volcanii*) can be simultaneously performed to improve confidence of downstream identification of neosynthesized proteins by mass spectrometry.

5. No reducing agent, such as dithiothreitol (DTT) or β-mercaptoethanol, should be added to avoid reduction of the L-AHA azide group.

6. Do not overdry pellets, otherwise the proteins will be difficult to solubilize.

7. Various amounts of 2-chloroacetamide powder can be fractionated into 1.5 mL black cups and stored at RT. Prior to use add the necessary volume of 10× PBS to such aliquot and mix well (make sure the reagent is completely dissolved). Use only freshly solubilized 2-chloroacetamide.

8. The end concentration of DBCO derivate may be optimized empirically. For *H. volcanii* we typically used 1 mM DBCO reagents as it provided the best signal–noise ratio in our hands.

9. Streptavidin–biotin complexes are extremely stable. The elution procedure should be selected according to the downstream analytical procedure. The experimenter should be aware about the pros and contras of the different elution procedures. The following procedures are exemplary elution procedures that were qualitatively well performing in our hands. Alternatively, on beads protease digest can be directly performed and further processed for mass spectrometry. However, note that in this condition biotinylated-AHA peptides will remain attached to the affinity purification matrix. Therefore additional labeling, using SILAC or $^{15}N$, is essential to distinguish neosynthesized proteins from background (e.g., [4, 5, 8]).

10. As alternative HRP-conjugated streptavidin can be used and detected by chemiluminescence. Please refer to manufacturer manual for experimental conditions.

## Acknowledgments

We are indebted of the scientists who have pioneered click chemistry, BONCAT, and other methodological aspects which have strongly inspired the establishment of this protocol. We are grateful to Prof. Dr. Karl-Dieter Entian (University of Frankfurt) for comments and suggestions. We would like to thank Dr. Robert Knüppel, Michael Jüttner and our colleagues from the chair of Biochemistry III and Biochemistry I for sharing protocols, materials, equipment, and discussion. Dr. Astrid Bruckmann (University of Regensburg) for assistance with 2D SDS-PAGE. Thanks to Prof. Dr. Sonja-Albers (University of Freiburg), Prof. Dr. Thorsten Allers (University of Nottingham), and Prof. Dr. Anita Marchfelder (University of Ulm) for kindly sharing strains and protocols. Work in the Ferreira-Cerca laboratory is supported by the chair of Biochemistry III "House of the Ribosome" – University of Regensburg, by the DFG-funded collaborative research center CRC/SFB960 "RNP biogenesis: assembly of ribosomes and nonribosomal RNPs and control of their function" (project AP1/B13) and by an individual DFG grant to S.F.-C. (FE1622/2-1; Project Nr. 409198929).

## References

1. Dermit M, Dodel M, Mardakheh FK (2017) Methods for monitoring and measurement of protein translation in time and space. Mol BioSyst 13:2477–2488. https://doi.org/10.1039/c7mb00476a

2. Ingolia NT, Hussmann JA, Weissman JS (2019) Ribosome profiling: global views of translation. Cold Spring Harb Perspect Biol 11:a032698. https://doi.org/10.1101/cshperspect.a032698

3. Zhao J, Qin B, Nikolay R et al (2019) Translatomics: the global view of translation. Int J Mol Sci 20:212. https://doi.org/10.3390/ijms20010212

4. Bagert JD, Xie YJ, Sweredoski MJ et al (2014) Quantitative, time-resolved proteomic analysis by combining bioorthogonal noncanonical amino acid tagging and pulsed stable isotope labeling by amino acids in cell culture. Mol Cell Proteomics 13:1352–1358. https://doi.org/10.1074/mcp.M113.031914

5. Bagert JD, van Kessel JC, Sweredoski MJ et al (2016) Time-resolved proteomic analysis of quorum sensing in Vibrio harveyi †electronic supplementary information (ESI) available: figures and tables. See DOI: 10.1039/c5sc03340c click here for additional data file. Chem Sci 7:1797–1806. https://doi.org/10.1039/c5sc03340c

6. Cox J, Mann M (2011) Quantitative, high-resolution proteomics for data-driven systems biology. Annu Rev Biochem 80:273–299. https://doi.org/10.1146/annurev-biochem-061308-093216

7. Gygi SP, Rist B, Aebersold R (2000) Measuring gene expression by quantitative p roteome analysis. Curr Opin Biotechnol 11:396–401. https://doi.org/10.1016/S0958-1669(00)00116-6

8. Rothenberg DA, Taliaferro JM, Huber SM et al (2018) A proteomics approach to profiling the temporal translational response to stress and growth. iScience 9:367–381. https://doi.org/10.1016/j.isci.2018.11.004

9. Chen X, Wei S, Ji Y et al (2015) Quantitative proteomics using SILAC: principles, applications, and developments. Proteomics 15:3175–3192. https://doi.org/10.1002/pmic.201500108

10. Ong S-E, Blagoev B, Kratchmarova I et al (2002) Stable isotope labeling by amino acids in cell culture, SILAC, as a simple and accurate

approach to expression proteomics. Mol Cell Proteomics 1:376. https://doi.org/10.1074/mcp.M200025-MCP200

11. Ong S-E, Mann M (2006) A practical recipe for stable isotope labeling by amino acids in cell culture (SILAC). Nat Protoc 1:2650–2660. https://doi.org/10.1038/nprot.2006.427

12. Dieterich DC, Link AJ, Graumann J et al (2006) Selective identification of newly synthesized proteins in mammalian cells using bioorthogonal noncanonical amino acid tagging (BONCAT). Proc Natl Acad Sci U S A 103:9482–9487. https://doi.org/10.1073/pnas.0601637103

13. Landgraf P, Antileo ER, Schuman EM, Dieterich DC (2015) BONCAT: metabolic labeling, click chemistry, and affinity purification of newly synthesized proteomes. In: Gautier A, Hinner MJ (eds) Site-specific protein labeling: methods and protocols. Springer, New York, New York, NY, pp 199–215

14. Glenn WS, Stone SE, Ho SH et al (2017) Bioorthogonal noncanonical amino acid tagging (BONCAT) enables time-resolved analysis of protein synthesis in native plant tissue. Plant Physiol 173:1543–1553. https://doi.org/10.1104/pp.16.01762

15. Hatzenpichler R, Scheller S, Tavormina PL et al (2014) In situ visualization of newly synthesized proteins in environmental microbes using amino acid tagging and click chemistry. Environ Microbiol 16:2568–2590. https://doi.org/10.1111/1462-2920.12436

16. Hatzenpichler R, Connon SA, Goudeau D et al (2016) Visualizing in situ translational activity for identifying and sorting slow-growing archaeal–bacterial consortia. Proc Natl Acad Sci U S A 113:E4069–E4078. https://doi.org/10.1073/pnas.1603757113

17. Saleh AM, Wilding KM, Calve S et al (2019) Non-canonical amino acid labeling in proteomics and biotechnology. J Biol Eng 13:43–43. https://doi.org/10.1186/s13036-019-0166-3

18. Shin J, Rhim J, Kwon Y et al (2019) Comparative analysis of differentially secreted proteins in serum-free and serum-containing media by using BONCAT and pulsed SILAC. Sci Rep 9:3096–3096. https://doi.org/10.1038/s41598-019-39650-z

19. Kiick KL, Saxon E, Tirrell DA, Bertozzi CR (2002) Incorporation of azides into recombinant proteins for chemoselective modification by the Staudinger ligation. Proc Natl Acad Sci U S A 99:19–24. https://doi.org/10.1073/pnas.012583299

20. Agard NJ, Baskin JM, Prescher JA et al (2006) A comparative study of bioorthogonal reactions with Azides. ACS Chem Biol 1:644–648. https://doi.org/10.1021/cb6003228

21. Leigh JA, Albers S-V, Atomi H, Allers T (2011) Model organisms for genetics in the domain archaea: methanogens, halophiles, Thermococcales and Sulfolobales. FEMS Microbiol Rev 35:577–608. https://doi.org/10.1111/j.1574-6976.2011.00265.x

22. Pohlschroder M, Schulze S (2019) Haloferax volcanii. Trends Microbiol 27:86–87. https://doi.org/10.1016/j.tim.2018.10.004

23. Cerletti M, Paggi RA, Guevara CR et al (2015) Global role of the membrane protease LonB in archaea: potential protease targets revealed by quantitative proteome analysis of a lonB mutant in Haloferax volcanii. J Proteome 121:1–14. https://doi.org/10.1016/j.jprot.2015.03.016

24. Cerletti M, Paggi R, Troetschel C et al (2018) LonB protease is a novel regulator of Carotenogenesis controlling degradation of phytoene synthase in Haloferax volcanii. J Proteome Res 17:1158–1171. https://doi.org/10.1021/acs.jproteome.7b00809

25. Costa MI, Cerletti M, Paggi RA et al (2018) Haloferax volcanii proteome response to deletion of a rhomboid protease gene. J Proteome Res 17:961–977. https://doi.org/10.1021/acs.jproteome.7b00530

26. Kirkland PA, Humbard MA, Daniels CJ, Maupin-Furlow JA (2008) Shotgun proteomics of the haloarchaeon Haloferax volcanii. J Proteome Res 7:5033–5039. https://doi.org/10.1021/pr800517a

27. McMillan LJ, Hwang S, Farah RE et al (2018) Multiplex quantitative SILAC for analysis of archaeal proteomes: a case study of oxidative stress responses. Environ Microbiol 20:385–401. https://doi.org/10.1111/1462-2920.14014

28. Schulze S, Adams Z, Cerletti M et al (2020) The archaeal proteome project advances knowledge about archaeal cell biology through comprehensive proteomics. Nat Commun 11:3145–3145. https://doi.org/10.1038/s41467-020-16784-7

29. Allers T, Ngo H-P, Mevarech M, Lloyd RG (2004) Development of additional selectable markers for the halophilic archaeon Haloferax volcanii based on the leuB and trpA genes.

Appl Environ Microbiol 70:943–953. https://doi.org/10.1128/AEM.70.2.943-953.2004

30. Blattner FR, Plunkett G, Bloch CA et al (1997) The complete genome sequence of *Escherichia coli* K-12. Science 277:1453. https://doi.org/10.1126/science.277.5331.1453

31. Hummel H, Böck A (1987) Thiostrepton resistance mutations in the gene for 23S ribosomal RNA of Halobacteria. Biochimie 69:857–861.

https://doi.org/10.1016/0300-9084(87)90212-4

32. Schindelin J, Arganda-Carreras I, Frise E et al (2012) Fiji: an open-source platform for biological-image analysis. Nat Methods 9:676

33. Knüppel R, Trahan C, Kern M et al (2021) Insights into synthesis and function of KsgA/Dim1-dependent rRNA modifications in archaea. Nucleic Acids Res 49(3):1662–1687. https://doi.org/10.1093/nar/gkaa1268

# Chapter 15

# Thermofluor-Based Analysis of Protein Integrity and Ligand Interactions

## Sophia Pinz, Eva Doskocil, and Wolfgang Seufert

## Abstract

Thermofluor is a fluorescence-based thermal shift assay, which measures temperature-induced protein unfolding and thereby yields valuable information about the integrity of a purified recombinant protein. Analysis of ligand binding to a protein is another popular application of this assay. Thermofluor requires neither protein labeling nor highly specialized equipment, and can be performed in a regular real-time PCR instrument. Thus, for a typical molecular biology laboratory, Thermofluor is a convenient method for the routine assessment of protein quality. Here, we provide Thermofluor protocols using the example of Cdc123. This ATP-grasp protein is an essential assembly chaperone of the eukaryotic translation initiation factor eIF2. We also report on a destabilized mutant protein version and on the ATP-mediated thermal stabilization of wild-type Cdc123 illustrating protein integrity assessment and ligand binding analysis as two major applications of the Thermofluor assay.

**Key words** Thermofluor, Thermal shift assay, Differential scanning fluorimetry, SYPRO Orange, Protein stability, Ligand binding, ATP, Cdc123, eIF2

## 1 Introduction

Recombinant proteins are widely used for biochemical analyses, and frequently the question comes up whether the purified or stored protein is still stable. Methods suitable to give an answer, such as CD spectroscopy or differential scanning calorimetry, typically require large protein amounts and expensive specialized instruments, which are not available in many laboratories. In contrast, Thermofluor is a low-cost and straightforward technique well suited as a routine protein quality control in most molecular biology laboratories. Such quality control is a must for batch-to-batch comparisons and to improve experimental reproducibility.

Thermofluor, a thermal shift assay also known as differential scanning fluorimetry (DSF), has become a versatile technique for the measurement of protein stability. Thermofluor makes use of an environmentally sensitive fluorescent dye, mostly SYPRO Orange

Karl-Dieter Entian (ed.), *Ribosome Biogenesis: Methods and Protocols*, Methods in Molecular Biology, vol. 2533, https://doi.org/10.1007/978-1-0716-2501-9_15, © The Author(s) 2022

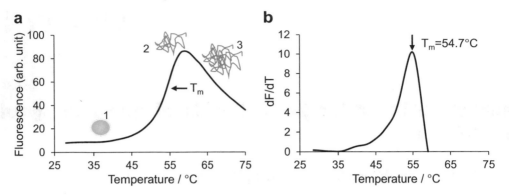

**Fig. 1** A typical Thermofluor profile. Data shown were obtained with SpCdc123-his6 in the presence of 5× SYPRO Orange. (**a**) At low temperatures the protein is well-folded (gray sphere). The fluorescent dye SYPRO Orange is quenched in the aqueous environment. Thus, only basal SYPRO Orange fluorescence emission is measured at 555 nm upon excitation at 470 nm (1). As the protein gradually unfolds (gray ravel), SYPRO Orange binds to exposed hydrophobic regions. This leads to a strong increase in fluorescence emission (2). The protein's melting temperature ($T_m$, arrow) is given by the inflection point where 50% of the protein is unfolded. Following the peak of fluorescence intensity (protein is completely unfolded), a decrease of intensity is observed (3). This is probably due to protein aggregation, which removes protein from the solution and prevents SYPRO Orange from interacting with hydrophobic patches. (**b**) First derivative of the fluorescence as a function of temperature. The protein's melting temperature ($T_m$, arrow) is easily identified as the peak of the curve (*see* **Note 13**)

[1, 2], to monitor the thermal unfolding of proteins. The dye is quenched in an aqueous environment, but undergoes a pronounced increase in fluorescent quantum yield upon binding to exposed hydrophobic regions of the protein as the protein unfolds (Fig. 1). The gradual increase of temperature as well as the concomitant detection of the fluorescent signal can be performed by standard real-time PCR instruments. Data fitting using the real-time PCR instrument's accompanying software quickly provides the melting temperature ($T_m$) of the protein under various conditions. The $T_m$ serves as a measure of protein stability [1, 3] and the shape of the curve as an indicator for protein integrity ( [2, 4] and Fig. 2).

Upon its first description in 2001 for high throughput drug discovery [5], dyes such as 1-anilino-8-naphthalenesulfonate (ANS) or dapoxyl sulfonic acid were used, but eventually the dye with the most favorable characteristics for Thermofluor turned out to be SYPRO Orange [1, 6]. It has a high increase in quantum yield, and its excitation and emission maxima of ~500 nm and ~600 nm, respectively [1, 6], are compatible with standard filter sets of most real-time PCR instruments [2].

The simplicity and economical protein requirement make Thermofluor very attractive for the routine quality control of purified recombinant proteins. Thermofluor allows to easily evaluate any adverse effects on the protein of choice that might occur during

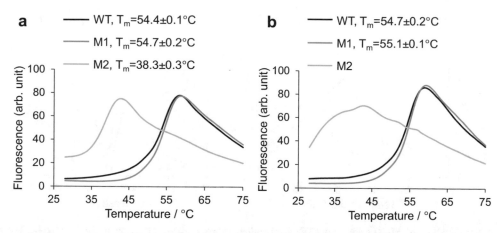

**Fig. 2** Thermal destabilization of a mutant protein. Thermofluor was performed using 5x SYPRO Orange and 2 μg (2 μM) SpCdc123-his6 wild-type (WT, black line) or two SpCdc123-his6 mutants: mutant 1 (M1, dark gray line) and mutant 2 (M2, light gray line). In the thermal denaturation profiles shown, fluorescence emission is plotted versus temperature to monitor protein unfolding. (**a**) Proteins in imidazole-containing buffer (50 mM Tris–HCl pH 8.0, 500 mM NaCl, approximately 160 mM imidazole) before dialysis. (**b**) Proteins in imidazole-free buffer (50 mM Tris–HCl pH 7.5, 500 mM NaCl) after dialysis (*see* **Note 3**). Shown is one representative curve per condition. The $T_m$ (calculated from duplicate reactions) was derived as the peak of the first derivative of the fluorescence as a function of temperature, calculated by the melting curve analysis of the Rotor-Gene Q Software 2.3.4. Mutant 1 is similarly stable as wild-type SpCdc123-his6. Both proteins are essentially unaffected by imidazole. Mutant 2 is less stable than wild-type SpCdc123-his6. In imidazole-free buffer, it does no longer show a defined unfolding transition. Together the data indicate that amino acid replacements can affect protein stability and sensitize a protein toward buffer composition

affinity purification, protein concentration, buffer exchange (Fig. 2), freezing or prolonged storage. In particular for mutant proteins, Thermofluor quickly shows whether or not amino acid exchanges do influence protein stability (Fig. 2). Thermofluor analysis therefore provides valuable data for the interpretation of downstream assays.

Ligand interaction usually stabilizes the native protein [1, 7, 8], thus leading to an increase in melting temperature. This can be employed, on the one hand, for ligand screenings in drug design [5, 8–10], and on the other hand, to characterize the binding of natural ligands, such as nucleotides, to proteins [11, 12] (Fig. 3). Even an approximation of $K_d$ values is possible [9, 13–15], which provides useful preinformation for biophysical methods like isothermal titration calorimetry (ITC) that consume larger quantities of protein. Thermodynamic parameters obtained from Thermofluor assays correlate well with those determined by other biophysical methods [4, 9, 16, 17]. Not only ligands but also solvents and additives affect the stability and thus the $T_m$ of proteins. Accordingly, Thermofluor is a popular method for the determination of optimal buffer conditions for protein purification, storage and structural studies such as crystallization or NMR [2, 3, 16, 18–20].

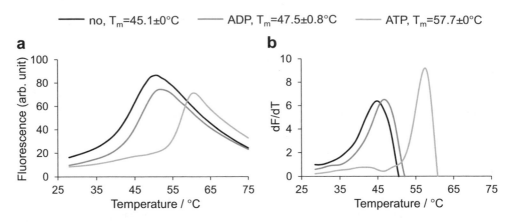

**Fig. 3** Stabilization of hD123 through ATP. Thermofluor was performed using 2 μg hD123(1–290)-his6 (2.3 μM) and 5× SYPRO Orange without nucleotide (no, black line), or with 1 mM ADP (ADP, dark gray line) or 1 mM ATP (ATP, light gray line). One representative curve is shown. (**a**) In the thermal denaturation profiles shown, fluorescence emission is plotted *versus* temperature to monitor the unfolding of hD123 (1-290)-his6. (**b**) The first derivative of the fluorescence as a function of temperature was exported from the Rotor-Gene Q Software 2.3.4 and plotted using Microsoft Excel. The $T_m$ is represented as the peak of the curve. The $T_m$ values shown in the legend were calculated as an average of duplicates from three independent experiments. The data indicate that ATP-binding stabilizes hD123 by more than 10 degrees

Recombinant proteins are critical tools in biochemical studies such as the analysis of ribosome biogenesis and mRNA translation. Recently it has become clear that the well-studied eukaryotic translation initiation factor 2 (eIF2) requires a dedicated assembly factor [21]. This protein called Cdc123 is conserved among eukaryotic organisms and indispensable for the viability of yeast and human cells [21–24]. Protein structure analysis revealed that Cdc123 is related to ATP-grasp enzymes [25]. Here we use Cdc123 as an example to present Thermofluor protocols for the analysis of protein stability and nucleotide binding. We show data illustrating a mutant protein that became unstable after removal of imidazole by dialysis, while generating a proper unfolding curve before dialysis (Fig. 2). Furthermore, as an example of a nucleotide-binding assay, we show that Cdc123 is stabilized strongly by ATP, and to some extent also by ADP (Fig. 3). While several of the technical aspects discussed here are specific to the real-time PCR machine Rotor-Gene Q 2plex Platform (Qiagen), the method can be applied to any standard real-time PCR instrument [2, 3, 9, 10, 13, 15] typically available in molecular biology laboratories.

## 2    Materials

1. SYPRO Orange Protein Gel Stain, 5000× concentrate in DMSO (e.g., Thermo Scientific) (*see* **Note 1**), diluted 1:5 in DMSO to yield a 1000× working dilution in DMSO (*see* **Note 2**). The 1000× SYPRO Orange stock is stored at 4 °C.

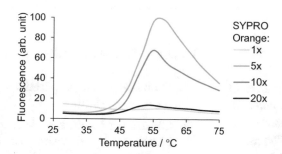

**Fig. 4** Fluorescence dye optimization. Melting curves are shown using different SYPRO Orange concentrations as described in Subheading 3.1. Thermofluor was performed using 2 μg his6-SpCdc123 (2 μM) together with 1× (light gray line), 5× (gray line), 10× (dark gray line), or 20× (black line) SYPRO Orange. The gain was set to 9.33. In the thermal denaturation profiles shown, fluorescence intensity is plotted versus temperature to monitor the unfolding of his6-SpCdc123. The melting curve with the best dynamic rage was obtained with 5× SYPRO Orange

2. Purified recombinant proteins dialyzed against 2× Thermofluor (TF) buffer (*see* **Note 3**).

   We used Cdc123 from *Schizosaccharomyces pombe* (Sp), carrying a six histidine affinity-tag (his6) at the N- or C-terminus, as indicated: his6-SpCdc123 (39.1 kDa) (Fig. 4) and SpCdc123-his6 (37.9 kDa) (wild-type (wt), mutant 1 (M1) with 2 amino acid exchanges, and mutant 2 (M2) with an additional third exchange) (Figs. 1 and 2). In addition, a C-terminally truncated version of the human homolog hD123 (hD123(1-290)-his6; 34.8 kDa) (Fig. 3) was used. All proteins were expressed in *E. coli* BL21-CodonPlus and purified on an ÄKTA system using Ni-NTA columns (GE Healthcare). An imidazole gradient (20–350 mM) was used for elution of the proteins from the column.

3. 2× Thermofluor (TF) buffer (*see* **Note 4**): 50 mM Tris/HCl pH 7.5, 400 mM NaCl.

4. 500 mM magnesium acetate.

5. Ultrapure water.

6. 100 mM ATP (pH adjusted with NaOH, e.g., Thermo Fisher Scientific) stored at −20 °C in small aliquots to avoid refreezing.

7. Real-time PCR instrument such as Rotor-Gene Q 2plex Platform (Qiagen) with Rotor-Gene Q Software 2.3.4; 0.1 ml 4-strip PCR-tubes and caps, or plates, as suitable for the real-time PCR instrument.

## 3   Methods

Unless indicated otherwise, all steps are performed on ice.

### 3.1   Optimization of Protein Amount and SYPRO Orange Concentration (See Note 5 and Fig. 4)

1. Each reaction is prepared in duplicate. The final volume of each reaction is 25 µl.

2. Clear the protein sample from aggregates and precipitates (*see* **Note 6**) by filtration or centrifugation (4 °C, 20 min, 16,000 rcf [max speed]).

3. Protein master mixes for 2 µg and 5 µg protein per reaction are prepared, each for 9 reactions, according to Table 1.

4. 1000× SYPRO Orange in DMSO is diluted in $H_2O$ to 5×, 25×, 50× and 100× SYPRO Orange (for 1×, 5×, 10×, and 20× SYPRO Orange in the final reaction). Prepare dilutions in $H_2O$ fresh each time.

5. Distribute 20 µl of each protein mix from **step 3** to 8 × 0.1 ml PCR tubes (*see* **Note 7**).

6. For duplicate reactions, add 5 µl of each SYPRO Orange dilution from **step 4** to 2 aliquots of each protein mix from **step 5**. Mix by pipetting up and down three times.

7. Close the tubes, place in a 72-well rotor of a real-time PCR instrument (Rotor-Gene Q 2plex Platform, Qiagen) and shake the liquid to the bottom of the tubes (*see* **Note 8**).

8. Run the melt program with the 470 nm source and 555 nm detector filter (*see* **Note 9**) using different gain settings (*see* **Note 10**). Ramp from 28 °C to 75 °C (*see* **Note 11**) rising by 1 °C each step. Wait for 90 s of premelt conditioning on first step. Wait for 15 s for each step afterward.

9. Melting curves as shown in Fig. 4 are obtained. Choose the condition with the lowest protein amount that gives a good signal to noise ratio and sharp unfolding transition (*see* **Notes 5** and **12**).

### Table 1
**Protein mix for optimization of SYPRO Orange and protein concentration**

| In final reaction (25 µl) | Stock | 1× | 9× |
|---|---|---|---|
| 2 µg or 5 µg protein in 2× Thermofluor buffer | $x$ µg/µl | $y$ µl | |
| 1× Thermofluor buffer | 2× | 12.5–$y$ µl | |
| 20 mM magnesium acetate | 500 mM | 1 µl | 9 µl |
| $H_2O$ to 20 µl | | 6.75 µl | 60.8 µl |

**Table 2**
**Buffer mix for protein stability assay**

| In final reaction (25 μl) | Stock | 1× | 9× |
|---|---|---|---|
| 20 mM magnesium acetate | 500 mM | 1 μl | 9 μl |
| 5× SYPRO Orange (conc. as optimized) | 1000× | 0.125 μl | 1.13 μl |
| $H_2O$ to 12.5 μl | | 11.38 μl | 102.4 μl |

**3.2 Protein Stability Assay**

1. Each reaction is prepared in duplicate. The final volume of each reaction is 25 μl. This example is calculated for the analysis of three different proteins (wild-type SpCdc123-his6 and two mutants).

2. Clear the protein sample from aggregates and precipitates (*see* **Note 6**) by filtration or centrifugation (4 °C, 20 min, 16,000 rcf [max speed]).

3. Per reaction, complete 2 μg protein to 12.5 μl with 2× TF buffer. A master mix for 3 reactions is prepared for each protein.

4. The buffer-mix is prepared as a master mix for 9 reactions as described in Table 2.

5. 12.5 μl protein-mix from **step 3** or 2× TF buffer is distributed in duplicate to 0.1 ml PCR tubes (*see* **Note 7**). 2× TF buffer serves as a negative control to measure background fluorescence.

6. 12.5 μl buffer-mix from **step 4** is added to the proteins and buffer control and mixed by pipetting three times up and down. The final reaction condition is 2 μg protein (= 2 μM SpCdc123-his6), 25 mM Tris pH 7.5, 200 mM NaCl, 20 mM magnesium acetate, 5× SYPRO Orange.

7. Continue as described in Subheading 3.1 **steps 7** and **8**.

8. Analyze the data using the instrument's accompanying software (Rotor-Gene Q Software 2.3.4) to obtain the $T_m$. The first derivative of the fluorescence is plotted as a function of temperature ($dF/dT$). The maximum peak of the curve represents the $T_m$ (*see* **Note 13**).

9. The result for wild-type SpCdc123-his6 and two mutants is shown in Fig. 2. The data indicate that mutant M2 is thermally destabilized and sensitive toward buffer exchange.

**3.3 Nucleotide Binding Assay**

1. Proceed as described in Subheading 3.2, except that in addition to Subheading 3.2 **step 4** two more buffer mixes are prepared containing 1 mM ATP or ADP (Table 3). Accordingly, a protein master mix for 7 reactions is prepared as described in Subheading 3.2 **step 3**.

**Table 3**
**Buffer mix for nucleotide binding assay**

| In final reaction (25 μl) | Stock | 1× | 9× |
|---|---|---|---|
| 20 mM magnesium acetate | 500 mM | 1 μl | 9 μl |
| 5× SYPRO Orange (or conc. as optimized) | 1000× | 0.125 μl | 1.13 μl |
| 1 mM ATP or ADP | 100 mM | 0.25 μl | 2.25 μl |
| H$_2$O to 12.5 μl | | 11.13 μl | 100.1 μl |

2. The melting curves of wild-type hD123 (hD123(1-290)-his6) in the absence of nucleotide and in the presence of ADP and ATP are shown in Fig. 3. The data indicate that ATP stabilizes hD123 by more than 10 degrees.

# 4    Notes

1. SYPRO Orange is light sensitive and should therefore be kept in the dark.

2. To avoid DMSO concentrations above 2% in the final reaction, the SYPRO Orange working stock solution should be as highly concentrated as possible. The SYPRO Orange dye (Invitrogen) is provided as 5000× solution in 100% DMSO. We found a 1000× SYPRO Orange in DMSO working stock dilution to be optimal. For 5× SYPRO Orange in the final reaction, DMSO is at 0.05%, while pipetting volumes are still acceptable.

3. The dialysis serves to remove the imidazole, which is in the elution buffer of our Ni-NTA–purified recombinant proteins. Imidazole influences the $T_m$ and the imidazole concentrations differ in each gradient-eluted protein fraction. After dialysis against a defined buffer, $T_m$ values are well reproducible. Furthermore, the dialysis against 2× TF buffer has the advantage, that even if high protein volumes have to be added to the reaction (in case of low initial protein concentrations) it is easy to keep the final buffer composition identical in all conditions. Half of the final reaction volume corresponds to protein volume plus 2×TF buffer.

4. The Thermofluor buffer composition can be adjusted to the protein's needs [3, 16, 18–20]. Tris is used here because of additional downstream assays.

5. We recommend the optimization of protein and SYPRO Orange concentration. The SYPRO Orange concentration strongly influences the increase in fluorescence upon protein denaturation (Fig. 4). Too much or too little SYPRO Orange

relative to protein leads to reduced quantum yield (*see* Fig. 4 20× and 1× SYPRO Orange). Choose the lowest protein amount that uses the full dynamic range of the photomultiplier, a good signal to noise ratio and sharp unfolding transition. Another approach, starting with a fixed 10× SYPRO Orange concentration and adjusting only protein amount, will in many cases consume more protein than necessary. We found that for most proteins optimal conditions are at around 2 µg protein (0.08 mg/ml) and 5× SYPRO Orange. However, in some cases protein concentrations might have to be varied from 0.01 to 0.2 mg/ml and SYPRO Orange from 1× to 20× to obtain suitable conditions.

6. Removing denatured protein from the sample is essential, since it might otherwise produce high background fluorescence.

7. Place the liquid approximately 3/4th down the tube to leave enough space above to add the SYPRO Orange–containing mix.

8. After placing the tubes in the 72-well rotor and attaching the locking ring, shake all liquid to the bottom of the tubes. Otherwise, no fluorescent signal will be collected at the beginning of the run, until the centrifugal force of the rotor forces the liquid to the bottom of the tube.

9. The emission and excitation peaks of protein-bound SYPRO Orange are at approximately 500 nm and 600 nm, respectively [1]. Using the standard 470 ± 10 nm excitation and 557 ± 5 nm emission filters provided with the Rotor-Gene Q 2plex Platform (Qiagen), we obtained substantial fluorescence increases: around 13-fold for lysozyme (3.8 µg) in 10× SYPRO Orange or around 22-fold for his6-SpCdc123 (2 µg) in 5× SYPRO Orange.

10. The gain determines the sensitivity of the photomultiplier that converts fluorescence photons to electronic signals. The gain setting is a means to modulate the signal amplification. If the gain is too high, the signal will be oversaturated. If the gain is too low, the signal will disappear in the background noise. To use the complete dynamic range of the photomultiplier, it is best to acquire the data on three to four channels with different gains in parallel. In the optimal gain setting, fluorescence values will approach the maximum threshold. We usually work with gains between 7.67 and 9.33.

11. For very stable proteins (e.g., lysozyme $T_m = 72\ °C$) increase the temperature range of the melting curve.

12. If the protein fails to generate a melting curve, the protein (1) might be already denatured, which results in high fluorescence, (2) might contain intrinsically disordered regions, which

also results in high background fluorescence, or (3) might lack hydrophobic regions. The latter is often the case for small proteins, for example, ubiquitin (data not shown) and [2].

13. Here, the $T_m$ is determined by plotting the first derivative of the fluorescence as a function of temperature, where the $T_m$ is represented as the peak of the curve. Alternatively, the $T_m$, as midpoint of the unfolding transition, can be determined by nonlinear fitting to a Boltzmann equation [3, 17]. The data can be easily exported from the real-time PCR instrument's software as a text file and analyzed with a method and software of choice.

## Acknowledgments

This work was supported by the Deutsche Forschungsgemeinschaft (DFG) within the collaborative research center SFB960. We thank Wolfgang Mages and Lena Kreuzpaintner for purification of the his6-SpCdc123 protein used in Fig. 4.

## References

1. Niesen FH, Berglund H, Vedadi M (2007) The use of differential scanning fluorimetry to detect ligand interactions that promote protein stability. Nat Protoc 2:2212–2221

2. Boivin S, Kozak S, Meijers R (2013) Optimization of protein purification and characterization using Thermofluor screens. Protein Expr Purif 91:192–206

3. Huynh K, Partch CL (2015) Analysis of protein stability and ligand interactions by thermal shift assay. Curr Protoc Protein Sci 79: 28.9.1–28.9.14

4. Poklar N, Lah J, Salobir M, Macek P, Vesnaver G (1997) pH and temperature-induced molten globule-like denatured states of equinatoxin II: a study by UV-melting, DSC, far- and near-UV CD spectroscopy, and ANS fluorescence. Biochemistry 36:14345–14352

5. Pantoliano MW, Petrella EC, Kwasnoski JD, Lobanov VS, Myslik J, Graf E, Carver T, Asel E, Springer BA, Lane P, Salemme FR (2001) High-density miniaturized thermal shift assays as a general strategy for drug discovery. J Biomol Screen 6:429–440

6. Steinberg TH, Jones LJ, Haugland RP, Singer VL (1996) SYPRO orange and SYPRO red protein gel stains: one-step fluorescent staining of denaturing gels for detection of nanogram levels of protein. Anal Biochem 239:223–237

7. Cimmperman P, Baranauskiene L, Jachimoviciūte S, Jachno J, Torresan J, Michailoviene V, Matuliene J, Sereikaite J, Bumelis V, Matulis D (2008) A quantitative model of thermal stabilization and destabilization of proteins by ligands. Biophys J 95:3222–3231

8. Kranz JK, Schalk-Hihi C (2011) Protein thermal shifts to identify low molecular weight fragments. Meth Enzymol 493:277–298

9. Lo MC, Aulabaugh A, Jin G, Cowling R, Bard J, Malamas M, Ellestad G (2004) Evaluation of fluorescence-based thermal shift assays for hit identification in drug discovery. Anal Biochem 332:153–159

10. Ehrhardt MKG, Warring SL, Gerth ML (2018) Screening chemoreceptor–ligand interactions by high-throughput thermal-shift assays. In: Manson MD (ed) Bacterial chemosensing: methods and protocols. Springer, New York, New York, NY, pp 281–290

11. Williams TL, Yin YW, Carter CW (2016) Selective inhibition of bacterial Tryptophanyl-tRNA Synthetases by Indolmycin is mechanism-based. J Biol Chem 291:255–265

12. Carver TE, Bordeau B, Cummings MD, Petrella EC, Pucci MJ, Zawadzke LE, Dougherty BA, Tredup JA, Bryson JW, Yanchunas J Jr, Doyle ML, Witmer MR, Nelen MI, DesJarlais

RL, Jaeger EP, Devine H, Asel ED, Springer BA, Bone R, Salemme FR, Todd MJ (2005) Decrypting the biochemical function of an essential gene from Streptococcus pneumoniae using ThermoFluor technology. J Biol Chem 280:11704–11712

13. Matulis D, Kranz JK, Salemme FR, Todd MJ (2005) Thermodynamic stability of carbonic anhydrase: measurements of binding affinity and stoichiometry using ThermoFluor. Biochemistry 44:5258–5266

14. Vivoli M, Novak HR, Littlechild JA, Harmer NJ (2014) Determination of protein-ligand interactions using differential scanning fluorimetry. J Vis Exp 91:51809

15. Bai N, Roder H, Dickson A, Karanicolas J (2019) Isothermal analysis of ThermoFluor data can readily provide quantitative binding affinities. Sci Rep 9:2650

16. Ericsson UB, Hallberg BM, Detitta GT, Dekker N, Nordlund P (2006) Thermofluor-based high-throughput stability optimization of proteins for structural studies. Anal Biochem 357:289–298

17. Wright TA, Stewart JM, Page RC, Konkolewicz D (2017) Extraction of thermodynamic parameters of protein unfolding using parallelized differential scanning Fluorimetry. J Phys Chem Lett 8:553–558

18. Kozak S, Lercher L, Karanth MN, Meijers R, Carlomagno T, Boivin S (2016) Optimization of protein samples for NMR using thermal shift assays. J Biomol NMR 64:281–289

19. Seabrook SA, Newman J (2013) High-throughput thermal scanning for protein stability: making a good technique more robust. ACS Comb Sci 15:387–392

20. Reinhard L, Mayerhofer H, Geerlof A, Mueller-Dieckmann J, Weiss MS (2013) Optimization of protein buffer cocktails using Thermofluor. Acta Crystallogr Sect F Struct Biol Cryst Commun 69:209–214

21. Perzlmaier AF, Richter F, Seufert W (2013) Translation initiation requires cell division cycle 123 (Cdc123) to facilitate biogenesis of the eukaryotic initiation factor 2 (eIF2). J Biol Chem 288:21537–21546

22. Bieganowski P, Shilinski K, Tsichlis PN, Brenner C (2004) Cdc123 and checkpoint forkhead associated with RING proteins control the cell cycle by controlling eIF2gamma abundance. J Biol Chem 279:44656–44666

23. Blomen VA, Májek P, Jae LT, Bigenzahn JW, Nieuwenhuis J, Staring J, Sacco R, van Diemen FR, Olk N, Stukalov A, Marceau C, Janssen H, Carette JE, Bennett KL, Colinge J, Superti-Furga G, Brummelkamp TR (2015) Gene essentiality and synthetic lethality in haploid human cells. Science 350:1092–1096

24. Wang T, Birsoy K, Hughes NW, Krupczak KM, Post Y, Wei JJ, Lander ES, Sabatini DM (2015) Identification and characterization of essential genes in the human genome. Science 350:1096–1101

25. Panvert M, Dubiez E, Arnold L, Perez J, Mechulam Y, Seufert W, Schmitt E (2015) Cdc123, a cell cycle regulator needed for eIF2 assembly, is an ATP-grasp protein with unique features. Structure 23:1596–1608

# Chapter 16

# In Vitro Assembly of a Fully Reconstituted Yeast Translation System for Studies of Initiation and Elongation Phases of Protein Synthesis

## Sandra Blanchet and Namit Ranjan

## Abstract

Protein synthesis is an essential and highly regulated cellular process. To facilitate the understanding of eukaryotic translation, we have assembled an in vitro translation system from yeast using purified components to recapitulate the initiation and elongation phases of protein synthesis. Here, we describe methods to express and purify the components of the translation system and the assays for their functional characterization.

**Key words** Translation, Ribosome, mRNA, tRNA, Yeast

## 1 Introduction

Protein synthesis in yeast is carried out by the 80S ribosomes that translate genetic information from messenger RNA (mRNA) into functional proteins with the help of aminoacyl-tRNAs (aa-tRNA) and a large number of specific translation factors. Translation entails four steps, initiation, elongation, termination, and ribosome recycling [1, 2]. During the initiation phase, the ribosome selects a start codon and an open reading frame for translation. Eukaryotic initiation factor 2 (eIF2), in its active GTP-bound form, binds to initiator methionyl-tRNA (Met-tRNA$_i^{Met}$) to form a ternary complex that delivers the tRNA to the small ribosomal subunit (40S). The 40S subunit together with eIF2–GTP–Met-tRNA$_i^{Met}$, eIF1, eIF1A, and eIF3 forms the 43S preinitiation complex (43S PIC), which then interacts with the mRNA that is recruited by the eIF4/ PABP complex to form the 48S complex (48S PIC). Following scanning and start codon recognition, eIF2 hydrolyzes GTP using eIF5 as a GTPase activating protein, allowing the dissociation of eIF2–GDP and recruitment of eIF5B. After large ribosomal subunit (60S) joining, eIF5B hydrolyzes GTP, the initiation factors

Karl-Dieter Entian (ed.), *Ribosome Biogenesis: Methods and Protocols*, Methods in Molecular Biology, vol. 2533, https://doi.org/10.1007/978-1-0716-2501-9_16, © The Author(s) 2022

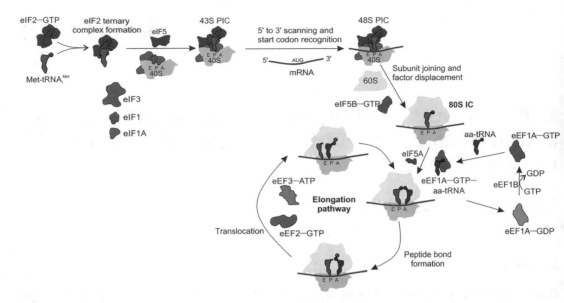

**Fig. 1** Schematic of components required to in vitro reconstitute yeast mRNA translation initiation and elongation using a short unstructured mRNA, which overcomes the requirement of eIF4F complex

dissociate and the 80S initiation complex (80S IC) is ready to enter elongation (Fig. 1). eIF2–GDP is recycled to its active GTP-bound form with the help of the nucleotide exchange factor eIF2B, whereas the nucleotide exchange in eIF5B occurs spontaneously [2–4]. In the subsequent step of elongation, the eukaryotic elongation factor eEF1A binds aa-tRNA in a GTP-dependent manner and delivers the aa-tRNA to the A site of the ribosome. Codon recognition by the aa-tRNA triggers GTP hydrolysis by eEF1A, releasing the factor, and enables the aa-tRNA to accommodate in the A site. Then, peptide bond forms between the peptidyl-tRNA in the P site and the aa-tRNA in the A site. In most cases, peptide bond formation occurs spontaneously at the peptidyl transferase center of the ribosome, but with some amino acids, for example, strings of consecutive prolines, it requires the help of eIF5A. eEF1A–GDP is recycled to its active GTP-bound form with the help of nucleotide exchange factor eEF1B. Following peptide bond formation, the ribosome moves along the mRNA by one codon in a process called translocation, which is facilitated by eEF2 in the GTP-bound state and the fungal-specific eEF3 in its ATP-bound state. Once the stop codon is reached, translation is terminated with the help of the release factors eRF1 and eRF3 (Fig. 1) [1, 5]. Ribosome recycling, which requires Rli1, Ligatin and can also be promoted by eIF3j [6–8], results in the disassembly of the ribosome posttermination complex into ribosomal subunits, tRNA, and mRNA.

In this chapter, we describe the reconstitution of yeast translation system to study the initiation and elongation phases. In detail, we provide updated purification protocols for individual translation factors, ribosomes, and aa-tRNAs. Furthermore, we describe several assays for testing the activity of the purified components, the efficiency of the initiation complex formation and of peptide bond formation. This in vitro translation system utilizes an unstructured model mRNA, which overcomes the requirement for mRNA capping and for auxiliary cap-binding proteins.

# 2    Materials

## 2.1    Media

1. YPD media: 10 g/L yeast extract, 20 g/L peptone, 2% glucose (1.8% agar-agar for plates).

2. Selective media: 5.1 g/L $(NH_4)_2SO_4$, 1.7 g/L yeast nitrogen base, 2% glucose, 0.67 g/L minimal media powder (-LEU -URA or -LEU) with 1.8% agar-agar for plates.

3. LB-media: 10 g/L tryptone; 10 g/L NaCl; 5 g/L yeast extract.

## 2.2    Antibiotics, DNase, and IPTG

1. 100 mg/mL ampicillin sodium salt.

2. 34 mg/mL chloramphenicol.

3. 2 units/μL DNase.

4. 1 mM puromycin.

5. 1 M Isopropyl β-D-1-thiogalactopyranoside (IPTG).

## 2.3    Buffers

1. **Buffer 1:** 10× Ribo Buffer A: 200 mM HEPES–KOH pH 7.5, 1 M KOAc, 25 mM Mg(OAc)$_2$.

2. **Buffer 2:** 1× Buffer 1, 1 mg/mL heparin sodium salt, 2 mM DTT.

3. **Buffer 3:** 1× Buffer 1, 400 mM KCl, 1 M sucrose, 2 mM DTT.

4. **Buffer 4:** 1× Buffer 1, 400 mM KCl, 1 mg/mL heparin sodium salt, 2 mM DTT.

5. **Buffer 5:** 50 mM HEPES–KOH pH 7.5, 500 mM KCl, 2 mM $MgCl_2$, 2 mM DTT.

6. **Buffer 6:** Same as buffer 5 with 5 mM $MgCl_2$, 0.1 mM ethylenediaminetetraacetic acid (EDTA) pH 8.0, 5% or 30% sucrose.

7. **Buffer 7:** 50 mM HEPES–KOH, 100 mM KCl, 250 mM sucrose, 2.5 mM $MgCl_2$, 2 mM DTT.

8. **Buffer 8:** 20 mM HEPES–NaOH pH 7.5, 150 mM NaCl, 5% glycerol, 4 mM ß-mercaptoethanol (ß-me).

9. **Buffer 9:** Same as buffer 8 with 1 M NaCl.

10. **Buffer 10:** 20 mM HEPES–KOH pH 7.5, 200 mM KCl, 2 mM DTT.

11. **Buffer 11:** Same as buffer 8 without NaCl and glycerol.

12. **Buffer 12:** 20 mM HEPES–NaOH pH 7.5, 500 mM NaCl, 5% glycerol, 4 mM ß-me.

13. **Buffer 13:** Same as buffer 12 with 150 mM NaCl.

14. **Buffer 14:** Same as buffer 13 with 30 mM L-glutathione reduced.

15. **Buffer 15:** Same as buffer 12 with 1 M NaCl.

16. **Buffer 16:** 20 mM HEPES–KOH pH 7.5, 100 mM KCl, 2 mM DTT.

17. **Buffer 17:** 50 mM HEPES–NaOH pH 7.5, 400 mM NaCl, 5% glycerol, 4 mM ß-me.

18. **Buffer 18:** 20 mM HEPES–NaOH pH 7.5, 500 mM NaCl, 30 mM L-glutathione reduced. 5% glycerol, 4 mM ß-me.

19. **Buffer 19:** 20 mM HEPES–NaOH pH 7.5, 275 mM NaCl, 5% glycerol, 4 mM ß-me.

20. **Buffer 20:** 20 mM HEPES–KOH pH 7.5, 200 mM KCl, 2 mM DTT.

21. **Buffer 21:** 20 mM HEPES–KOH pH 7.5, 500 mM KCl, 10% glycerol, 3 mM ß-me.

22. **Buffer 22:** Same as buffer 21 with 30 mM L-glutathione reduced.

23. **Buffer 23:** 20 mM HEPES–KOH pH 7.5, 200 mM KCl, 10% glycerol, 2 mM DTT.

24. **Buffer 24:** 20 mM HEPES–KOH pH 7.5, 100 mM KCl, 5% glycerol, 2 mM DTT.

25. **Buffer 25:** 20 mM 3-($N$-morpholino)propane sulfonic acid (MOPS)–KOH pH 6.7, 500 mM KCl, 10% glycerol, 3 mM ß-me.

26. **Buffer 26:** Same as buffer 25 with 30 mM L-glutathione reduced.

27. **Buffer 27:** 20 mM HEPES–KOH pH 7.5, 200 mM KCl, 10% glycerol, 2 mM DTT.

28. **Buffer 28:** 20 mM HEPES–KOH pH 7.5, 100 mM KCl, 5% glycerol, 2 mM DTT.

29. **Buffer 29:** 75 mM HEPES–KOH pH 7.6, 100 mM KCl, 100 µM GDP, 10 mM ß-me.

30. **Buffer 30:** 20 mM HEPES–KOH pH 7.6, 500 mM KCl, 20 mM imidazole, 10% glycerol, 0.1 mM $MgCl_2$, 10 µM GDP, 10 mM ß-me.

31. **Buffer 31:** Same as buffer 30 with 250 mM imidazole.

32. **Buffer 32:** 20 mM HEPES–KOH pH 7.6, 100 mM KCl, 10% glycerol, 0.1 mM $MgCl_2$, 10 µM GDP, 2 mM DTT.

33. **Buffer 33:** Same as buffer 32 with 1 M KCl.

34. **Buffer 34:** 20 mM HEPES–KOH pH 7.6, 100 mM KOAc, 0.1 mM $Mg(OAc)_2$, 10% glycerol, 2 mM DTT.

35. **Buffer 35:** 20 mM HEPES–KOH pH 7.6, 2 mM DTT, 10 µM GDP.

36. **Buffer 36:** 20 mM Tris–HCl pH 7.5, 350 mM KCl, 5 mM $MgCl_2$, 1 mM PMSF, 10% glycerol, 20 mM imidazole, 0.5 mM ß-me.

37. **Buffer 37:** Same as buffer 36 with 450 mM KCl.

38. **Buffer 38:** Same as buffer 37 with 250 mM imidazole.

39. **Buffer 39:** 20 mM Tris–HCl pH 7.5, 75 mM KCl, 10% glycerol, 2 mM DTT.

40. **Buffer 40:** 50 mM Tris–HCl pH 7.5, 5 mM $MgCl_2$, 50 mM $NH_4Cl$, 0.2 mM PMSF, 10% glycerol, 0.1 mM EDTA pH 8.0, 1 mM DTT.

41. **Buffer 41:** 20 mM Tris–HCl pH 7.5, 50 mM KCl, 0.1 mM EDTA pH 8.0, 0.2 mM PMSF, 25% glycerol, 1 mM DTT.

42. **Buffer 42:** Same as buffer 41 with 500 mM KCl.

43. **Buffer 43:** 20 mM Tris–HCl pH 7.5, 0.1 mM EDTA pH 8.0, 200 mM KCl, 25% glycerol, 1 mM DTT.

44. **Buffer 44:** 50 mM potassium phosphate pH 8.0, 1 M KCl, 0.2 mM PMSF, 1% Tween 20, 10 mM imidazole.

45. **Buffer 45:** Same as buffer 44 with 20 mM imidazole.

46. **Buffer 46:** Same as buffer 44 with 500 mM imidazole.

47. **Buffer 47:** 20 mM Tris–HCl pH 7.5, 100 mM KCl, 0.1 mM EDTA pH 8.0, 10% glycerol, 0.2 mM PMSF, 1 mM DTT.

48. **Buffer 48:** 20 mM HEPES–KOH pH 7.5, 500 mM KCl, 20 mM imidazole, 10% glycerol, 2 mM ß-me.

49. **Buffer 49:** 20 mM HEPES- KOH pH 7.5, 100 mM KCl, 250 mM imidazole, 10% glycerol, 2 mM ß-me.

50. **Buffer 50:** 20 mM HEPES- KOH pH 7.5, 100 mM KCl, 10% glycerol, 2 mM DTT.

51. **Buffer 51:** 20 mM Tris–HCl pH 7.5, 100 mM KCl, 1 mM DTT.

52. **Buffer 52:** 20 mM HEPES- KOH pH 7.5, 100 mM KCl, 2 mM DTT.

53. **Buffer 53:** Same as buffer 52 with 250 mM imidazole.

54. **Buffer 54:** YT buffer: 30 mM HEPES–KOH pH 7.5, 100 mM KOAc, 3 mM $MgCl_2$.

55. **Buffer 55:** YT9 buffer: 30 mM HEPES–KOH pH 7.5, 100 mM KOAc, 9 mM $MgCl_2$.

56. **Buffer 56:** YT0 buffer: 30 mM HEPES–KOH pH 7.5, 100 mM KOAc.

57. **Buffer 57:** 30 mM Bis-Tris pH 6.0, 10 mM $MgCl_2$, 300 mM NaCl.

58. **Buffer 58:** Same as buffer 57 with 1 M NaCl.

59. **Buffer 59:** $HAKM_7$: 30 mM HEPES–NaOH pH 7.5, 70 mM $NH_4Cl$, 30 mM KCl, 7 mM $MgCl_2$.

60. **Buffer 60:** HPLC purification buffer: A 20 mM $NH_4OAc$, 10 mM $MgCl_2$, 400 mM NaCl, 5% ethanol.

61. **Buffer 61:** HPLC purification buffer B: 20 mM $NH_4OAc$, 10 mM $MgCl_2$, 400 mM NaCl, 15% ethanol.

62. **Buffer 62:** HPLC-buffer A: 0.1% trifluoroacetic acid (TFA).

63. **Buffer 63:** HPLC-buffer B: 0.1% TFA; 65% acetonitrile.

*2.4 Strains and Plasmids*

| Protein | Expression host | Genotype/Description | References |
|---------|-----------------|----------------------|------------|
| eIF1 | *E. coli* | $P_{T7}$; eIF1 cloned NdeI/XhoI; $Ap^R$ | Kind gift from Dr. Ralf Ficner |
| eIF1A | *E. coli* | $P_{tac}$; GST-tag; eIF1A cloned BamHI/XhoI; ApR | This work |
| eIF5 | *E. coli* | $P_{tac}$; GST-tag; eIF5 cloned BamHI/XhoI; ApR | This work |
| eIF5B | *E. coli* | $P_{tac}$; GST-tag; eIF5B cloned BamHI/XhoI; ApR | This work |
| eIF2 | *S. cerevisiae* | *MATα leu2-3 leu2-112 ura3-52 ino1 gcn2Δ pep4::LEU2 sui2Δ HIS4-lacZ* pAV1089 [SUI2 SUI3 His-tagged GCD11 URA3] | [9] |
| eIF3 | *S. cerevisiae* | *MATa/α ura3-52/ura3-52 trp1/trp1 leu2-Δ1/leu2-Δ1 his3-Δ200/his3-Δ200 pep:: HIS4/pep::HIS4 prb1-Δ 1.6/prb1-Δ1.6 can1/can1 GAL⁺*(pLPY-PRT1His-TIF34HA-TIF35Flag)/ (pLPY-TIF32-NIP1) | [10] |
| eIF5A (*see* **Note 1**) | *E. coli* | $P_{tac}$; GST-tag; eIF5A cloned BamHI/XhoI; ApR | This work |

(continued)

| Protein | Expression host | Genotype/Description | References |
|---|---|---|---|
| DYS1-LIA1 | *E. coli* | $P_{tac}$; His-tag; DYS1 and LIA1 cloned PacI/SwaI; ApR | This work |
| eEF2 | *S. cerevisiae* | *MAT*a *ade2 leu2 ura3 his3 leu2 trp1 eft1::HIS3 eft2:: TRP1* pEFT2-6xHis LEU2 CEN | [11] |
| eEF1A and Ribosomal subunits (YAS2488) | *S. cerevisiae* | *MAT*a *leu2-3112 his4-539 trp1 ura3-52 cup1::LEU2/ PGK1pG/MFA2pG* | [12] |

# 3  Methods

### 3.1  Purification of Ribosomal Subunits from S. Cerevisiae

1. Streak the YAS2488 strain on a YPD plate and incubate for 2 days at 30 °C (*see* **Note 2**). Inoculate a preculture of 200 mL YPD media overnight in a shaker at 30 °C with 180 rpm. Inoculate 100 L YPD culture with the preculture at a starting $OD_{600}$ of 0.1 and grow until mid-log phase in a bioreactor. Harvest the cells, wash the pellets with MilliQ water and suspend the cell pellets in 1 mL/g of cells in buffer 2. Prepare frozen cell droplets by dropping the lysate using a syringe or serological pipette in liquid nitrogen. Grind the cell droplets using an ultracentrifugal mill prechilled with liquid nitrogen. Collect the powder and store in −80 °C freezer.

2. Thaw 200 g (~400 mL lysate) of grinded powder, add 100 μL DNase to the lysate and incubate for 30 min on ice. Add one EDTA-free Protease Inhibitor tablet dissolved in 1× buffer 1. Centrifuge at 25,364 × *g* at 4 °C for 30 min to clear the lysate. Collect the supernatant carefully without disturbing the pellets and note the exact volume. At this point, bring the KCl concentration to 500 mM and filter the lysate using 1 μm glass fiber filters or equivalent. Chill Ti45 ultracentrifuge tubes. Add 7 mL of sucrose cushion (buffer 3) into each tube. Carefully layer 55 mL of cleared lysate onto each sucrose cushion. Centrifuge at 235,418 × *g* for 2 h at 4 °C. Immediately remove the lipids layer on top of each tube and carefully swipe the tubes to get rid of leftover lipids and extra supernatant. The ribosomal pellet should be transparent. Add 1 mL of buffer 4 to each tube and incubate on ice for 15 min. Dissolve the pellets by gently pipetting using a P1000 pipette. Pool the ribosome solution and bring the final volume to 10 mL with buffer 4. Stir at a moderate speed with a micro-stir bar for 1 h at 4 °C.

3. Add 200 μL of sucrose cushion (buffer 3) in chilled MLA 130 tubes and carefully layer 1 mL of ribosome solution in each tube, on top of the sucrose cushion. Centrifuge at 603,000 × $g$ for 30 min at 4 °C. Discard the supernatant by inverting the tubes. Add 400 μL of buffer 5 to each tube and incubate on ice for 15 min. Dissolve the pellets carefully, pool the solution in a 15 mL falcon tube and bring the total volume to 6 mL with buffer 5. Add 60 μL of 100 mM puromycin and incubate for 15 min on ice and then 10 min at 37 °C.

4. Gradient preparation and ribosome layering: Prepare 5%–30% sucrose gradient in SW32 tubes. Pipet 25 mL of 30% sucrose solution (buffer 6) at the bottom and carefully layer 15 mL of 5% sucrose solution (buffer 6) on top. Close the gradient tube with caps without any bubbles. Prepare the gradient using Gradient Master. Remove the caps from the gradient tubes and take 1 mL out from the top of each SW32 tube. Carefully layer 1 mL of ribosome solution on each SW32 gradient tube. Centrifuge at 106,750 × $g$ for 16 h at 4 °C.

5. Gradients are fractionated either using a peristaltic pump connected to an FPLC system or gradient fractionation system. Collect the fractions from the bottom of the tube and measure $OD_{260}$ of each fraction. The first peak with higher sucrose concentration corresponds to the 60S subunits peak and the second large peak corresponds to the 40S subunits peak. Pool the fractions corresponding to 40S and 60S subunits and concentrate using a 100 kDa MWCO Vivaspin concentrator. Exchange to buffer 7 using the same concentrator. Measure the $OD_{260}$ of concentrated 40S and 60S subunits solutions and calculate the concentrations using the extinction coefficients $2 \times 10^7 \, M^{-1} \, cm^{-1}$ for 40S subunits and $4 \times 10^7 \, M^{-1} \, cm^{-1}$ for 60S subunits [13].

6. Quality control for rRNA integrity: Prepare solutions containing 3 pmol of 40S or 60S subunits with 60% formamide and 1x loading dye (50 mM Tris–HCl pH 7.6, 0.25% bromophenol blue, 60% glycerol). Load on a 1% agarose gel premixed with SYBR gold dye. Run the gel at 70 V (10 V/cm of gel) for 1 h (dye should reach two-thirds of the gel). Visualize 28S and 18S rRNA for 60S and 40S subunits under UV gel scanner. 5S and 5.8S are too small to be visualized on the gel.

### 3.2 Purification of Initiation Factors

Unless specified otherwise, all purifications are performed using an FPLC system.

1. eIF1

Express eIF1 from pETT22b plasmid (no tag) in BL21 *E. coli* cells. Inoculate a preculture of 200 mL LB with 100 μg/mL carbenicillin and grow at 37 °C overnight. Next day, inoculate 6 L of LB with 100 µg/mL carbenicillin with the overnight preculture at a starting $OD_{600}$ of 0.1 and grow in a shaker at 37 °C with 180 rpm. Induce expression with 0.5 mM IPTG when $OD_{600}$ reaches 0.8 and incubate at 37 °C for additional 3–4 h. Harvest the cells at 7000 rpm for 10 min at 4 °C and store at −80 °C. Resuspend the cell pellet in buffer 8 (3 mL/g of cells) complemented with 100 µL of DNase and one protease inhibitor tablet. Homogenize the cell suspension on ice and use Emulsiflex to lyse the cells. Centrifuge at 180,800 × $g$ for 1 h at 4 °C. Collect the supernatant and filter it through 1 µm glass fiber filters or equivalent. Equilibrate the HiTrap SP column with buffer 8. Load the sample onto the column in buffer 8. Wash the column with buffer 8. Elute with a linear gradient from 0% to 100% of buffer 9 over 60 mL. Collect 2 mL fractions, analyze on a 15% SDS-PAGE and pool the fractions containing eIF1. Dilute the pool to decrease the salt concentration to 150 mM NaCl with buffer 11. Equilibrate the HiTrap Heparin column with buffer 8. Load the diluted sample and wash the column with buffer 8. Elute eIF1 with a linear gradient from 0% to 100% of buffer 9 over 60 mL. Collect 2 mL fractions, analyze on a 15% SDS-PAGE and pool the fractions containing eIF1. Concentrate eIF1 and load on a HiLoad 26/600 Superdex75 pg size-exclusion chromatography column preequilibrated with buffer 10. Collect 2 mL fractions, analyze on a 15% SDS-PAGE and pool the fractions containing eIF1. Concentrate the eIF1 using a 5 kDa MWCO Vivaspin concentrator. Check the final concentration at the spectrophotometer ($OD_{280}$, extinction coefficient 3105 $M^{-1}$ $cm^{-1}$), flash-freeze aliquots, and store at −80 °C.

2. eIF1A

Express eIF1A from pGEX-6P1 plasmid (GST tag) in BL21 *E. coli* cells. Inoculate a pre-culture of 200 mL LB with 100 µg/mL carbenicillin and grow at 37 °C overnight. Next day, inoculate 6 L of LB with 100 µg/mL carbenicillin with the overnight preculture at a starting $OD_{600}$ of 0.1 and let it grow in a shaker at 37 °C with 180 rpm. Reduce the temperature from 37 °C to 16 °C when $OD_{600}$ reaches 0.4, induce expression with 0.5 mM IPTG when $OD_{600}$ reaches 0.8 and grow for additional 16 h. Harvest the cells at 7000 rpm for 10 min at 4 °C. Resuspend the cell pellets (30–50 g) in 2 mL/g with buffer 12 complemented with 100 µL of DNase and one protease inhibitors tablet. Homogenize the cell suspension on ice and use Emulsiflex to lyse the cells. Centrifuge at 180,800 × $g$ for 1 h at 4 °C. Collect the supernatant and filter using 1 µm glass fiber filters or equivalent. Equilibrate the GSTrap column with buffer 13. Load the lysate and wash the column with buffer 13. Elute eIF1A with

100% of buffer 14 and collect 2 mL fractions. Analyze the fractions on a 15% SDS-PAGE. Pool the elution fractions and add PreScission protease (1 μM final) to cleave the tag while dialyzing overnight at 4 °C against 2 L of buffer 13. Load the dialyzed sample on a Resource Q column and elute with 0 to 100% buffer 15 over 60 mL. Analyze the fractions on a 15% SDS-PAGE, pool the fractions containing eIF1A. Concentrate eIF1A and load on a HiLoad 26/600 Superdex75 pg size-exclusion chromatography column preequilibrated with buffer 16. Collect 2 mL fractions, analyze on a 15% SDS-PAGE and pool the fractions containing eIF1A. Concentrate proteins using a 5 kDa MWCO Vivaspin concentrator. Check the final concentration at the spectrophotometer ($OD_{280}$, extinction coefficient 10,095 $M^{-1}$ $cm^{-1}$), flash-freeze aliquots, and store at −80 °C.

3. eIF5

Express eIF5 from pGEX-6P1 plasmid (GST tag) in BL21 *E. coli* cells. Inoculate a preculture of 200 mL LB with 100 μg/mL carbenicillin and grow at 37 °C overnight. Next day, inoculate 6 L of LB with 100 μg/mL carbenicillin with the overnight preculture at a starting $OD_{600}$ of 0.1 and let it grow in a shaker at 37 °C with 180 rpm. Reduce the temperature from 37 °C to 16 °C when $OD_{600}$ reaches 0.4, induce expression with 0.5 mM IPTG when $OD_{600}$ reaches 0.8 and grow for additional 16 h. Harvest the cells at 7000 rpm for 10 min at 4 °C. Resuspend the cell pellets (30–50 g) in 2 mL/g with buffer 17 complemented with 100 μL of DNase and one protease inhibitors tablet. Homogenize the cell suspension on ice and use Emulsiflex to lyse the cells. Centrifuge at 180,800 × $g$ for 1 h at 4 °C. Collect the supernatant and filter using 1 μm glass fiber filters or equivalent. Equilibrate the GSTrap column with buffer 17. Load the lysate and wash the column with buffer 17. Elute eIF5 with 100% of buffer 18 and collect 2 mL fractions. Analyze the fractions on a 15% SDS-PAGE. Pool the elution fractions and add PreScission protease (1 μM final) to cleave the tag while dialyzing overnight at 4 °C against 2 L of buffer 19. Perform a second GSTrap column and eIF5 remains now in the flow-through as the GST tag is cleaved. Concentrate eIF5 and load on a HiLoad 26/600 Superdex75 pg size-exclusion chromatography column preequilibrated with buffer 20. Collect 2 mL fractions, analyze on a 15% SDS-PAGE and pool the fractions containing eIF5. Concentrate proteins using a 10 kDa MWCO Vivaspin concentrator. Check the final concentration at the spectrophotometer ($OD_{280}$, extinction coefficient 30,285 $M^{-1}$ $cm^{-1}$), flash-freeze aliquots, and store at −80 °C.

4. eIF5A

Express eIF5A from pGEX-6P1 plasmid (GST tag) in Rosetta 2 cells. Inoculate a preculture of 200 mL LB with 100 μg/mL carbenicillin and 34 μg/mL chloramphenicol, and grow at 37 °C overnight. Next day, inoculate 6 L of LB with 100 μg/mL carbenicillin with the overnight preculture at a starting $OD_{600}$ of 0.1 and let it grow in a shaker at 37 °C with 180 rpm. Induce eIF5A expression with 0.5 mM IPTG when $OD_{600}$ reaches 0.8 and incubate at 37 °C for additional 3–4 h. Harvest the cells at 7000 rpm for 10 min at 4 °C. Resuspend the cell pellets (30–50 g) in 2 mL/g with buffer 21, complemented with 100 μL of DNase and one protease inhibitors tablet. Homogenize the cell suspension on ice and use Emulsiflex to lyse the cells. Centrifuge at 180,800 × $g$ for 1 h at 4 °C. Collect the supernatant and filter using 1 μm glass fiber filters or equivalent. Equilibrate the GSTrap column with buffer 21. Load the lysate and wash the column with buffer 21. Elute eIF5A with buffer 22 and collect 2 mL fractions. Analyze the fractions on a 15% SDS-PAGE. Pool the elution fractions and add PreScission protease (1 μM final) to cleave the tag while dialyzing overnight at 4 °C against 2 L of buffer 23. After dialysis, load eIF5A on a HiLoad 26/600 Superdex75 pg size-exclusion chromatography column preequilibrated with buffer 24. Collect 2 mL fractions, analyze on a 15% SDS-PAGE and pool the fractions containing eIF5A. Concentrate proteins using a 5 kDa MWCO Vivaspin concentrator. Check the final concentration at the spectrophotometer ($OD_{280}$, extinction coefficient 3105 $M^{-1}$ $cm^{-1}$), flash-freeze aliquots, and store at −80 °C.

5. eIF5B-397C

Express eIF5B-397C from pGEX-6P1 plasmid (GST-tag) in BL21 *E. coli* cells. Inoculate a preculture of 200 mL LB with 100 μg/mL carbenicillin and grow at 37 °C overnight. Next day, inoculate 6 L of LB with 100 μg/mL carbenicillin with the overnight preculture at a starting $OD_{600}$ of 0.1 and let it grow in a shaker at 37 °C with 180 rpm. Induce eIF5B-397C expression with 0.5 mM IPTG when $OD_{600}$ reaches 0.8 and incubate at 37 °C for additional 3–4 h. Harvest the cells at 7000 rpm for 10 min at 4 °C. Resuspend the cell pellets (30–50 g) in 2 mL/g with buffer 25, complemented with 100 μL of DNase and one protease inhibitors tablet. Homogenize the cell suspension on ice and use Emulsiflex to lyse the cells. Centrifuge at 180,800 × $g$ for 1 h at 4 °C. Collect the supernatant and filter using 1 μm glass fiber filters or equivalent. Equilibrate the GSTrap column with buffer 25. Load the lysate and wash the column with buffer 25. Elute eIF5B-397C with 100% of buffer 26 and collect 2 mL fractions. Analyze the fractions on a 15% SDS-PAGE. Pool the elution fractions and add PreScission protease (1 μM final) to cleave the tag while dialyzing overnight at 4 °C against 2 L of buffer 27. After dialysis, load eIF5A on a HiLoad 26/600 Superdex200 pg size-exclusion chromatography column preequilibrated with buffer 28. Collect 2 mL fractions for each, analyze on a 15% SDS-PAGE and pool the fractions containing eIF5B-397C. Concentrate proteins using a 30 kDa MWCO Vivaspin concentrator. Check the final concentration at the spectrophotometer ($OD_{280}$, extinction coefficient 46,215 $M^{-1}$ $cm^{-1}$), flash-freeze aliquots, and store at −80 °C.

6. eIF2

Streak eIF2 strain on a selective media (-LEU -URA) plate and incubate for 2 days at 30 °C. Inoculate a preculture of 200 mL selective media (-LEU -URA) overnight in a shaker at 30 °C with 180 rpm. Inoculate 100 L selective media (-LEU -URA) with the preculture at a starting $OD_{600}$ of 0.1 and grow until mid-log phase in a bioreactor. Harvest the cells, wash the pellets with MilliQ water and suspend the cell pellets in 1 mL/g of cells in buffer 29. Prepare frozen cell droplets by dropping the lysate using a syringe or serological pipette in liquid nitrogen. Grind the cell droplets using an ultracentrifugal mill prechilled with liquid nitrogen. Collect the powder and store in −80 °C freezer. Thaw the grinded yeast cell powder (~200 mL lysate in buffer 29) on ice and add one protease inhibitor tablet. Centrifuge at 180,800 × $g$ for 30 min at 4 °C. Collect the supernatant into a fresh beaker and note down the volume. Stir the supernatant on ice or in the cold room. While stirring, gradually add grinded solid ammonium sulfate to 75% saturation (48.3 g ammonium sulfate/100 mL of lysate) and stir for 1 h. Centrifuge at 235,418 × $g$ for 1 h at 4 °C. Discard the supernatant and resuspend the pellet in at least 200 mL of buffer 30. Filter the lysate through 1 μm glass fiber filters or equivalent. Equilibrate HisTrap columns with buffer 30. Load the sample onto the columns, wash the columns with buffer 30 and elute the proteins with 100% buffer 31. Collect 2 mL fractions, analyze on a 15% SDS-PAGE and pool the fractions containing eIF2. Dilute the pooled fractions five times by slowly adding buffer 35 with constant mixing to avoid precipitation. Equilibrate the Heparin column with buffer 32. Load the diluted sample immediately onto the Heparin column and wash with buffer 32. Elute eIF2 with a linear gradient from 0% to 100% of buffer 33 over 60 mL. Collect 2 mL fractions, analyze on a 15% SDS-PAGE and pool the fractions containing eIF2. Decrease the salt concentration of the pool to 100 mM KCl. Spin the sample for 20 min at 13,200 rpm at 4 °C. Equilibrate the HiTrap Q column with buffer 32. Load the diluted sample and wash the column with buffer 32. Elute eIF2 with a linear gradient from 0% to 100% of buffer 33 over 60 mL. Collect 2 mL fractions, analyze on a 15% SDS-PAGE and pool the fractions containing eIF2. Concentrate the eIF2 protein with a 10 kDa MWCO cutoff concentrator and exchange the buffer with buffer 34. Check the final concentration at the spectrophotometer ($OD_{280}$, extinction coefficient 59,010 $M^{-1}$ $cm^{-1}$), flash-freeze aliquots, and store at $-80\,^\circ$C.

7. eIF3

Streak eIF3 strain on a selective media (-LEU -URA) plate and incubate for 2 days at 30 $^\circ$C. Inoculate a preculture of 200 mL selective media (-LEU -URA) overnight in a shaker at 30 $^\circ$C with 180 rpm. Inoculate 100 L selective media (-LEU -URA) with the preculture at a starting $OD_{600}$ of 0.1 and grow until mid-log phase in a bioreactor. Harvest the cells, wash the pellets with MilliQ water and suspend the cell pellets in 1 mL/g of cells in buffer 36. Prepare frozen cell droplets by dropping the lysate using a syringe or serological pipette in liquid nitrogen. Grind the cell droplets using an ultracentrifugal mill prechilled with liquid nitrogen. Collect the powder and store in $-80\,^\circ$C freezer. Thaw the grinded yeast cell powder (~200 mL lysate in buffer 36) on ice and add one protease inhibitor tablet. Centrifuge at 88,180 $\times$ $g$ for 15 min at 4 $^\circ$C. Collect the supernatant and filter through 1 μm glass fiber filters or equivalent. Equilibrate two HisTrap columns with buffer 36. Load the lysate on the columns; wash the columns with buffer 36 then with buffer 37. Elute the proteins with 100% buffer 38. Collect 2 mL fractions, analyze on a 15% SDS-PAGE and pool the fractions containing eIF3 subunits. Load eIF3 on a Hi Load 26/600 Superdex200 pg size-exclusion chromatography column preequilibrated with buffer 39. Collect 2 mL fractions, analyze on a 15% SDS-PAGE and pool the fractions containing eIF3. Concentrate the eIF3 with a 10 kDa MWCO Vivaspin concentrator. Check the final concentration at the spectrophotometer ($OD_{280}$, extinction coefficient 365,210 $M^{-1}$ $cm^{-1}$), flash-freeze aliquots, and store at $-80\,^\circ$C.

8. eEF1A

Streak the YAS2488 strain on a YPD plate and incubate for 2 days at 30 $^\circ$C. Inoculate a preculture of 200 mL YPD media overnight in a shaker at 30 $^\circ$C with 180 rpm. Inoculate 100 L YPD culture with the preculture at a starting $OD_{600}$ of 0.1 and grow until mid-log phase in a bioreactor. Harvest the cells, wash the pellets with MilliQ water and suspend the cell pellets in 1 mL/g of cells in buffer 40. Prepare frozen cell droplets by dropping the lysate using a syringe or serological pipette in liquid nitrogen. Grind the cell droplets using an ultracentrifugal mill prechilled with liquid nitrogen. Collect the powder and store in $-80\,^\circ$C freezer. Thaw grinded yeast cell powder (~200 mL lysate in buffer 40) on ice and add one protease inhibitor tablet. Check the pH of the lysate and adjust it to pH 7.7 by adding dropwise untitrated 1 M Tris to avoid protein precipitation. Centrifuge the lysate at 180,800 × $g$ for 1 h at 4 °C. Collect the supernatant and filter it through 1 μm glass fiber filters or equivalent. Connect HiTrap Q column on top of HiTrap SP column as a tandem and equilibrate with buffer 41. Load the lysate onto the columns in tandem. Disconnect HiTrap Q column and wash HiTrap SP column with buffer 41 (eEF1A will bind to HiTrap SP and most impurities will bind to HiTrap Q). Elute the protein from the HiTrap SP column with a linear gradient of buffer 42 from 0% to 100% over 30 mL. Collect 2 mL fractions, analyze on a 15% SDS-PAGE and pool the fractions containing eEF1A. Load eEF1A on a Hi Load 26/600 Superdex200 pg size-exclusion chromatography column preequilibrated with buffer 43. Collect 2 mL fractions, analyze on a 15% SDS-PAGE and pool the fractions containing eEF1A. Concentrate the eEF1A pool with a 10 kDa MWCO Vivaspin concentrator. Check the final concentration at the spectrophotometer ($OD_{280}$, extinction coefficient 45,295 $M^{-1}$ $cm^{-1}$), flash-freeze aliquots, and store at −80 °C (*see* **Note 3**).

9. eEF2

Streak eEF2 strain on a selective media (-LEU) plate and incubate for 2 days at 30 °C. Inoculate a preculture of 200 mL selective media (-LEU) overnight in a shaker at 30 °C with 180 rpm. Inoculate 100 L selective media (-LEU) with the preculture at a starting $OD_{600}$ of 0.1 and grow until mid-log phase in a bioreactor. Harvest the cells, wash the pellets with MilliQ water and suspend the cell pellets in 1 mL/g of cells in buffer 44. Prepare frozen cell droplets by dropping the lysate using a syringe or serological pipette in liquid nitrogen. Grind the cell droplets using an ultracentrifugal mill prechilled with liquid nitrogen. Collect the powder and store in −80 °C freezer. Thaw grinded yeast cell powder (~200 mL lysate in buffer 44) on ice and add one protease inhibitor tablet. Check the pH of the lysate and adjust it to pH 7.7 by dropwise addition of untitrated 1 M Tris to avoid protein precipitation. Centrifuge the lysate at 18,900 × $g$ for 20 min at 4 °C. Collect the supernatant carefully, it should be as clear as possible. Centrifuge a second time in ultracentrifuge at 235,418 × $g$ for 1 h at 4 °C. Collect the supernatant and filter it through 1 μm glass fiber filters or equivalent. Equilibrate two HisTrap columns with buffer 44 and load the lysate onto the columns. Wash the columns with buffer 45. Elute the protein with 100% buffer 46. Collect 2 mL fractions, analyze on a 12% SDS-PAGE and pool the fractions containing eEF2. Load eEF2 on a Hi Load 26/600 Superdex200 pg size-exclusion chromatography column preequilibrated with buffer 47. Collect 2 mL fractions, analyze on a 12% SDS-PAGE and pool the fractions containing eEF2. Concentrate the pool of eEF2 using 30 kDa MWCO Vivaspin concentrator. Measure the final concentration at the spectrophotometer ($OD_{280}$, extinction coefficient 74,300 $M^{-1}$ $cm^{-1}$), flash-freeze aliquots, and store at $-80\ °C$ (*see* **Note 4**).

### 3.3 In Vitro Hypusination of eIF5A

#### 3.3.1 Purification of eIF5A Hypusination Enzymes Deoxyhypusine Synthase (Dys1) and Deoxyhypusine Hydroxylase (Lia1) (See Note 5)

Coexpress the proteins from pQLinkH plasmid (His tag) in BL21 *E. coli* cells. Inoculate a preculture of 200 mL LB with 100 μg/mL carbenicillin and grow at 37 °C overnight. Next day, inoculate 6 L of LB with 100 μg/mL carbenicillin with the overnight preculture at a starting $OD_{600}$ of 0.1 and grow it in a shaker at 37 °C with 180 rpm. Induce the expression with 0.5 mM IPTG at 0.8 $OD_{600}$ and incubate at 37 °C for additional 4 h. Harvest the cells at 7000 rpm for 10 min at 4 °C. Resuspend the cell pellet in 3 mL/g buffer 48, add one protease inhibitor tablet and 100 μL of DNase solution. Homogenize the cell suspension on ice and use Emulsiflex to lyse the cells. Centrifuge at 180,800 × $g$ for 30 min at 4 °C. Collect the supernatant and filter it through glass fiber filters or equivalent. Equilibrate two Protino Ni-IDA 2000 columns separately with buffer 48. Load the lysate over two tandem columns. Separate the columns and wash them with buffer 48. Elute each column with buffer 49 and collect 1 mL fractions in 1.5 mL Eppendorf tubes. Analyze the fractions on a 15% SDS-PAGE and pool the fractions containing Dys1 and Lia1. Dialyze the pool against 2 L of buffer 50 overnight at 4 °C with stirring. Next day, perform a second dialysis with fresh 2 L of buffer 50 for 2–3 h at 4 °C. Concentrate the pool using a 10 kDa MWCO Vivaspin concentrator. Measure the final concentration at the spectrophotometer ($OD_{280}$), flash-freeze aliquots, and store at $-80\ °C$ (*see* **Note 6**).

#### 3.3.2 In Vitro Hypusination [14, 15]

This is performed in a two-step process. In the first step, the synthesis of deoxyhypusine is catalyzed by deoxyhypusine synthase Dys1 using the reaction described in Table 1.

Mix components as indicated in Table 1 and incubate at 37 °C for 1 h. Exchange the buffer on a NAP-column equilibrated with buffer 51. Load the sample and collect the flow-through. Add 1 mL of buffer 51 and collect the eluent. Repeat the elution step once more. Analyze the eluents on a 15% SDS-PAGE and pool the fractions containing eIF5A.

In the second step, the deoxyhypusine hydroxylase Lia1 catalyzes the final step of hypusination.

Mix the components indicated in Table 2 and incubate at 37 °C for 2 h. Purify modified eIF5A from the enzyme mix using Protino Ni-IDA 2000 column. Equilibrate the column with buffer 52. Load the reaction sample and wash the column two times with

**Table 1**
**In Vitro Hypusination Step 1**

| Components | Final concentration | Unit |
|---|---|---|
| Glycine-NaOH, pH 9.2 | 0.2 | M |
| DTT | 1.0 | mM |
| BSA | 2.5 | mg/mL |
| NAD | 1.0 | mM |
| Spermidine | 7.5 | μM |
| eIF5A | 9.0 | μM |
| Dys1/Lia1 | 0.2 | μM |

**Table 2**
**In Vitro Hypusination Step 2**

| Components | Final concentration | Unit |
|---|---|---|
| Tris–HCl, pH 7.5 | 20 | mM |
| DTT | 6 | mM |
| BSA | 1 | mg/mL |
| eIF5A from reaction 1 | 6 | μM |
| Dys1/Lia1 | 6 | μM |

4 mL of buffer 52. Elute three times with 3 mL buffer 53 with a fraction size of 1 mL. Analyze the fractions on a 15% SDS-PAGE and pool the fractions containing eIF5A.

Load eIF5A on a Superdex75 10/300 GL size exclusion chromatography column preequilibrated with buffer 52. Collect fractions of 250 μL, analyze on a 15% SDS-PAGE and pool the fractions containing eIF5A. Concentrate the pool using a 5kDA MWCO Vivaspin concentrator. Measure the final concentration at the spectrophotometer ($OD_{280}$), flash-freeze aliquots, and store at −80 °C.

**3.4   RNA Synthesis and Purification**

Prepare initiator tRNA ($tRNA_i^{Met}$) by in vitro transcription using T7 RNA polymerase. A plasmid containing a 92 nucleotides-long DNA with the T7 promoter (underlined) and the initiator tRNA sequence was purchased from Eurofins.

5′<u>TAATACGACTCACTATA</u>AGCGCCGTGGCGCAGTGG
AAGCGCGCAGGGCTCATAACCCTGATGTCCTCGGA
TCGAAACCGAGCGGCGCTACCA3′.

**Table 3**
**In Vitro Transcription Setup**

| Components | Final concentration | Unit |
|---|---|---|
| Transcription buffer | 1 | $x$ |
| DTT | 10 | mM |
| NTP mix | 3 | mM |
| Pyrophosphate, inorganic (PPase) | 0.005 | U/µL |
| RNase inhibitor | 0.1 | U/µL |
| Amplified DNA | 0.5–1.0 | µg/µL |
| T7 RNA polymerase | 0.05 | U/µL |

Amplify the DNA using the following forward and reverse primers for in vitro transcription.

Forward primer: 5′TAATACGACTCACTATAAGCGCCG3′.

Reverse primer: 5′T$^m$G$^m$GTAGCGCCGCTCGGTTTC3′ (*see* **Note 2**).

Perform in vitro transcription using the reaction components as described in Table 3:

Purify the transcription product on a HiTrap Q column. Load the transcription product on a HiTrap Q column preequilibrated with buffer 57. Elute the product with a linear gradient from 0% to 100% buffer 58 over 120 mL. Collect 2.5 mL fractions, analyze on a 12% UREA-PAGE and pool the fractions containing tRNA$_i^{Met}$. Precipitate tRNA$_i^{Met}$ by adding 1/10 volume of 200 mM KOAc pH 5 and 2.5 volumes of ice-cold ethanol at −20 °C overnight. The next day, centrifuge at 3901 × $g$ for 60 min at 4 °C to pellet tRNA$_i^{Met}$. Dry and dissolve the pellet in water.

Perform the aminoacylation reaction at 37 °C for 30 min using the components indicated in Table 4.

Quench the reaction by adding 1/10 volume of 200 mM KOAc pH 5. Extract Met-tRNA$_i^{Met}$ by adding 1 volume of phenol (RNA grade) and collect the upper aqueous phase after 10 min centrifugation at 3901 × $g$ at room temperature. Precipitate Met-tRNA$_i^{Met}$ by adding 1/10 volume of 200 mM KOAc pH 5 and 2.5 volumes of ice-cold ethanol at −20 °C overnight. The next day, centrifuge at 3901 × $g$ for 60 min at 4 °C to pellet Met-tR-NA$_i^{Met}$. Dry and dissolve the pellet in water. Purify Met-tRNA$_i^{Met}$ by HPLC using a LiChrospher WP 300 RP-18 (5 µM) reverse phase column preequilibrated with buffer 60. Load the product and elute with a linear gradient from 0% to 100% buffer 61 over 255 mL. Collect 3 mL fractions and count the radioactivity of each fraction. Pool the fractions containing radioactivity and precipitate as before. Finally, dissolve the pellet in water and measure

**Table 4**
**Aminoacylation Reaction Setup**

| Components | Final concentration | Unit |
|---|---|---|
| Buffer 59, HAKM$_7$ | 1 | $x$ |
| MgCl$_2$ | 4 | mM |
| DTT | 2 | mM |
| ATP | 3 | mM |
| [$^3$H]-Methionine | 15 | μM |
| tRNA$_i$$^{Met}$ | 1 | μM |
| Yeast extract | 1 | % |

concentration by dividing obtained [$^3$H] radioactivity by the specific activity of [$^3$H]-Methionine to obtain the pmol of methionine incorporated. Divide obtained pmol by the volume of water used to dissolve the final pellet to obtain the final concentration of [$^3$H] Met-tRNA$_i$$^{Met}$ [16].

Perform aminoacylation of individual tRNA$^{Val}$ and tRNA$^{Phe}$ using the components indicated in Table 4 with [$^{14}$C]Valine or [$^{14}$C]Phenylalanine, respectively. Purify aa-tRNA by HPLC as described for Met-tRNA$_i$$^{Met}$.

The mRNA used was purchased from IBA; the unstructured 5′ UTR is underlined, the initiation codon is indicated in bold and is followed by the valine and phenylalanine codons.

5′GGUCUCUCUCUCUCUCUCUCUAUGGUUUUUUCU-CUCUCUCUC3′.

### 3.5 Nucleotide Binding and Dissociation Assay for eIF5B-397C and eEF1A

To monitor the nucleotide binding and dissociation ability of eIF5B-397C and eEF1A, we used a fluorescence change that is observed upon mant-GTP binding to and dissociation from eIF5B-397C or eEF1A [17]. The experiments were carried out in a stopped-flow apparatus. Fluorescence of mant was excited at 363 nm and measured after passing KV408 long-pass filters. We collected 5–7 individual traces for each experiment, averaged them and plotted against time.

For nucleotide binding assay, prepare 800 μL of 1 μM eIF5B-397C or 0.2 μM eEF1A and 800 μL of 1 μM mant-GTP in YT buffer (buffer 54). In a stopped-flow apparatus, rapidly mix the protein with mant-GTP solutions. Follow the time course of reaction for 10 s (eIF5B-397C) or 100 s (eEF1A) by monitoring the fluorescence change.

For nucleotide dissociation assay, incubate 0.2 μM eIF5B-397C or eEF1A with 5 μM mant-GTP in YT buffer (buffer 54) with 3 mM PEP and 1% PK, for 10 min at 26 °C. Prepare 800 μL of

1 mM GTP in YT buffer (buffer 54). In a stopped-flow apparatus, collect the traces over 10 s (eIF5B-397C) or 100 s (eEF1A) by rapidly mixing equal volumes of reactants and monitoring the time courses of fluorescence change.

### 3.6 eIF2–GTP–Met-tRNAi^Met Ternary Complex Formation Assay

Incubate 4 µM eIF2 (2× over tRNA) in YT buffer conditions with 3 mM PEP, 1% PK, 1 mM DTT, 2 mM GTP for 10 min at 26 °C. Start the reaction by adding 2 µM of [$^3$H]Met-tRNA$_i$$^{Met}$ and incubate at 26 °C. Collect 10 µL samples before the addition of Met-tRNA$_i$$^{Met}$ at (0 time) and after different incubation times points. Spot them on 0.2 µM nitrocellulose filters presoaked in YT buffer (buffer 54) and wash with 5 mL of YT buffer. Transfer the filters into a polyethylene scintillation vials, add 10 mL of Quickszint 361 (Zinsser Analytic) scintillation cocktail to each tube, mix well and count the radioactivity in a scintillation counter.

### 3.7 80S Initiation Complex Formation

#### 3.7.1 Method 1: Size-Exclusion Chromatography

Prepare the ternary complex by incubating 4 µM of eIF2 with 3 mM PEP, 1% PK, 1 mM DTT, 1 mM GTP in YT buffer (buffer 54) in a 80 µL reaction volume for 10 min at 26 °C. Add [$^3$H]Met-tRNA$_i$$^{Met}$ to 2 µM and incubate for additional 5 min at 26 °C. Separately, prepare 80 µL of 48S IC by mixing 1 µM 40S subunits with 5 µM mRNA (5× over 40S), 5 µM eIF1 (5× over 40S), 2 µM eIF3 (2× over 40S), 2.5 µM eIF1A (2.5× over 40S), 2.5 µM eIF5 (2.5× over 40S), 2 mM DTT, 0.25 mM spermidine, and 1 mM GTP in YT buffer. Incubate for 5 min at 26 °C. Add 1.5 µM 60S subunit (1.5× over 40S) and 3 µM eIF5B (2× over 60S) and incubate for additional 5 min at 26 °C. Mix the ternary complex to 48S IC and load on a Biosuite450 (WATERS) size-exclusion chromatography column preequilibrated by YT buffer (buffer 54) on a HPLC. Run the sample at 0.8 mL/min for 25 min in YT buffer (buffer 54) and follow the absorbance at 290 nm. Collect 0.5 min fractions (0.4 mL) and count the radioactivity for each fraction. Pool the fractions containing 80S IC, count the radioactivity, calculate the concentration (obtained [$^3$H] radioactivity divided by the specific activity of [$^3$H]-Methionine to obtain the pmol of methionine incorporated. Divide obtained pmol by the volume of 80S IC to obtain the final concentration), flash-freeze aliquots, and store at −80 °C.

#### 3.7.2 Method 2: Sucrose Cushion Centrifugation

This method allows preparing larger quantities of complexes; all concentrations are doubled compare to Method 1. Prepare 500 µL of ternary complex by incubating 8 µM of eIF2 with 3 mM PEP, 1% PK, 1 mM DTT, 2 mM GTP for 10 min at 26 °C in YT buffer. Add 4 µM [$^3$H]Met-tRNA$_i$$^{Met}$ and incubate for additional 5 min at 26 °C. Separately, prepare 500 µL of 48S IC by mixing 2 µM 40S with 10 µM mRNA (5× over 40S subunits), 10 µM eIF-mix (mixture of initiation factors eIF1, eIF1A, eIF3, eIF5) (5× over 40S), 2 mM DTT, 0.25 mM spermidine and 1 mM GTP in YT buffer (buffer 54). Incubate for 5 min at 26 °C, then add 3 μM 60S subunits (1.5× over 40S) and 6 μM eIF5B (2× over 60S) and incubate for 5 min at 26 °C. Mix the ternary complex with the 48S IC and adjust the MgCl$_2$ to a final concentration of 9 mM to stabilize the 80S IC.

On ice, add 300 μL of 1 M sucrose (prepared in buffer 55 containing 9 mM MgCl$_2$ (YT9 buffer)) into TLS-55 centrifuge tubes and carefully layer 1 mL of 80S IC reaction on top without disturbing the sucrose. Centrifuge in a TLS-55 rotor at 259,000 × *g* for 2 h at 4 °C. Invert the tubes to remove the supernatant and carefully wipe off excess of liquid without perturbing the pellet. Place the tubes on ice and dissolve the pellets in buffer 55 containing 9 mM MgCl$_2$. Resuspend the pellet gently, count the radioactivity, calculate the concentration (as in Method 1), flash-freeze aliquots, and store at −80 °C.

**3.8  Peptide Bond Formation Assay**

Prepare the ternary complex eEF1A–GTP–[$^{14}$C]Val-tRNA$^{Val}$ by incubating 1 μM eEF1A, 0.1 μM eEF1Bα, 3 mM PEP, 1% PK, 1 mM DTT, 0.5 mM GTP in YT buffer (buffer 54) for 15 min at 26 °C. Add 0.2 μM [$^{14}$C]Val-tRNA$^{Val}$ (5 eEF1A:1 aa-tRNA) and incubate for 5 min at 26 °C. Then add 2 μM modified eIF5A to the ternary complex. Separately, prepare 1 μM 80S IC in YT buffer containing 3 mM MgCl$_2$ by diluting 80S IC by YT0 buffer (buffer 56). Mix equal volumes of 80S IC containing [$^3$H]Met-tRNA$_i^{Met}$ with the eEF1A–GTP–[$^{14}$C]Val-tRNA$^{Val}$ ternary complex. After the desired incubation times quench the reaction by adding KOH to a final concentration of 0.5 M. Release the peptides by alkaline hydrolysis for 45 min at 37 °C, separate the reaction products by LiChrospher 100 RP-8 (5 μm) reversed-phase HPLC using buffer 62 and buffer 63, and quantified by double-label ([$^3$H] and [$^{14}$C]) radioactivity counting [17]. To form tripeptides, additionally prepare the eEF1A–GTP–[$^{14}$C]Phe-tRNA$^{Phe}$ ternary complex by incubating 1 μM of eEF1A, 0.1 μM of eEF1Bα, 3 mM PEP, 1% PK, 1 mM DTT, 2 mM GTP for 15 min at 26 °C, in YT buffer (buffer 54). After incubation add 0.2 μM of [$^{14}$C]Phe-tRNA$^{Phe}$ (5 eEF1A:1 aa-tRNA) and incubate for additional 5 min at 26 °C. Then add 1 μM eEF2 and 4 μM eEF3 to ternary complex. Mix equal volumes of ribosomes containing dipeptidyl-tRNA with the ternary complex. After the desired incubation times, quench the reaction and analyze the peptide products as described above for the dipeptides.

# 4  Notes

1. eIF5A contains the uncommon amino acid hypusine, which is derived from lysine in two modifying steps (deoxyhypusine synthase and deoxyhypusine hydroxylase).

2. Use fresh plates; plates older than 2 weeks result in decreased ribosome yields.

3. eEF1A is sensitive to freezing and thawing as it loses activity. Prepare small aliquots.

4. Do not concentrate eEF2 above 100 μM to avoid precipitation and activity loss.

5. $T^m$ and $G^m$ are $2'$-$O$ methylated nucleotides to reduce the occurrence of $3'$ heterogeneity due to the addition of nontemplated nucleotides by T7 polymerase.

6. The purification of these proteins does not require the use of an FPLC system.

## Acknowledgments

We thank Prof. Marina Rodnina for critical reading of the manuscript, and Olaf Geintzer, Tessa Hübner, Theresia Niese for expert technical assistance. We thank Profs. Ralf Ficner, Alan Hinnebusch, Jon R. Lorsch, and Terri G. Kinzy for plasmids to express and purify translation factors. This work is supported by the Deutsche Forschungsgemeinschaft (DFG) in the framework of the Schwerpunktprogram (SPP1784), and by the Max Planck Society.

## References

1. Dever TE, Green R (2012) The elongation, termination, and recycling phases of translation in eukaryotes. Cold Spring Harb Perspect Biol 4:a013706

2. Rodnina MV, Wintermeyer W (2009) Recent mechanistic insights into eukaryotic ribosomes. Curr Opin Cell Biol 21:435–443

3. Acker MG, Lorsch JR (2008) Mechanism of ribosomal subunit joining during eukaryotic translation initiation. Biochem Soc Trans 36:653–657

4. Jackson RJ, Hellen CU, Pestova TV (2010) The mechanism of eukaryotic translation initiation and principles of its regulation. Nat Rev Mol Cell Biol 11:113–127

5. Andersen CB, Becker T, Blau M, Anand M, Halic M, Balar B, Mielke T, Boesen T, Pedersen JS, Spahn CM, Kinzy TG, Andersen GR, Beckmann R (2006) Structure of eEF3 and the mechanism of transfer RNA release from the E-site. Nature 443:663–668

6. Pisarev AV, Skabkin MA, Pisareva VP, Skabkina OV, Rakotondrafara AM, Hentze MW, Hellen CU, Pestova TV (2010) The role of ABCE1 in eukaryotic posttermination ribosomal recycling. Mol Cell 37:196–210

7. Shoemaker CJ, Green R (2011) Kinetic analysis reveals the ordered coupling of translation termination and ribosome recycling in yeast. Proc Natl Acad Sci U S A 108:E1392–E1398

8. Skabkin MA, Skabkina OV, Dhote V, Komar AA, Hellen CU, Pestova TV (2010) Activities of Ligatin and MCT-1/DENR in eukaryotic translation initiation and ribosomal recycling. Genes Dev 24:1787–1801

9. Pavitt GD, Ramaiah KV, Kimball SR, Hinnebusch AG (1998) eIF2 independently binds two distinct eIF2B subcomplexes that catalyze and regulate guanine-nucleotide exchange. Genes Dev 12:514–526

10. Phan L, Schoenfeld LW, Valasek L, Nielsen KH, Hinnebusch AG (2001) A subcomplex of three eIF3 subunits binds eIF1 and eIF5 and stimulates ribosome binding of mRNA and tRNA(i)Met. EMBO J 20:2954–2965

11. Jorgensen R, Carr-Schmid A, Ortiz PA, Kinzy TG, Andersen GR (2002) Purification and crystallization of the yeast elongation factor eEF2. Acta Crystallogr D Biol Crystallogr 58:712–715

12. Acker MG, Kolitz SE, Mitchell SF, Nanda JS, Lorsch JR (2007) Reconstitution of yeast

translation initiation. Methods Enzymol 430: 111–145

13. Munoz AM, Yourik P, Rajagopal V, Nanda JS, Lorsch JR, Walker SE (2016) Active yeast ribosome preparation using monolithic anion exchange chromatography. RNA Biol 14(2): 188–196. https://doi.org/10.1080/15476286.2016.1270004:0

14. Wolff EC, Lee SB, Park MH (2011) Assay of deoxyhypusine synthase activity. Methods Mol Biol 720:195–205

15. Park JH, Wolff EC, Park MH (2011) Assay of deoxyhypusine hydroxylase activity. Methods Mol Biol 720:207–216

16. Rodnina MV, Semenkov YP, Wintermeyer W (1994) Purification of fMet-tRNA(fMet) by fast protein liquid chromatography. Anal Biochem 219:380–381

17. Ranjan N, Rodnina MV (2017) Thiomodification of tRNA at the wobble position as regulator of the kinetics of decoding and translocation on the ribosome. J Am Chem Soc 139:5857–5864

# INDEX

Karl-Dieter Entian (ed.), *Ribosome Biogenesis: Methods and Protocols*, Methods in Molecular Biology, vol. 2533,
https://doi.org/10.1007/978-1-0716-2501-9, © The Editor(s) (if applicable) and The Author(s) 2022

Printed in the United States
by Baker & Taylor Publisher Services